*A unique example of* ***great expertise*** *combined with* ***great common sense!***

*A book that every woman considering breast augmentation should read!*

*Page after page of* ***valuable information based on an expert's knowledge*** *and a load of common sense.*

*If more women read this book BEFORE having an augmentation, we would hear about fewer problems AFTERWARDS.*

***Priceless****, practical advice and methods.*

*A book that some surgeons will probably wish you hadn't read!*

*More PRACTICAL INFORMATION about breast augmentation than anything currently available.*

***A fresh, provocative approach*** *— especially coming from a surgeon!*

*A POWERFUL TOOL for any woman considering augmentation.*

*At first glance, maybe more than you want to know — unless you really want* ***the best breast result!***

***Raises the bar*** *in breast augmentation Olympics!*

*Brings home the REAL-LIFE REALITY that* ***we are responsible for our own fate.***

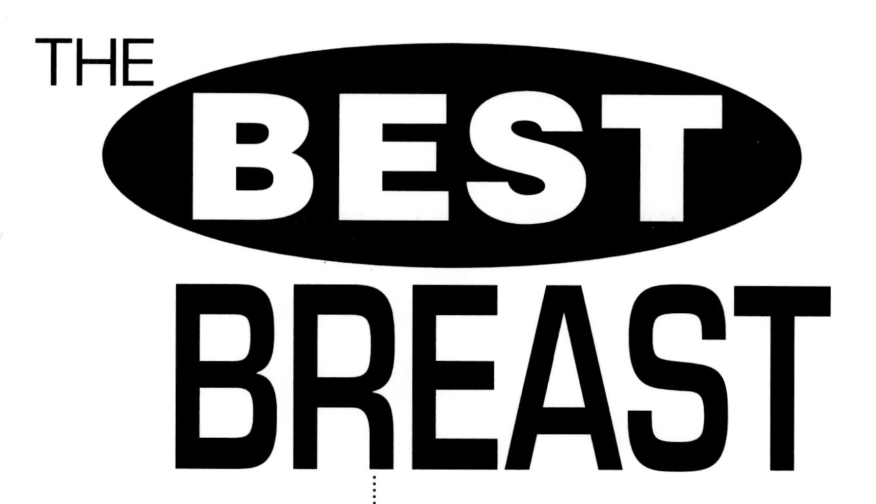


the ULTIMATE discriminating woman's guide to breast augmentation

JOHN B. TEBBETTS, M.D.
TERRYE B. TEBBETTS

CosmetXpertise
Dallas, Texas

**The BEST BREAST**

The ultimate discriminating woman's guide to breast augmentation.



Published by CosmetXpertise.



Library of Congress Catalog Card Number: 99 - 74355

ISBN: 0-9670311-0-9

---

Design, layout and illustration: Kim Hoggatt Krumwiede

Printed in the United States of America.

If you are **considering breast augmentation** surgery,

*If you are* ***discriminating,***
*and like to know the*
***facts before making decisions**,*

If you want to base your decisions on
**FACTS** and **KNOWLEDGE**
instead of hype and fluff,

If you believe in the
***value of common sense combined with KNOWLEDGE,***

If you want **one resource that contains the most information about breast augmentation**,

I*f you want information based on experience from* ***two of the world's experts in the field of breast augmentation*** *— a surgeon and a woman who cares for augmentation patients every day,*

If you decide to have breast augmentation and you'd like to get the **BEST** BREAST,

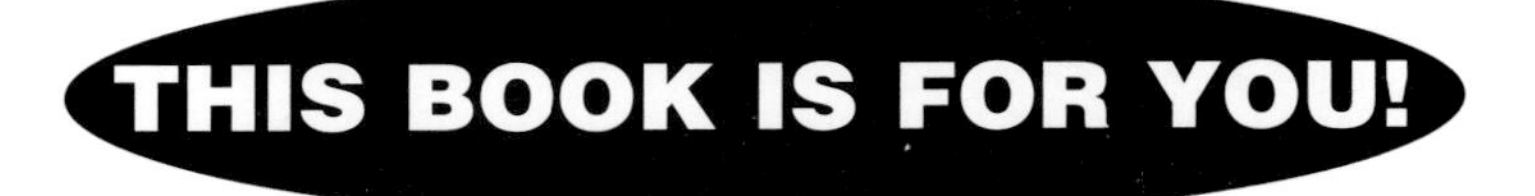

# [FOREWORD]

***Where is the wisdom we have lost in knowledge? Where is the knowledge we have lost in information?***

*-T.S. Eliot*

**This book is for women considering breast augmentation.** In 1998, more than a quarter of a million women in the United States had breast augmentation surgery. Worldwide, more than 3 million women have breast implants. The vast majority of these women are pleased with their results, but some are not. Why not? In many cases, prospective augmentation patients make poor decisions based on minimal information, impulse, and self-derived logic — then question the less-than-optimal results.

Your best chance for the best breast is the first operation. The questions you ask and the decisions you make **BEFORE** that first operation will largely determine the results. The more seriously you **pursue information and knowledge before making decisions**, the better the decisions and the better the chance of an optimal result.

Even in this age of exploding technology and information exchange, there was no single, comprehensive information resource for prospective breast augmentation patients — until now. This book is a comprehensive guide derived from 30 years' combined experience treating augmentation patients, designing surgical techniques and implants. Information becomes knowledge when combined with a logical, common sense, stepwise approach to making decisions that will help you in your quest for the best breast. This book provides information, knowledge, and common sense tools to help you make the important decisions.

**Decisions without knowledge are often flawed.**

**The more you know,<br>the better decisions you'll make.**

**The better decisions you make, the more likely you'll have a good result...the BEST breast.**

# [TABLE OF CONTENTS]

PAGE

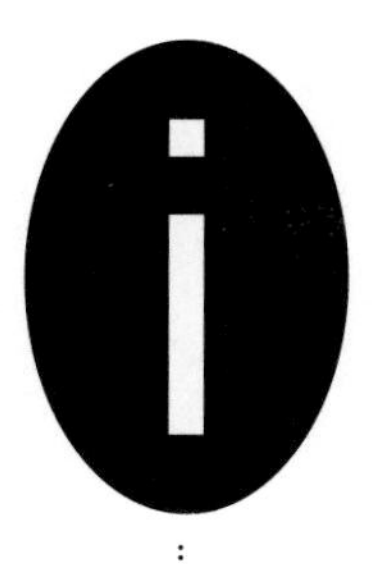

# INTRODUCTION

***"It's normal to want to feel normal. It's also normal to want to be the best you can be."***

***The BEST BREAST is the NATURAL FEMALE BREAST — until nature misses a beat, takes a toll, or a woman decides that it's not.***

**It's normal** to want to feel normal. It's also normal **to want to be the BEST that you can be.**

## WHAT IS NORMAL? WHAT IS BEST?

***What is normal?*** If you asked a hundred women, you might get 100 different answers. What is normal is personal to each individual — something that's most important to that person alone. Wanting to feel normal and be the best you can be are human traits that motivate and reward on a very personal level.

Every woman's breasts are special. Special in ways that may differ among women, but special in a personal way to each woman. Breasts change significantly during a woman's lifetime. During adolescence, the breasts usually enlarge. With pregnancy, the breasts enlarge, cycle during nursing, become smaller after pregnancy, and change in shape. Aging also changes the shape and position of a woman's breasts, and is usually not consistent during these changes. A woman's breasts never match. Enlargement during puberty and pregnancy is not predictable, and the effects of pregnancy on the breast can vary widely. A woman's tissue characteristics and the size of her breasts affect changes in the appearance of her breasts as she ages.

A woman may view her breasts differently at different times in her life, so the best breast at one time may not necessarily be the best breast at another time. In this book, we define the best breast for any woman as a personal decision, defined by that one woman's personal feelings, wishes, her tissues, and what her body will allow her to have. In this book, we will help you understand the choices available for breast augmentation, provide facts about those choices, and guide you in your decision-making process.

***The best breast is the natural female breast — until nature misses a beat, takes a toll or a woman decides that it's not.*** The only totally natural breast is a totally natural breast. An augmented breast is not totally natural, and you should not expect it to be. If you want a totally natural breast, you should probably not have a breast augmentation. On the other hand, if the benefits outweigh the tradeoffs, and the risks of breast augmentation are acceptable to you, augmentation provides options that can improve what you can't improve or restore what you can't restore.

## PRACTICAL ANATOMY OF THE BREAST

The **basic components of the breast** are:
1) a **skin envelope**, and 2) **breast tissue** filler (parenchyma).

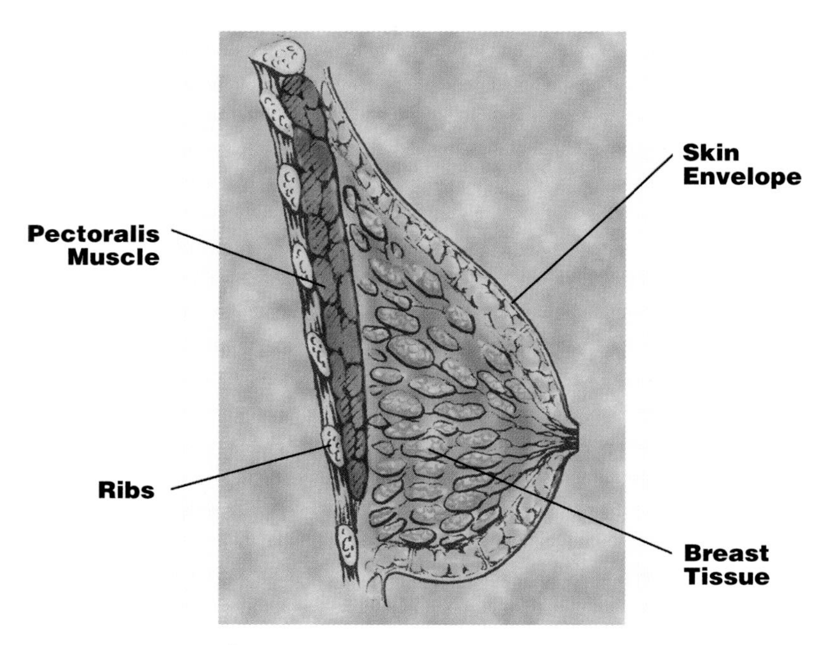


**Figure 1-1.**

In simple terms, the breast consists of a *skin envelope* that surrounds and contains the *breast tissue*. The breast tissue lies on top of a the *pectoralis muscle*. Beneath the muscle layer are the *ribs* that form the *chest wall* (Figure 1-1).

The skin envelope is the main support of the breast. Attachments are present between the back of the breast tissue and the front of the muscle, but these attachments don't contribute significant support to the breast. The larger the breast, with or without pregnancy, with or without an implant, the more gravity pulls downward on the breast tissue, stretching the lower skin envelope and allowing the breast to sag.

**Following augmentation**, the components of the breast are: 1) the **skin envelope**, 2) the **breast tissue**, and 3) the **implant**.

## WOMEN WHO CONSIDER AUGMENTATION

Three groups of women frequently consider breast augmentation:

**1**

Women in whom ***nature "missed a beat"*** during breast development (Figure 1-2),

**Figure 1-2.**

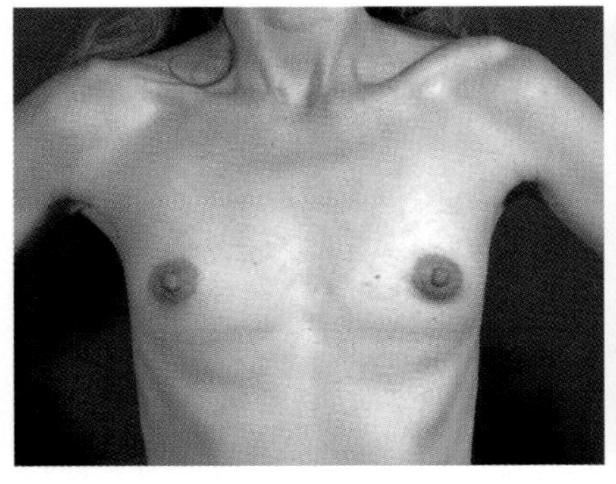

**Inadequate Breast Development During Puberty**

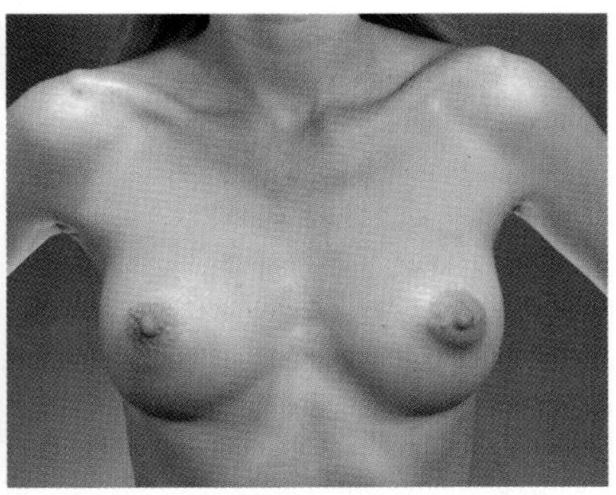

**Following Breast Augmentation**

## 2

Women in whom ***nature "took a toll" during pregnancy*** and nursing (Figure 1-3), and

**Figure 1-3.**

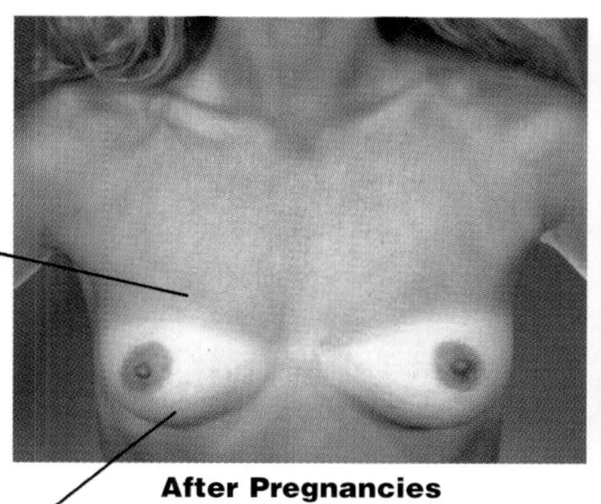


**After Pregnancies**

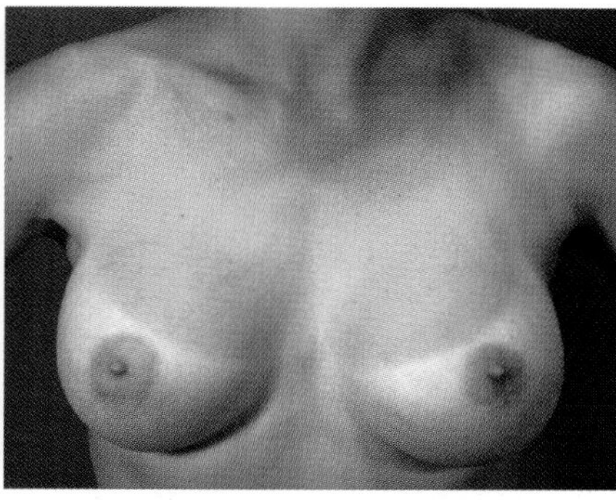

**Following Breast Augmentation**

## 3

Women who, for personal reasons, would like to ***improve the appearance or shape of their breasts*** (Figure 1-4).

**Figure 1-4.**

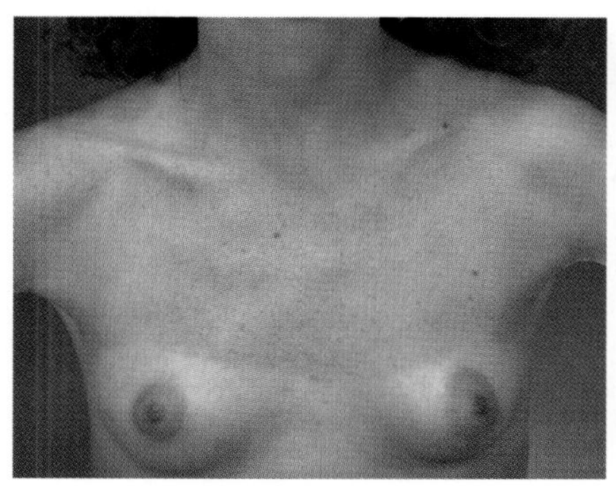

**Unsatisfactory Appearance To Patient**

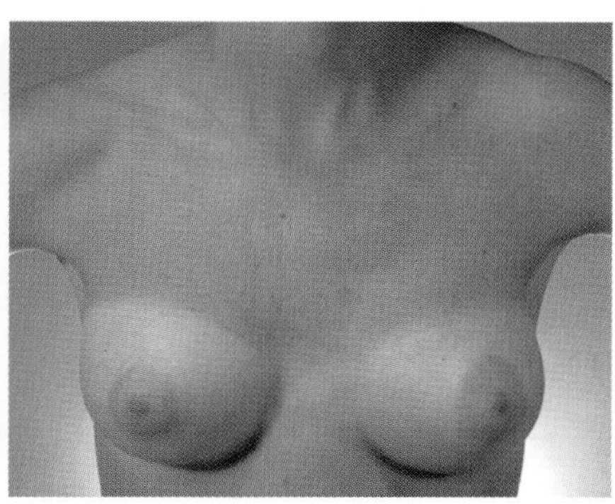

**Following Breast Augmentation**

## ABNORMAL DEVELOPMENT DURING PUBERTY: WHEN NATURE MISSES A BEAT

When breast development is *inadequate during puberty*, the breasts are disproportionately small compared to the rest of a woman's figure (Figure 1-5). Some women refer to this disproportion as a "bowling pin" figure, with the hips and lower body appearing wider than the narrower upper body. Buying clothing can be difficult. If it fits the bottom, it doesn't fit the top. Pushing up what you have is an option, provided you have enough to push up. Fillers are also an option, but a constant nuisance, and the balance provided by push up or fillers disappears when clothing is removed. Fillers and enhancers never feel like they belong to you. They never become a natural part of your body image.

**Figure 1-5.**

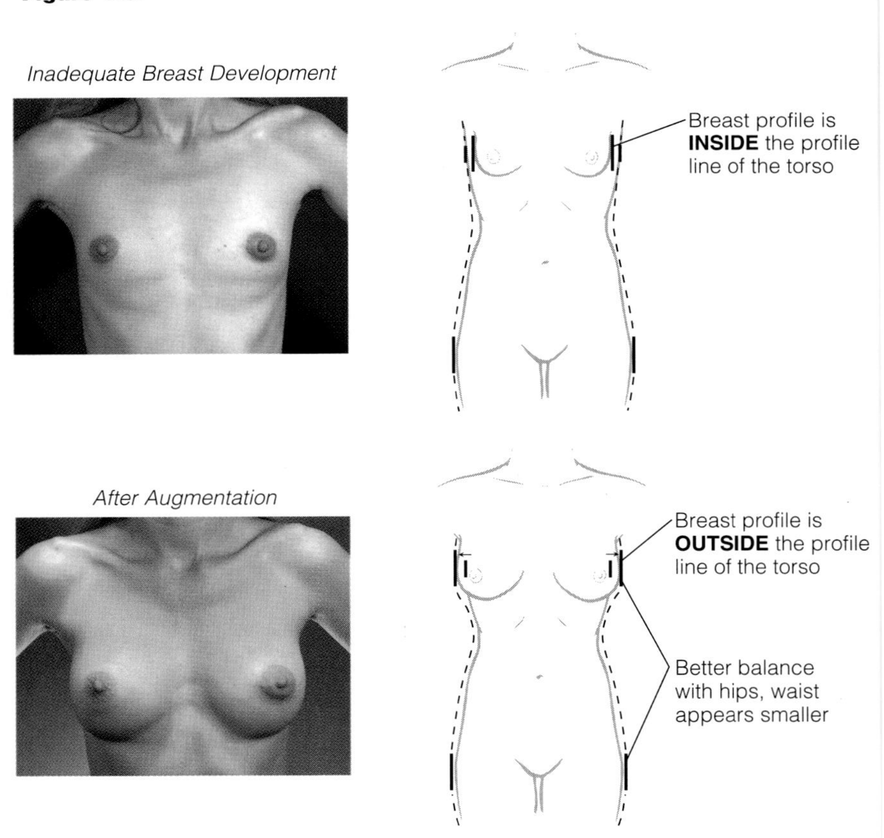

**Inadequate breast development** during puberty produces breasts that **don't appear normal**.

The **abnormal appearance** can be a **deformity or an imbalance** with the rest of a woman's figure.

If the breasts *develop abnormally during puberty,* the shape of the breast can be abnormal (Figure 1-6) and can affect how a woman feels about herself. No woman has two breasts that are the same, but sometimes the normal amount of variation in breast shape and size is too much (Figure 1-4- significant asymmetry). Imagine the difficulty trying to buy clothing, dressing to feel normal, and how you might feel when clothing is removed.

*Before* *After*

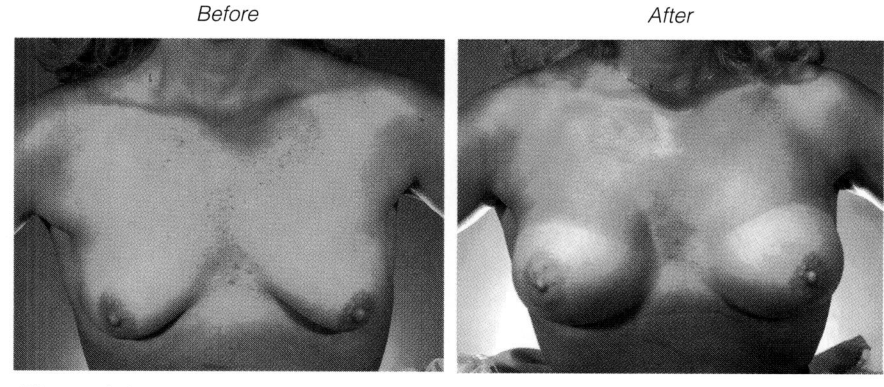

**Figure 1-6.**

## CHANGES FOLLOWING PREGNANCY

Hundreds of women who consult us for breast augmentation *following pregnancy* have said, "I had no idea what pregnancy and nursing would do to my breasts. Not that it isn't worth it, I just had no idea. I loved it when they were full, but now they're saggy and almost gone!" The effects of pregnancy and nursing on the breast are variable but usually predictable. During pregnancy, tissue inside the breast enlarges and the skin envelope stretches. As the skin stretches, usually more in the lower breast, the larger, heavier breast is pulled downward by gravity, regardless of how much it is supported by a bra. During nursing, the breast cycles up and down, repeatedly stretching the skin. Following pregnancy and nursing, the tissue inside the breast (the breast parenchyma) usually decreases substantially in size, often to a size less than before the pregnancy, but the skin almost never shrinks back to its original size.

A stretched and **enlarged skin envelope** with **less breast tissue** to fill it is common **following pregnancy**.

The **RESULT** is an **empty upper breast** and a **sagging** appearance in the ***lower breast***.

*More skin* with *less filler* is typical following pregnancy and nursing. The stretched skin envelope with insufficient tissue to fill it produces predictable changes in breast appearance. The breast tissue filler predictably falls to the bottom of the envelope, leaving the upper breast appearing empty. Most women describe the empty upper breast and fuller lower breast as "saggy." Many women who consult us for augmentation following pregnancy ask for more fill in the upper breast to help restore a breast form closer to the breast they had before pregnancy.

## WOMEN WHO WANT TO IMPROVE APPEARANCE OF THEIR BREASTS

The third group of women who seek augmentation usually want to improve the shape and/or size of their breasts for a variety of personal reasons. These are normal women who want to feel better, who want to be the best they can be. Some developed very unattractive breasts during puberty. Others have so much variation between the breasts that they have difficulty with clothing options (Figure 1-4). Still others want to improve the balance between the upper and lower portions of their body. Each woman's reasons are personal. Every woman has the right to want to optimize any aspect of her appearance.

## THE IMPORTANCE OF REALISTIC EXPECTATIONS

**Your expectations** for augmentation **must be realistic** for you to be **HAPPY** with the results.

The goal of augmentation is to improve the size and shape of your breasts. To the extent that the results meet your goals, you can have a more positive self-image, and these feelings may allow you to project a more open, positive image to others. But the only predictable change is larger breasts. This is an operation on the breasts, not on the brain. Positive psychological effects are common, but are not necessarily predictable. Certainly, your breast augmentation cannot be expected to have any predictable effect on other people. Some will notice; some may not — depending on your choices of clothing and breast exposure. Love life may improve, but it may not. The breasts are only one of the many factors that affect the quality of one's love life! A better figure doesn't necessarily guarantee a model more modeling jobs or an actress more roles. The decision to have a breast augmentation should be based on realistic, personal objectives that you discuss with your surgeon.

Your surgeon can only work with what you bring — your ***tissues*** and your ***expectations***.

The better you communicate with your surgeon, the more thoroughly your surgeon presents your options. The more expertly your surgeon executes your choices, the more likely you will have a result that pleases both of you.

## THE IMPORTANCE OF INFORMATION AND KNOWLEDGE

A patient motivated us to write this book with the following challenge, "Knowing everything that 20 years of experience has taught you, help me and other patients with the tough questions we all face. To make the best decisions about augmentation, what do I need to know, how do I go about learning it, and what is the logical sequence of making informed decisions? Walk me step-by-step through a thorough, logical approach to making good decisions about breast augmentation."

Based on our experience in treating thousands of breast augmentation patients over the past 20 years, we are convinced that patients need more information to guide them through the research and decision-making process when considering this operation. You can't be helped by what you don't know. The more you know, both good and bad, the more realistically you can evaluate your options, the more equipped you are to deal with surgeons and the surgical experience, and the more likely you are to enjoy the benefits and minimize the risks and tradeoffs of augmentation.

**KNOWLEDGE** is the basis of a **logical approach** to **good decision making**.

Based on our experience with patients, we believe in a simple premise. The more you know, the better you can make informed decisions. The more thoroughly you research and understand your options, the better your decisions. The better your decisions, the more likely you are to achieve your goals with minimal risks and tradeoffs. The better you communicate your desires and questions to your surgeon, the more likely you'll make good team decisions. Knowledge, common sense, and communication skills are important.

## HOW THIS BOOK IS ORGANIZED

We have organized this book for flexibility. For the most complete information in the most logical sequence, read from beginning to end. If you want an overview without details, read the emphasized text in each chapter, and use the appropriate checklists. Refer back to specific chapters for more details. To make the information more practical and useful, we've included removable cards in the back of the book that include the most critical information and checklists.

Visualize your quest for the best breast as a staircase (Figure 1-7). Each chapter of this book represents one step on the staircase. The steps are divided into four main parts that approach augmentation in a logical sequence:

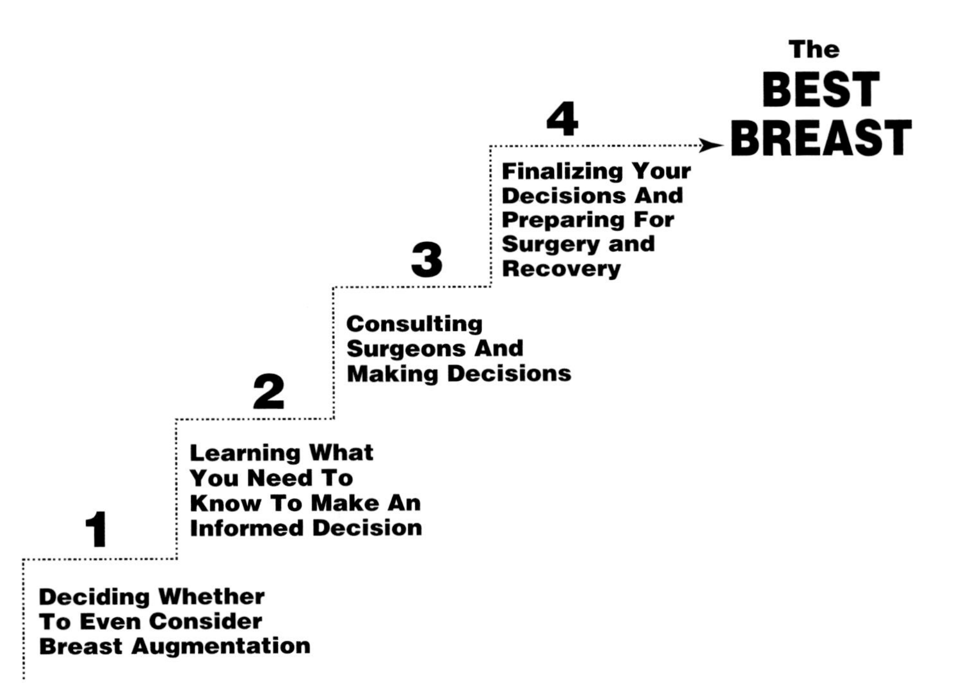


**Figure 1-7.**

## PART 1
## Deciding Whether to Even Consider Breast Augmentation

To decide whether you even want to consider augmentation, you will need some information. In Part 1, we'll present some hard choices and hard facts. If they aren't acceptable, you don't need to waste your time and additional resources.

## PART 2
## Learning What You Need to Know to Make an Informed Decision

Most patients don't even know what they need to know to start considering augmentation. You need knowledge before you ever consult a surgeon. We think it's critical for you to build a base of knowledge so that you can make the most of the time and money you spend consulting surgeons. A little homework in preparation for your consultations is invaluable. You'll learn how to ask the right questions, how to separate substance from hype, and how to evaluate the surgeons you consult.

## PART 3
## Consulting Surgeons and Making Decisions

In Part 3, you'll learn how to locate qualified surgeons with appropriate credentials, how to gather and assess information from surgeons, how to define your expectations before seeing the surgeon, and how to get the most out of your consultations.

## PART 4
## Finalizing Your Decisions and Preparing for Surgery and Recovery

Finally, we will put it all together. In Part 4, we'll help you with the final choices — picking the surgeon, the implant, the pocket location, the incision location, and the time to have your surgery. After the choices, you will learn how best to prepare for surgery physically, mentally and financially, what to expect during recovery, and how to live with your new breasts in the future.

**Our purpose is to help you climb the stairs and meet your goals for the BEST BREAST.** If you are considering breast augmentation, we want you to know as much as we can possibly share with you, based on our experiences as a team who provides information and surgical care to breast augmentation patients. Our hope is that sharing our combined knowledge and experience will help you. Logically, one step at a time.

## *Let's get started!*

### SUMMING UP:

- **The best breast is the natural female breast — until nature misses a beat, takes a toll, or a woman decides that it's not.**

- The **basic components of the breast** are
  1) a **skin envelope** and
  2) **breast tissue filler** (parenchyma).

  *Following augmentation*, the components of the breast are
  1) the **skin envelope**,
  2) the **breast tissue**, and
  3) the **implant.**

- **Your expectations for augmentation must be REALISTIC for you to be happy with the results.**

- **Your surgeon can only work with what you bring — *YOUR TISSUES AND YOUR EXPECTATIONS.***

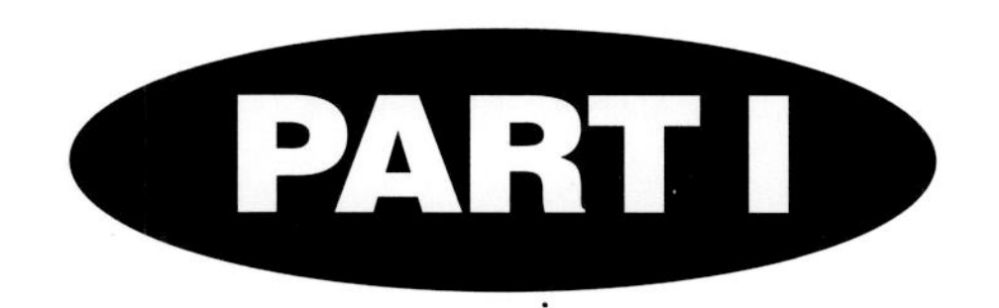


# BREAST AUGMENTATION: Should You Even Consider It?

[CHAPTER ONE]

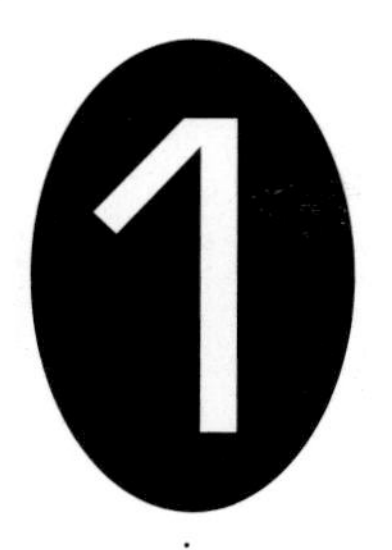

# How Can This Book **HELP ME**?

***"If there were one best answer to each question, all breast augmentation would be done the same."***

## QUESTIONS .... AND MORE QUESTIONS .....

If you are considering breast augmentation, you probably have a lot of questions. Questions that need answers before you decide to have an augmentation. Most patients begin thinking about this procedure and, hopefully, soon realize that they have more questions than answers.

How much **does it cost?**

How **big** should I be?

What is the ***best*** place to put the ***incision***?

What is the BEST type of IMPLANT?

How do I find a **good surgeon**?

*How does that surgeon do the procedure?*

How long will I be off work?

When can I return to *normal activities* and *exercise*?

How long until my breasts **LOOK NATURAL**?

**Surely, there is ONE best answer to each of these questions.**

## YOU ARE AN INDIVIDUAL—*different* FROM OTHER WOMEN

In reality, the answer to each of these questions is the same, "It depends." **If there were one best answer to each question, all breast augmentations would be done the same**. You are an individual, different from every other woman. Your tissues are different, your breasts are different, and your desires and expectations are probably different. Ask yourself, "Do I want a rubber stamp, standard augmentation, or would I prefer that every aspect of my augmentation be tailored to my specific desires and my tissues?" If given a choice, do you buy the same size and style of dress that you think other women would buy or wear? Of course not, and it's not logical to think that the best choices in breast augmentation for your friend who had the procedure are necessarily the best choices for you.

***If a surgeon does all breast augmentations the same***, the surgeon is probably doing a lot of them ***wrong***.

**No two** *women are* **the same**.

*Their* ***tissues*** *are not the same.*

The **BEST BREAST** for each woman is **NOT *the same***.

***How do you know what's best for you?***
*You begin by asking the* **RIGHT QUESTIONS**.

This book helps you ask the RIGHT QUESTIONS
**based on knowledge**.

## HELPING YOU ASK THE RIGHT QUESTIONS

If someone you know has had an augmentation, have you seen the result? Do you like it? Even if you do, are your tissues exactly the same as her tissues before she had the operation? If not, your result won't be the same either. If you see pictures in a magazine of breasts that you like, can you take the pictures to the surgeon (like you would take pictures of a hairstyle to your hair stylist) and expect to get the breast that is pictured? Not if you or the surgeon is very sophisticated. Is the woman pictured your age? Did her breasts start out looking like your breasts? Are your pregnancy histories similar? Is the picture taken to enhance the look of the breasts? Has the picture been retouched? If a surgeon asks you to bring a picture and casually assures you that you will get that breast, or if the surgeon asks you to stuff trial implants or bags into a bra the size you'd like to be, beware! Using pictures to help understand what you like is logical, but you should thoroughly understand all the factors that make you different from the woman in the picture, and understand and accept what your individual tissues will allow you to have. The same is true for trial implants or bags of fluid in a bra. The bra is not your tissue. It doesn't respond to the presence of an implant in the same way that your tissues will respond. Did your surgeon discuss all of these issues with you? More importantly, did your surgeon discuss how your choices now may affect your breasts in the future as you get older? How do you know what you need to know? How do you go about researching all of the important information? How do you ask the right questions in the right order?

How can this book help? By asking some basic questions and providing information to help you answer the questions in a logical sequence. ***As you read and review this chapter, ask yourself, "Are these the logical questions I should be asking? Are the topics presented in an order that seems logical and helpful to me?"*** If these questions and topics sound reasonable to you, you'll find this book useful. Let's look at an overview of the questions we'll ask and the information we'll cover, and you can determine how the information can best help you.

## ASKING THE RIGHT QUESTIONS IN THE RIGHT ORDER

This book helps you ask the right questions in a logical order. Each chapter adds **information** that builds your **knowledge**.

What does augmentation really do?

Is augmentation medically safe? Do I understand the medical evidence?

What are basic questions I should ask before proceeding?

Am I just being vain?

Can I correct the problem any other way?

Am I willing to do my homework and make this my own decision?

Am I willing to realistically accept the tradeoffs and risks?

Can I handle the costs financially?

How can I locate qualified surgeons?

How do I prepare for my visit with a surgeon?

How do I "interview" a surgeon?

How do I judge a good result — and a bad one — when I see it?

How do I define what I want, and how do I reconcile my desires with reality?

How do I "grade" the surgeons I consult?

How do I finalize my decisions and prepare for surgery?

What is recovery like, and how do I care for my breasts later?

If you want the best breast, you need to know the answers to each of these questions. This book will help you with the answers.

## WHAT DOES AUGMENTATION REALLY DO?

Breast augmentation enhances ***what you already have*** and ***what you already are***.

*Breast augmentation works with* YOUR TISSUES *and* YOUR WISHES *to improve what you have.*

It fills the skin envelope of your breast (*what you already have*) to enlarge and improve the shape of your breast and usually helps you feel better about you (*what you already are*). Now that we know what it does, where do we start? You'll need a lot of information, but the information is more useful if you learn in a logical, stepwise process.

## HOW CAN THIS BOOK HELP ME?

By now, you should have definite feelings for how this book can help you. If the questions sound logical, the topics sound intriguing, and the order of our information sounds logical, ***you'll find this book helpful***.

[CHAPTER TWO]

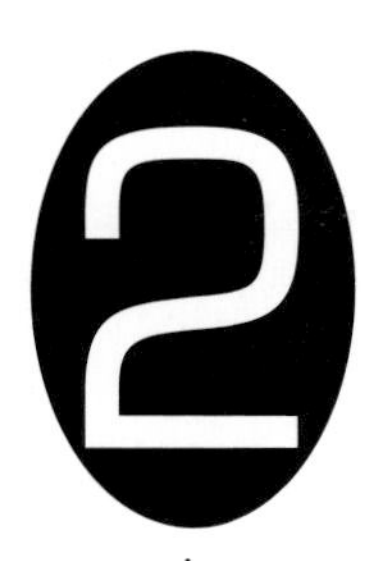

# STEP 1: Does It MAKE SENSE to Even Think About It?

***"One good way to start thinking about breast augmentation is to ask yourself some very basic, important questions."***

One good way to start thinking about breast augmentation is to ask yourself some very basic, important questions. Is the procedure medically safe? Are there specific issues in my medical history that I should consider before proceeding? Am I just being vain? Can I achieve the changes I want any other way? If the answers to this first series of questions are positive, then it's time to ask yourself some "Am I?, Can I?" types of questions. Am I willing to do my homework and make my own decisions? Am I willing to realistically accept the tradeoffs and risks? Can I handle the costs or the financial burden? Am I willing to use common sense when making my decisions? Am I willing to remove my implants if necessary? Answering these questions is the first step. If you can't take the first step successfully, you probably shouldn't try to climb the stairs.

## IS IT SAFE? THE MEDICAL EVIDENCE

To judge whether something is safe medically, you need to know a little about medical science. Medicine is not an exact science. The answers to most medical questions are rarely black and white. Instead, most answers are usually shades of gray. Good decisions in medicine are based on 1) weighing evidence scientifically (does the data prove the hypothesis in a scientific study?) and 2) clinical experience (the sum of a physician's experience treating patients). Part science and part art, plastic surgery relies on scientific evidence and experience.

**NO PROCEDURE in plastic surgery is perfect.**

Perfection isn't an option — only improvement.

**What is "BEST" and what is "RIGHT" are always shades of gray. Don't expect many black and white answers.**

***No procedure*** is without tradeoffs and risks (the grays).

Whether something is reasonable depends on whether the potential benefits outweigh the potential tradeoffs and risks. Whether something is safe is relative. The best decisions are based on scientific evidence and your comfort level with the tradeoffs and risks.

## Current Scientific Studies and Evidence

Somewhere, someone can always tell you a personal horror story about almost any experience in life, even having a baby. Does that stop us from having babies? No. We weigh the pros and cons and make a personal decision. Most potential gains involve some risks. For most "pros," some "cons" usually exist. Breast augmentation is no exception.

Sound medical decisions are usually based on scientifically tested and proven evidence, reinforced by substantial clinical experience treating patients (on-the-job training). What is "scientifically tested and proven" evidence? First, a well-designed scientific study is performed (tough to do), and then the evidence is reviewed by professional peers (other plastic surgery experts in the field). If the study is scientifically sound after review, it is usually published in well-respected medical journals. That process takes time. When you hear, read, or see something in the media about breast implants or augmentation, it may or may not be true, especially when a technique or device is new. The question to ask is, "How long has it been tested? Do we really know yet?" It takes time to treat and follow enough patients to know if something is good. Good scientific studies that answer the important questions are very time consuming. Compiling meaningful clinical experience takes years. When we try to answer the following important questions, our answers are based on the best scientific evidence available and on 20 years of clinical experience treating and following breast augmentation patients.

## The Most Compelling Answers to Date...

To date, one of the most conclusive, compelling, and reassuring sources of information is the report of the National Science Panel appointed by U.S. District Judge Sam Pointer, the presiding judge over the class action breast implant litigation. This panel was appointed by Judge Pointer to evaluate all existing scientific evidence and determine whether silicone gel breast implants cause any type of autoimmune diseases, connective tissue diseases, or immune system dysfunctions. Four disciplines were represented on the panel by world-recognized experts in each discipline: Immunology, epidemiology, toxicology, and rheumatology. Their conclusions?

***Immunology*** — "The main conclusion that can be drawn from existing studies is that women with silicone breast implants do not display a silicone-induced systemic abnormality in the types or functions of cells of the immune system."

***Epidemiology*** — "No association was evident between breast implants and any of the individual connective tissue diseases, all definite connective tissue diseases combined, or the other autoimmune/rheumatic conditions."

***Toxicology*** — "In conclusion, the preponderance of evidence from animal studies indicates little probability the silicone exposure induces or exacerbates systemic disease in humans."

***Rheumatology*** — "Furthermore, many of the rheumatologic complaints reported are common in the general population as presenting complaints in physician's offices. No distinctive features relating to silicone breast implants could be identified."

This panel of ***unbiased experts unequivocally concluded*** that **BREAST IMPLANTS DO NOT CAUSE ANY OF THESE DISEASES**.

Their findings point out one of the greatest hoaxes ever perpetrated on American women by the FDA and plaintiff lawyers—banning a device that does not cause disease, depriving American women of their rights to valid information and valid choices with regard to breast implants, and making plaintiff lawyers wealthier in the process!

## *Do breast implants cause breast cancer?* NO

Appendix 1 at the back of this book summarizes pertinent medical studies that have been published in respected, peer-reviewed medical journals with regard to breast implants and breast cancer. Each of these studies reaches a similar conclusion: ***Breast implants do not cause breast cancer.*** Approximately 10-11 percent of women in the United States, with or without breast implants, will develop breast cancer during their lifetimes. The best scientific studies compared similar large groups of women with and without breast implants and found that the occurrence of breast cancer was not significantly different in women with implants compared to women without implants.

## *Do breast implants cause autoimmune disease?* NO

Autoimmune diseases are conditions that cause the body's own immune system to malfunction and result in certain symptoms, conditions, or groups of symptoms and conditions that have been categorized as diseases. Examples of autoimmune conditions include scleroderma, rheumatoid arthritis, lupus, and fibromyalgia. One of the most respected organizations in the world that deals with these diseases is the American College of Rheumatology. The following statement was issued by the American College of Rheumatology regarding breast implants and the risk of autoimmune diseases:

## American College of Rheumatology Statement on Silicone Breast Implants

### Approved by Board of Directors on Oct. 22, 1995

The American College of Rheumatology recognizes that many women who have received silicone breast implants have musculoskeletal complaints that are also very common in the general population. Many rheumatologists have examined women with implants who have scleroderma, lupus, fibromyalgia, or other well-defined disorders. The problem has been to determine whether any cause-and-effect relationship exists between silicone implants and the musculoskeletal symptoms. Previous data were solely based on anecdotal evidence. In 1994, the American College of Rheumatology stated the importance and great need for scientific analysis of this question.

Two large studies now have been completed. The first was conducted on all women in a single county in Minnesota who received implants between 1964 and 1991. At a mean follow-up of 7.8 years, there was no association between breast implants and connective tissue or rheumatic disease (NEJM 330:1697-702, 1994). The second study was a follow-up of the Nurses Health Study. Among this very large cohort, after 14 years of follow-up, no evidence existed for an association between silicone breast implants and connective tissue diseases (NEJM 332:1666-70, 1995).

The American College of Rheumatology believes that these studies provide compelling evidence that silicone implants expose patients to no demonstrable additional risk for connective tissue or rheumatic disease. Anecdotal evidence should no longer be used to support this relationship in the courts or by the FDA. Clinicians, scientists, academicians, and editors who have been harassed by plaintiffs' attorneys for their involvement in scientific research efforts related to silicone implant deserve the continued support of their institutions and professional societies.

> In future cases involving rheumatic diseases possibly associated with an environmental agent, we call upon the FDA and other regulatory agencies to allow professional societies, such as the American College of Rheumatology, to foster appropriate and scientifically developed epidemiological studies. Anecdotal reports, while of importance to call attention to a potential problem, should not be utilized to formulate decisions and regulations.
>
> The American College of Rheumatology is the most respected, professional organization of rheumatologists. It includes practicing physicians, research scientists and health professionals who are dedicated to healing, preventing disability, and eventually curing the more than 100 types of arthritis and related disabling and sometimes fatal disorders of the joints, muscles and bones.

Appendix 2 summarizes pertinent medical studies about autoimmune disease that have been published in respected, peer-reviewed medical journals.

A certain percentage of women, based on hereditary or environmental factors, will develop autoimmune diseases during their lifetimes. Logically, some women who have breast implants will develop autoimmune diseases. This does not mean that the breast implants *caused* the autoimmune disease.

## What We Currently Tell Patients About Autoimmune Disease

If you have a family history of autoimmune disease, you should understand that, although you may be genetically destined to develop the disease at some point, there may be factors that could stress your autoimmune system and possibly cause you to develop the disease sooner (though we have no scientific proof of that risk). Emotional stress or physical stress of any kind, even having a surgical procedure, might theoretically stress your system excessively. At the very least, if you have a family history of autoimmune disease, we want you to consult a board certified rheumatologist or immunologist and get a written opinion regarding the safety of your having breast augmentation. Before having an augmentation, you should ask yourself, "If I knew that I might be prone to develop an autoimmune disease because of heredity or other factors, if a breast augmentation might cause me to develop it sooner, is it worth it to me to have a breast augmentation?"

## Internet references

If you want to dig deeper into scientific studies and additional information, check out the Internet references.

FDA Information and Position Statement re: Breast Implants:
**www.fda.gov/oca/breastimplants/bitac.html**

American Society of Aesthetic Plastic Surgery:
**www.surgery.org**

American Society of Plastic and Reconstructive Surgeons:
**www.plasticsurgery.org**

Our website:
**plastic-surgery.com**

The book website:
**thebestbreast.com**

**Do breast implants cause any other known diseases? NO**

At this time, there is ***no credible, scientific evidence that breast implants cause any type of disease***, regardless of the type of breast implant.

This does not mean that there could not be a disease or diseases of which we are unaware that are affected by breast implants. It simply means that, currently, no such disease has been documented scientifically.

For over 30 years, breast implants have been used in the United States in over two million women. Complications from breast implant surgery certainly occur in a small percentage of patients, and these complications can produce significant problems if they are not treated promptly and correctly. Later in this book, we will address the specific risks of complications so that you can determine whether those risks are reasonable.

## *If breast implants don't cause any of these diseases, why all the lawsuits? Why do I hear about all these breast implant disasters?*

When humans get diseases, it's human nature to ask, "Why me? What caused this?" The physical and emotional stress of disease causes most people to lose their feeling of "normal" and frightens them. Regardless of the disease, most of us instinctively want to blame it on something. When potential financial gain is added to the equation, regardless of the disease or condition, a plaintiff lawyer feeding frenzy is predictable. "Would you like some money? We can probably get some for you!" Whether from a plaintiff lawyer or a con man (not a totally incidental comparison), these words can be hard to resist. Our judicial system has been called an example to the world—good in some ways, for sure, but not so good in other ways.

In medical cases in this country, there is no requirement that evidence introduced in the courtroom must be based on quality, scientific evidence. Any lawyer can hire any "expert" whose testimony becomes evidence, whether or not the expert's opinion has been tested in peer-reviewed, published scientific studies. Needless to say, there are plenty of "experts" who, in exchange for money, will testify to almost anything regarding a medical situation. Fortunately, recent federal court decisions have emphasized the importance of basing judgement on scientific data, an encouraging sign for the future. Until that happens, remember: The facts in a case don't necessarily need to be scientifically "right" or justifiable to get an award. The plaintiff lawyer only needs to convince a jury. How many juries would you want making your medical decisions for you?

Companies that are sued face a dilemma that is great for the plaintiff lawyer and not so great for the company. Fighting the suit with a trial is often more expensive than settling the suit by paying a monetary settlement (some have called it legalized bribery), so the company makes a business decision to settle. Legalized extortion? Certainly sounds like it to us. Judgements that are not based on scientific evidence ultimately cost all of us. The company pays. The company does not have as much money left for research and development of better products. The company is forced to raise the price of its product (breast implants). A higher priced, less state-of-the-art product is the result. ***How good is that for you?***

Are all lawsuits bogus and without merit? Certainly not. Plastic surgeons aren't perfect. We make mistakes. If a surgeon makes mistakes that are below the standard of usual and customary medical practices, then the surgeon should be held accountable for malpractice. There should not be a double standard. If we want tort reform to reduce frivolous cases without merit, surgeons must perform to an acceptable level and be held responsible for our actions when we do not. We also must be willing to police ourselves by holding our colleagues accountable to an acceptable standard of care.

## *Team decisions and accountability*

During my career, I have been asked to review a large number of breast implant cases in which "disasters" occurred. What was to blame? The implant? Almost never! In almost every case, problems were directly related to **BAD TEAM DECISIONS** by the patient and the surgeon. What do we mean by "team" decisions? The team consists of you and your surgeon. Both of you are responsible for decisions you should make jointly. Let me tell you about a case that illustrates the point.

Julie (a fictitious name but a real patient) came to see us after having an augmentation and after four reoperations for excessive breast firmness due to capsular contracture, each time placing larger and larger implants. Her surgeon (she let the same surgeon reoperate four times and had never sought a second opinion until now!) continued to honor her wishes to try to achieve softer breasts and get larger implants! Bad team decisions! Her breasts were like rocks, and only thin skin, stretched from excessively large implants, covered her implants. We told Julie, "Enough is enough. More operations will only mean more potential complications, costs, risks, and possible permanent deformity. The best option is to remove the implants. You are one of a very small percentage of patients who persistently form tight capsules around your implants. We can't change your body's response, and we can't continue to surgically assault your tissues."

Julie's response? "No way. Not a chance. No way I'm giving up my implants. I know I can find someone who'll operate on me again!" True, no doubt. Also true: Bad decision by Julie. When the inevitable complications occur, who is the last person Julie will blame? Julie! You guessed it! She'll almost never blame herself. Instead, the surgeon and the implant will get the blame. The surgeon probably deserves some blame; the implant does not. The last surgeon who operates on Julie will get most of the blame, but it's Julie and the first surgeon who made the bad team decisions.

Most surgeons want to please their patients. Most patients want to keep their implants at any cost. Under certain circumstances, this combination can present problems. Going in, you should be aware of both good and bad results. You should know , "If bad happens, what will be done?" You and your surgeon should also set limits up front that define: "If bad happens, when do we stop? When do we remove implants?" Plan up front for the worst-case scenario, commit to limits prior to surgery, and disasters will be almost non-existent. Problems are rare, but if you beat a dead horse, you get a beaten, dead horse. You are responsible for your decisions. A qualified surgeon will help inform you, so that you can make good decisions, but remember, the decision is still yours. Do your research, think past dinner, and make your decisions carefully.

Disaster = Device (implant) alone?
***Almost never***.

Disaster = Device + poor surgeon judgement +
poor patient judgement
**BAD TEAM DECISIONS**

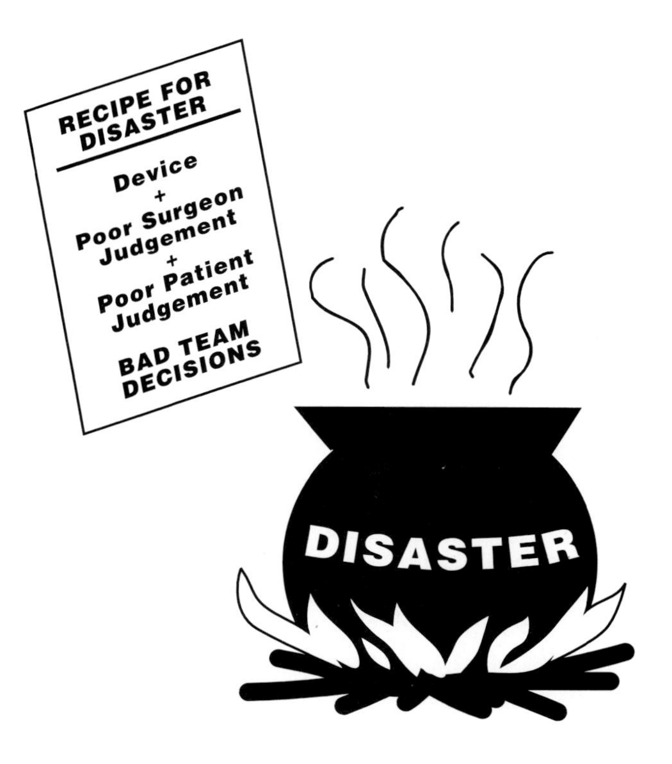


***Is augmentation medically safe?* YES, *provided you use good judgement and make good decisions.*** But if for any reason, you are not comfortable and convinced after considering the medical evidence, don't have an augmentation.

## WHAT IN MY MEDICAL HISTORY SHOULD I CONSIDER?

Few hard rules exist that specify who should or should not have an augmentation based on medical history alone. Here too, there are more grays than blacks or whites. Each case is different, and each surgeon approaches these issues differently. Here's what we tell our patients.

Recognizing that augmentation is a totally elective procedure (it's not medically necessary), if you have any of the following, we advise careful consideration about augmentation:

### 1) A strong family history of breast cancer

***Mother with breast cancer***—
you probably should ***reconsider***.

***Mother and grandmother with breast cancer*** —
**FORGET IT**. You definitely shouldn't have augmentation.

Any breast implant can interfere with mammograms to some degree. Mammograms are not 100 percent accurate even without a breast implant. From 5-15 percent of breast cancers do not show up on a mammogram. The techniques used to do the mammogram and the experience of the person interpreting the mammogram also affect accuracy. But if you know that you are at significantly increased risk of breast cancer due to a strong family history, a breast augmentation just doesn't make good sense.

### 2) A personal history of autoimmune disease such as scleroderma, rheumatoid arthritis, lupus, or fibromyalgia

Even though breast implants have been shown **NOT** to **CAUSE** these diseases, any stress (a surgical procedure, for example) could possibly affect the course of the disease. Why take a chance?

Interestingly, we have seen patients in consultation who had autoimmune diseases who brought written statements from their immunologists stating that the immunologist did not think that having an augmentation would affect their disease. A real chance for a bad decision? Do we *know absolutely* that just having an elective operation might not make the disease worse? If the disease did get worse, even if the implant didn't cause it, guess who (what) would get the blame? We didn't do the augmentation.

### 3) HIV

Since HIV is also a disease that affects the immune system, the same logic applies for HIV that applies for other autoimmune diseases.

Any avoidable event that could possibly stress the immune system, especially when it is not medically necessary, ***probably isn't a good idea***.

Add to that the increased risk of transmission to all of the medical personnel involved for a procedure that is not medically necessary. ***Make good sense?*** **NO.**

Having said no, I would hasten to add that exceptions exist for every generalization in medicine. Our medical knowledge and, hopefully, our control of this dread disease are improving. If this disease is controlled, if we can prove that augmentation wouldn't make the disease worse, and if we have better measures to protect the patient and personnel, a patient's quality-of-life issues deserve careful consideration.

### 4) Any other medical disease or condition

If you are not totally healthy, or if you have ever had any other disease or condition diagnosed by your family physician or internist, you should consult that physician about the advisability of having an augmentation. We require a written letter from the physician confirming their opinion that your having an augmentation is reasonable, safe, and will not interfere with the management of your other conditions.

## AM I JUST BEING VAIN?

Do you like feeling normal? For whatever personal reasons, do you feel that your breasts are less than normal or optimal? Do your breasts make dressing difficult? Do you have difficulty shopping for clothing? Do you like feeling that you are the best you can be, given what you have to work with, and what you can't do for yourself? If you answer yes to these questions, you are very normal. If being vain is a desire to feel normal and wanting to be the best you can be, so be it. But it's not. Fact is, almost all of us do things that someone else might consider vain— personal things that are our own business —that we do only for ourselves (and don't need to explain to anyone else) — things that make us feel better about ourselves. The key is doing those things responsibly.

Earlier, we discussed **three large groups of women who consider augmentation**:

**1**

The "***I never developed much to begin with***" group

**2**

The "***I lost everything I had after my baby***" group, and

**3**

The " ***I want to improve for personal reasons***" group.

All perfectly normal women with perfectly normal, personal reasons to consider augmentation? Maybe; maybe not. There are always weird exceptions in any large group of people. Weird situations make the sensational stories you see in the media. The vast majority of all women we see who are considering augmentation are perfectly normal and approach this decision responsibly.

## CAN I CHANGE ANY OTHER WAY?

### Devices—And Their Vices

Aren't "wonder" bras wonderful? Compared to what? If you've got something the bra can push where you want it to go, usually up and in, then they're more wonderful than without them. But what if you don't have much to push somewhere? If you have enough to push, and you're happy with that, why have an augmentation? "Wonder" bras are cheaper and involve fewer tradeoffs and risks. But if you don't have anything much to push, and you want something to push , how can you get it?

Fillers and enhancers simply fill and enhance. From washcloths to Kleenex, from balloons to commercially available breast enhancers, every imaginable material has probably been tucked into a bra at one time or another. The good news? Any of them can fill and enhance provided they stay put. The bad news? They don't always stay put, and even if they do, they can be a huge nuisance. They're hot, itch, move around, and move out of place. The worst news about fillers and enhancers? As one of my patients told me, "They are slightly less than special when I undress, especially in front of, or with the help of, my lover?"

**A true patient story ...**

Another patient was a tall, lithe, beautiful executive who happened to have a lovely figure except that she had virtually no breast tissue. She had considered all options and decided that the most state-of-the-art, shaped "enhancers" that fit inside her bra were the best answer. Everything went well until she was informed that she had been honored with her company's highest achievement award, and that the award would be presented at a black tie gala that required a new black dress. Unfortunately, the perfect dress was strapless. Undaunted and resourceful, this patient decided to solve her problem with a large amount of electrical tape. Preparations for the evening were something akin to wiring the Pentagon. After applying several rolls of electrical tape, everything was perfectly in place. Enhanced didn't even begin to describe the result!

As this beautiful, but somewhat nervous, executive stood accepting her award and anticipating her speech, she began perspiring heavily. The instant she stepped to the microphone to address her audience, something "enhanced" started to move. One sentence into the speech, something started sliding. With a deft grab of the award plaque, she clutched it to her chest and stopped the downwardly sliding enhancer with one hand, while she turned the page of her speech with the other. One minute later, the unthinkable—the other side started shifting to the side and sliding down! In one motion, she not so deftly swept the other elbow downward and up to get things hitched back up, then hugged the plaque to her chest with both arms. The next sentence became the last line of the speech, spoken as she unconsciously backed away from the microphone and hastily exited the stage. "I'm so honored and happy with this award that I may not let it go all night."

What about the water bra? As another patient told us, "Just imagine, if you're caught out in the desert, you have a built-in canteen! Wonder if it sloshes?" Another device, same problems. It's a thing.

***External devices aren't as good*** as something that you don't have to think about—something that you incorporate unconsciously into your body image, then **forget that it's there**.

Something that to many women seems ***more normal***.

## The Muscle Myth

Ever hear, "If you just work out enough and build up your pec (pectoralis major) muscles, you can enlarge your breasts." Muscle is not breast tissue, and no matter how much you exercise it, you can't make it look like or act like breast tissue.

To make a pectoralis muscle enlarge significantly, you've got to do serious, regular, body-building exercises. Assuming you have the time and motivation, what you get is a bigger, thicker pectoralis muscle. Since most normal women don't have big, thick pectoralis muscles, you don't notice the muscle when you look at the breast of most normal women. It's under there, but you don't see it. When you see a breast sitting on top of a big, thick pectoralis, you'll almost always notice it because it doesn't look like something you normally see. The bigger muscle almost never blends naturally with the lines of the breast, so instead of seeing larger breasts, what you see is larger pectoralis with still small breasts on top of it. Bottom line?

*You* **can't predictably make the breast appear larger** *(and you definitely can't make the breast appear natural)* **by exercising or building up the pectoralis muscle** — *or by any other exercises.*

### Other Magic Remedies?

Whenever you are dealing with an area of the body that affects one's sense of well being and relates to sex, you'll see every imaginable (and some you can't imagine) solution to any perceived problem relating to that area. Somehow, there seems to always be a definite, sure-fire cure for what ails you. The breast is no exception.

Drugs, herbs, lotions, massage — ***you name it*** — have been touted as a predictable way to enlarge women's breasts.
**We're not aware of a SINGLE ONE that really works**.

The only thing that predictably gets larger is the bank account of whoever sells it. Worse, some remedies, especially drugs, have effects or side effects that can be harmful if used improperly. Good examples are some types of hormones (steroids, estrogens, testosterone). Used properly for specific conditions under qualified medical supervision, each of these drugs works wonderfully for specific conditions. ***Used to enlarge the breasts?* NO. *Purely and simply, no.***

Maybe there is a better way to predictably enlarge the breasts other than augmentation, but we don't know a better, safer and more predictable method. Assuming you are convinced that you can't do it on your own, you'll logically need some help, but help is the key word. Part of the job is yours. Part of the responsibility is yours. All of the costs are yours. How much you are willing and able to do and the quality of the decisions you make will have a lot to do with the result now and in the future.

## WHAT OTHER PEOPLE THINK AND SAY...

In deciding whether to consider breast augmentation, you'll probably hear a lot of different opinions. Listen carefully, consider the content and source of the opinions, and filter out what you consider useful information. **Asking the following questions can be enlightening and helpful:**

**Am I capable** *of making my own, personal decisions?*

**Why would someone else want to make a decision for me or influence my decision?**
*Is my personal business their business?*

**Has this person had a breast augmentation?**
*If not, how does he or she know?*

**Did this person have a good result?**
*If so, why? How much does she know? Is she like me? What can I learn from her? What do I want to learn from her?*

**Did this person have a bad result?**

*Why? Did she do her homework? Did she and her surgeon(s) make good team decisions? If she had a problem, was it because of the implant? Is there any reason to expect that I would have the same problem? How much does she know? Is she like me? What can I learn from her? What do I want to learn from her?*

**Is this opinion based on facts and knowledge,** *or is it based on fluff?*

## The Media and Breast Augmentation

Breast augmentation is a popular topic. The media is interested in breast augmentation because you, their customers, are interested in breast augmentation. You'll hear about whatever the media thinks you want to hear about—good or bad—as long as the media thinks the topic will make a good story and that you'll read, watch, or listen. But most often, you'll hear about bad. In the media, if it bleeds, it leads (to quote a news anchor patient). What percentage of stories on the evening news are "good news" stories? I can't prove it, but I'd bet that over 90 percent of media stories about augmentation are ***problem based.*** How productive is time spent hearing about problems? Why not spend the time offering ***knowledge-based*** solutions to avoid the problems at the outset?

**WHAT PERCENTAGE OF MEDIA STORIES FOCUS ON PROBLEMS?**
*What you need are solutions!*

*Which is more* **PRODUCTIVE**, *hearing about* **PROBLEMS AND NEGATIVES,** *or* **LEARNING ABOUT SOLUTIONS TO AVOID PROBLEMS?**

**WHAT YOU DON'T NEED IS SENSATIONALISM!**
**WHAT YOU DO NEED IS SUBSTANCE!**

*Sensationalism can help you become the next sensational story! Substance helps you avoid becoming the next headline!*

Are magazines, television and radio a good source of information? Sometimes yes, sometimes no. It's your job to listen carefully, filter fact from fluff, consider the sources and the content, and then use good information appropriately. ***At the end of any time spent watching, reading, or listening to media presentations, ask yourself:***

**What did I learn that added to my knowledge?**
**What did I learn that will help me make better decisions?**

*Write down a list! I bet it will be a short one!*

***When you see information about augmentation in magazines or on TV, consider the following:***

**Media information is only as good as the sources.**

*If you don't know the sources, don't bet on the accuracy of the content.*

**If it's not stimulating, exciting, or new, you're not likely to hear about it.**

*How often have you seen stories about plastic surgery that focus on common sense and decision making skills?*

**How many important, long-term personal decisions do you base on something stimulating and new?**

*If a lot, how did the decisions work out long term?*

**To make good decisions about plastic surgery, you need far more information than you can find in magazines or on television.**

*How often does media take responsibility for the decisions that result from their information?*

**What most patients hope for and get is a routine, excellent result after an augmentation! How often do you hear this story in the media?**
*Balance is important, but sometimes the routine isn't exciting, stimulating or "new" enough to be reported.*

**Are confrontation and controversy more important than basic information about augmentation?**
*What percentage of your time is best spent on basic information versus controversy and confrontation?*

**What can the media never tell you? Just how good your surgeon is at planning and performing your augmentation! And that has a lot to do with your result!**
*Use media information responsibly, but don't neglect your homework!*

And, most important...

**You can't educate yourself with sound bites.**
*You need information and a willingness to use it!*

Breast augmentation is a complex topic. You need a lot of information to develop a broad perspective that helps you make good decisions. Most media articles and stories address one or two aspects of augmentation. Print space and television time don't allow adequate coverage of all the important issues! You'll get pieces of information that are important to the pie; you just never get the whole pie! You see steps on the stairs, but you never see the whole staircase.

### What Does This Say About Our Culture?

Why would a woman want to put some foreign object in her body just to have larger breasts? If I've heard this question once, I've heard it a hundred times! My answer?
It depends on your assumptions! If you assume that the only reason that women have breast augmentations is to have a

large chest (and many people make that assumption) and be noticed, then perhaps it says that our culture notices large breasts. After all, breasts have been a visual sexual symbol since the beginnings of civilization.

***To generalize that most women want augmentation to have a large, noticeable chest is tenuous, if not patently, absurd!***
I wouldn't want to try to sell that concept to most women I know!

***Another assumption is that women are intelligent individuals who are capable of making personal decisions based on valid information and their right to choose.***
Most of our patients fall into this category!

There's a lot of axe grinding with respect to augmentation. You've got folks who want to sell stories and television time. Their axe is to always tell you about the new, the wonderful, or the controversial. You've got unhappy patients whose axe is, unfortunately, a bad result or experience that they are just sure you'll have, too (regardless of whether your decisions are the same as theirs). You've got surgeons who make their living doing augmentations (We're in this category), so their axe is to tell you how good augmentation is! The only person you rarely hear axe grinding is the happy patient who would have an augmentation again in an instant but doesn't feel compelled to discuss it with anyone!

***How many "good news," "I am thrilled with the improvement," "I would do it again in an instant" stories have you seen, heard, or read?***
If you think it's because they are rare, just ask around!

## THE "AM I" AND "CAN I" QUESTIONS

If you can't answer ***YES*** to every question that follows, you might consider stopping on this first step of the stairs.

### *Am I willing to do my homework and make this my own decision?*

What homework? The more you learn and understand about breast augmentation, the more likely you are to make the right decisions that ultimately determine your result. The homework isn't heavy, and some women hardly do it at all. Some women also aren't happy with the results. Even if they are, some women don't really know whether they have a good result or not. If you care and you want to know, our goal is to help give you the tools.

**Your homework consists of reading this book and every piece of informational material that you accumulate from surgeons and other sources.**
*Make a list of issues and questions.*
*Get answers before making decisions.*

If the answers don't make sense, seek more information and other answers. Organize your questions, and ask them over and over to different surgeons until you are satisfied. Follow the steps outlined in this book, and you'll be far better prepared and informed than most prospective augmentation patients who don't do their homework. Most of all, you'll be more comfortable making decisions that can affect your result, and the decisions will be better ones.

Who else would make your decisions for you? Hopefully, no one. Hopefully, those close to you will be supportive and respect your intelligence, privacy, and decisions. What about everyone else? What will they think? Who cares? It doesn't matter, and it isn't their business. But for the sake of discussion, let's assume someone else feels they could (or should) make decisions for you. What about a boyfriend, husband, or significant other? Should they be interested? You bet. Interested in you (if they really care), and if they're normal, in your breasts as well. Should they become informed, provide input, ask questions? Yes, great! But make decisions for you? That's something else. ***Whenever a patient mentions the demands made by a significant other with respect to augmentation, we have two ready replies:***

**1)** We hope the statistics never apply to you, but the divorce rate is 50 percent in the United States, so you have a coin-toss chance that the person who enjoys your breasts with you now won't be the same person enjoying them with you in the future. If you're doing it for someone else and not specifically for you, how do you plan to deal with the next significant other wanting something different? Another operation?

***Make your own decisions for you and only for you.***
*If you're happy with the results, you can credit yourself. If not, you know whom to blame.*

**2)** Have you ever seen the person who wants to make your decision for you change his or her mind about anything? What do you do when that person has a change of heart after placing the order? This isn't McDonalds! We're not talking about fast food, a little more mustard, or cut the onions. It isn't even Neiman Marcus. We're not talking about a gown that can be altered or replaced with another gown. We're talking about making changes to your body that you'll live with from now on.

***Think long term. Don't make decisions that you're likely to want or need to change.***
*Nothing gets better when you need to change things later.*

## Am I Willing to Realistically Accept the Risks and Tradeoffs?

Later, we will go into a lot more detail about specific risks and tradeoffs. For now, let's just assume (because it's true) that every augmentation involves tradeoffs and risks. No matter who does it, no matter how well it's done, no matter what technique, incision location, pocket location or implant, there are tradeoffs and risks. The only question is whether you learn what they are, consider them, and, hopefully, avoid them, or whether you never know. Never knowing can be nice, but only if you are the luckiest person in the world—a person who magically (with minimal thought and preparation) gets the best result by a surgeon (whom you located fortuitously) who never has complications, using an implant that is perfect and lasts forever, and can control every aspect of your body's healing processes. Fairy tale. Never happens.

You need to know details about risks and tradeoffs before you can decide whether you are willing to accept them. We'll supply the details later. ***For now, just ask yourself:***

***Do I fully understand that this is not magic?***
It is surgery that involves factors that neither I nor any surgeon can fully control.

***Do I understand that nothing material, even a breast implant, lasts forever?***

***Do I accept that any surgery is serious, and that I will live with the results forever?***

***Do I understand that perfection is not an option, only improvement?***

***Can I accept that although risks are very low, bad things can happen?***

**If you can't answer YES to all of these questions**, breast augmentation may not be the best thing for you.

**STOP ON THE FIRST STAIRSTEP.**

## Can I Handle the Costs?

For a first-time augmentation (primary), costs can vary a lot, and we'll go into more detail later. For now, assume that you'll spend between $4,000 and $8,000 for an augmentation by a board-certified surgeon. Less than $4000, you're likely getting a "bargain" that may not be a bargain later. More than $8000, you're likely paying more than you need to pay to get a top-quality augmentation with a state-of-the-art implant. Like everything else, these costs will increase in the future.

**When it comes to price, think value.**
*If ever value is important, it's when you are hiring someone to operate on you!*

***Can I afford it? Not can I somehow get the money to get the implants, but "Can I really afford it?"***
*If not, DON'T DO IT until you CAN afford it.*

In our experience, patients who plan carefully and save for their augmentations are often happier than patients who stretch beyond their means to borrow money or spend money they don't have, then later have difficulty paying it back. A financial burden can detract from fully enjoying the result. Financing options that we'll discuss later are available, but financing is a reasonable option only when the payments fit your income and your budget.

If someone else pays for the augmentation, the question, "Can you afford it?" takes on an entirely new meaning and raises other issues. Under the correct circumstances, wonderful (a gift from your husband). Under other circumstances, not so wonderful. How good will it feel if later someone informs you that they own a piece of you? Is it worth it to afford it?

## Am I Willing to Use Common Sense? Can I Think Past Dinner?

These questions are certainly not meant to insult or demean. Neither question, however, should be taken lightly. The anticipation prior to augmentation and the positive effects after surgery are powerful and can affect even highly intelligent, accomplished, reasonable people. Once you decide to have implants, you want them now and you want to keep them forever.

**Throughout your quest for the BEST breast, common sense is invaluable.**
The more you use it, the easier and better your decisions.

If you don't feel confident that you have common sense and can use it no matter how appealing something becomes, be careful. Many patients and, regrettably, some surgeons focus on the here and now. Think past dinner? Dinner is here and now, tonight. Think at least five years ahead.

**Thinking past dinner means recognizing that what you do now, you will live with for the rest of your life.**
Choose for now and for when you're 60 or older.

We'll tell you how later. If you use common sense and think past dinner, you'll make better decisions. Can you do it? If the answer is yes, take a step upward.

## Am I Willing to Remove an Implant if Necessary?

Once you get the implants, if you're like 99 percent of patients, you'll want to keep them, no matter what. Our advice to our patients is, "Implants are wonderful for the overwhelming majority of patients. If for any reason they're not, especially if there's any hint that they could affect your health or well-being in the future, remove them. We both need to make that commitment before doing your augmentation." What makes implant removal necessary? Very rare incidences of infection and multiple recurrences of capsular contracture are reasons that I recommend implant removal to patients. More about that later.

Before having an augmentation, ***if you can't commit to removing your implants if it becomes necessary***, I would recommend you DON'T have an augmentation.

Many surgeons don't discuss this specific issue during consultations, but it's better to address the issue **before** surgery than to first hear about it **after** surgery.

## *So, does it* MAKE SENSE *to even think about* AUGMENTATION?

I hope you've got a better feeling for the answer to this question by now. If it makes sense to continue to think about it, the next step on the stairs is learning what you need to know and how to go about it.

[CHAPTER THREE]

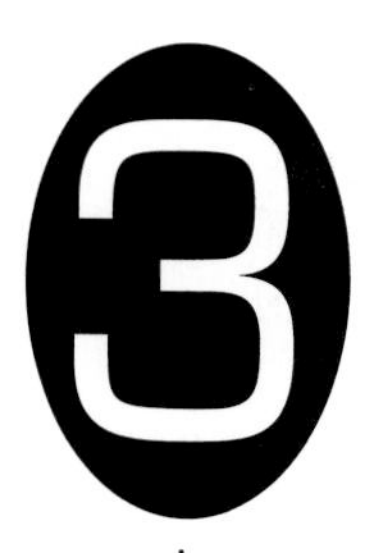

# FIRST THINGS FIRST: What You Need to Know and How to Go About Finding It

***"If you want to make the best decisions for your future, you'll consider at least 10 topics... before you think about the only three decisions that a less-informed patient considers."***

Before we go into detail about the many different options and choices in breast augmentation, let's start by making a ***shopping list of what you need to know***. Then we'll give you a guide for learning what you'll need to know. Armed with your shopping list and your guide, you can better explore each step in detail. Before you climb the stairs, we'll give you a look at the entire staircase.

## You need to know the answers to more than three questions.

When considering augmentation, many women focus only on three basic questions:

1) **What cup size am I going to be? (What size implant?)**
2) **Where will the incision be?**
3) **Will my implant be over the muscle or under the muscle?**

Why these three questions? For many patients, these are the only issues they ever hear from friends, other patients, and the media. Believe it or not, many patients only hear about the first two. They don't ask. They often don't know ***what*** to ask. Regrettably, some surgeons don't volunteer information about CHOICES and OPTIONS. Some surgeons are not committed to patient education. If you don't know, if you don't care to ask, and if your surgeon doesn't help as much as possible, the result can be less-than-optimal decisions.

**WEAK TEAM PREPARATION**
can lead to
**BAD TEAM DECISIONS**.

## We want good team decisions. Good team decisions begin with YOU.

If you aren't armed with knowledge, one member of the team is weak— you. Without the basics, why bother researching surgeons? You won't be able to distinguish fact from fluff. If you can't evaluate a surgeon, you'll likely not select the best surgeon for you. Then another member of the team is weak — the surgeon. Two weak team members increase the chances of weak or bad team decisions.

**If you want to make the best decisions for your future, you'll consider at least 10 topics...**
*before you think about the only three decisions that a less-informed patient considers.*

Let's start with a shopping list of 10 topics you need to research before you contact a surgeon:

### What You Need to Know BEFORE Consulting a Surgeon

1. What do I want, and what will my body allow me to have?
2. Implant types and options: Shape, smooth or textured shell, type of filler material
3. Possible complications, risks, and tradeoffs
4. Implant pocket location: Over muscle (retromammary) or partially under muscle (partial retropectoral)
5. Incision location options
6. Implant size
7. Options and tradeoffs: Sorting them out
8. Complications and tradeoffs: Things you and the surgeon can't control
9. Recovery: Ask about it up front, because what you hear can tell you a lot
10. How to organize your information to use it effectively

Learn about these topics before you call a surgeon's office.

## HOW TO GO ABOUT IT

In this chapter, we give you an overall outline of what you need to know to make good team decisions. In the chapters that follow in Part 2 of the book, we'll explore the details of every topic on this list to let you look at the stairs thoroughly before you start climbing. Having armed you with knowledge, in Part 3 we will move to the next logical steps — contacting and consulting surgeons and making decisions. Finally, in Part 4, you'll finalize decisions and prepare for surgery and recovery. Our reason for this sequence is:

It's best to know what you need to know, learn it, then apply what you know to surgeon selection and the decision-making process.

### The "How to Go About It" List

1. List what you need to know (the 10 topics).
2. Research each topic.
3. Armed with knowledge, prepare for surgeon consultations.
4. Consult surgeons and evaluate what they tell you (using what you have learned).
5. Choose your surgeon.
6. Select from your options and discuss the tradeoffs with your surgeon (TEAM DECISIONS).
7. Think about the choices you've made and the tradeoffs you've accepted. Be sure you're comfortable.
8. If you have any questions, or if anything is not clear, talk with your surgeon again. The time to clarify every detail is before, not after, your surgery.
9. Have your surgery and follow your surgeon's instructions for recovery.
10. Enjoy!

***Now that we understand the process, let's begin learning what we need to know!***

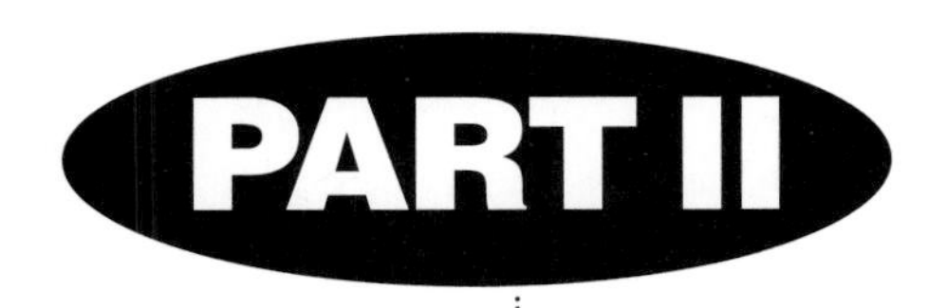


# ARMING YOURSELF WITH INFORMATION: Learning What You Need to Know to Make an Informed Decision

[CHAPTER FOUR]

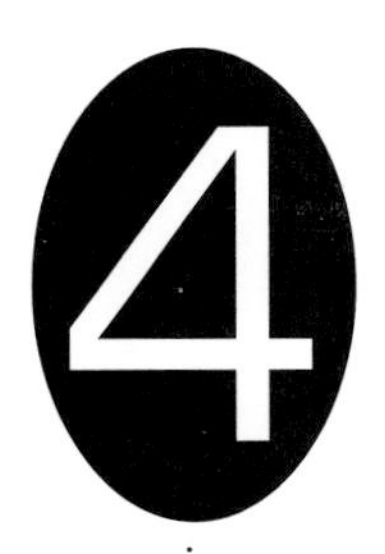

# RECONCILING DESIRES WITH REALITY: What Do I Want and What Will My Body Allow Me to Have?

***"If you and your surgeon don't recognize and acknowledge what your body tissues will allow you to have now and for the future, one or both of you may pay a penalty you don't want to pay."***

One of the first and most important steps on the staircase is understanding the importance of reconciling desires with reality: What you want with what your body will allow you to have.

## WHY DEFINE WHAT YOU WANT, AND HOW DEFINITIVE SHOULD YOU BE?

Let's start by assuming that you would like to have breasts that are beautiful or, at the least, better than they are now. But what is a "beautiful" breast? What is "better than they are now?" You probably have some feelings about the answers to these questions, but the feelings may be general, not well-defined. That's okay for starters. In fact, that's probably a good start. Think first in generalizations, then focus and define your desires more clearly as you learn more. You don't like what you have now, but how do you make a surgeon understand what you want?

The more clearly you **define your expectations**, and the better you **communicate your specific desires** to your surgeon, the more likely you'll **achieve your goals**.

## ONCE YOU'VE DEFINED IT, IS IT ACHIEVABLE? AT WHAT PRICE?

Assume we've defined our goals and expectations in detail. **Great!** We know what we want, but getting it can be another matter. Reality sets in. Is it achievable? What are the costs? Will circumstances allow me to get what I want? These questions always require answers.

Let's assume you'd like to have beautiful, full C cup or small D cup breasts with a naturally sloping upper breast (they look like breasts, not volleyballs), a nice hang to the lower breast without sagging, and nipples that point slightly upward, that will maintain that look forever as you grow older. But, you are 40 years old, have never had children, have virtually no breast tissue (your chest is absolutely flat), you are a workout fanatic with almost no body fat, and you hate wearing bras. Can you get what you want? Will your body allow you to have what you want? Is it doable with current implant options and surgical techniques? **NO WAY, NO HOW, NOT GONNA HAPPEN! YOUR BODY IS NOT GOING TO ALLOW YOU TO HAVE WHAT YOU WANT, AND IF YOU PUSH IT, YOUR BODY AND YOU WILL PAY THE PRICE!** If you get implants large enough to produce the D cup you want, your tissues won't support the weight, and your already thin tissues will sag and thin more!

**In breast augmentation, one of the most difficult steps on the staircase is reconciling what you want with what your body will allow you to have!**

*To* ***make the right choices,*** *you'll need to understand more about your* ***TISSUES****.*

Unfortunately, few surgeons and even fewer patients spend enough time with this step before doing an augmentation. A skilled, experienced surgeon can deliver almost anything you can dream up. With today's surgical techniques and implant options, you can create almost any size breast. What can be unfortunate is the price you pay, now or later.

**You come with only one set of tissues, and you can't replace those tissues.**

*If you choose options that exceed what those tissues will allow you to have, not just now, but later,* ***you'll pay****.*

**Many patients never know before their augmentation what price they may pay years later if they don't recognize and respect what their tissues will allow them to have.**

*Unless you like problems, more surgeries, more costs, more disappointments,* ***you don't want to ignore what your tissues will allow you to have***.

Is there any excuse for not knowing, not respecting, your tissues? Maybe not good excuses, but there may be some mitigating circumstances. Some surgeons, especially early in their careers, have not followed enough patients long enough to fully appreciate what happens to tissues over time and how implant options can affect the equation. Happy augmentation patients often do not return for long-term follow-up appointments, so the surgeon can't learn from what the surgeon doesn't see. The last thing that many younger patients want to think about is getting older (to be honest, even I don't like thinking about it, and I *am* older). But *you will get older*. Your tissues will change, and not for the better (visualize your grandmother's breasts). How your implant affects those tissues can change over time. If you ***make good team decisions now***, you have a much better chance of having nice grandmother breasts in the future.

## A CONCEPT AND A MISSION... TO AVOID PENALTIES IN THE FUTURE

One of the missions of this book is to raise the level of awareness of this important concept:

**If you and your surgeon don't recognize and acknowledge what your body tissues will allow you to have now and for the future, one or both of you may pay a penalty you don't want to pay.**

Any team decision that ignores this concept is a bad team decision. You can make it be a bad decision by asking for the wrong thing(s). Your surgeon can present or encourage choices that make a bad team decision. Or your surgeon can, with perfectly good intentions, try to deliver what you ordered without helping you understand the implications of your choices. Any one or combination of these can result in bad team decisions that penalize you and your surgeon in the future.

## WHERE DO WE START? WITH WHAT YOU DON'T LIKE, OR WITH WHAT YOU WANT?

Both, actually. Start with what you don't like; then list what you want. To help, here's a list of steps:

### Defining what you DON'T LIKE and what you WANT — A LIST

1. List the things you dislike about your breasts.
2. List how those dislikes affect your feeling of being normal, or how those dislikes affect your lifestyle.
3. List the basics of what you would like to have, based on what you know now.
4. Read the rest of this chapter to help you understand what your body may allow you to have.
5. Refine your list of what you'd like to have based on your new knowledge.
6. Look at your list carefully, and ask yourself if you're willing to live with your choices long term..
7. Finalize your list of "wants" that you'll discuss with surgeons you visit.
8. Don't let window shopping (looking at pictures in magazines and surgeon's "brag books") fool you about reality and the future. Think about your own tissues.

## LISTING YOUR DISLIKES

Make this easy. Pick simple things like these that we have heard from patients:

*My breasts are too small for my figure.*
*I wish the top of me matched the bottom.*
*I look like a bowling pin.*
*I can't fill up any bra.*
*I wish I could wear a T-shirt or blouse without a bra.*
*I'm tired of buying things to fit the bottom, then having to spend more money altering or filling the top.*
*Cleavage is not a word in my vocabulary.*
*If I could take what's on my butt and put it in my breasts, I'd be deadly.*
*Every bathing suit I buy must contain helpful devices.*
*I'm sick of males asking me why I just don't wear trunks instead of that girlish bathing suit.*
*If I'm not careful, I'll trip on them.*
*Hold a pencil underneath? Hell, I could hold a barbell!*
*My upper breasts look like ski slopes! No, they look worse than a ski slope.*
*I wish I had what I had before I was pregnant.*
*I liked what I had when I was pregnant (or nursing) a lot better than what I have now.*

I'm sure there are more, but you get the idea...

## LISTING WHAT YOU WANT BASED ON WHAT YOU KNOW NOW

These are examples listed according to how often we hear them from patients:

*Fuller upper breasts*
*More cleavage*
*X cup breast (choose the cup size)*
*Perkier breasts*
*Not huge, but proportionate to my figure*

*More fullness at the sides to balance my hips*
*A better shape to my breasts*
*Fix my weird nipples*
*Baywatch breasts — big and round*

Now that we know what we *don't like* and *what we would like to have*, let's learn more about the implications of our wants.

## HOW NOT TO DEFINE YOUR EXPECTATIONS

Although some methods of defining breast size are popular, they are not as accurate as we might like to believe. First, let's consider how not to define your desired breast.

### Cup size — especially cup size alone

Cup size is not even a consistent ***fashion*** measurement, let alone a ***medical*** term that can accurately and consistently define breast size.

But it's probably the most common yardstick women use. Any woman who has ever shopped for bras knows that a B is not a B is not a B. Although the labels say the same size, when you put them on, some fit and some don't. For the same woman, some B cup bras fit better than her usual C cup, and vice versa. Some B cup bras fit better than other B cup bras. Check your own bra drawer! How many cup sizes do you have?

We frequently hear from patients, "I'm sorta a B cup and I want to be a full C cup." Our response is simple. Tell me what a sorta B or a full C cup is! Can you go buy me a bra that is labeled sorta B or full C? If you can't define it, and you can't buy a bra labeled it, how do you expect a surgeon to create it?

**Cup size is extremely variable and inconsistent from one brand of bra to another.**

*If cup size is inconsistent, and you know it from buying your own bras, why would you want to rely on cup size to specify what you want?*

You can't define it because it isn't a consistent measurement from manufacturer to manufacturer, as much as they'd like you to think it is. If a surgeon guarantees you a cup size, that should tell you something about the surgeon. How can you deliver something that isn't consistently definable? What about the surgeon who *doesn't even know* that bra cup size is not consistent or definable?

How do we use cup size? We have no objection to using cup size as a general guideline, provided you recognize it is only a **general guide** that can't be ordered or delivered, and your surgeon doesn't talk to you about cup size **ONLY** when defining your desired outcome.

***We always ask our patients the following questions:*** What cup size were you before you were pregnant? Largest during pregnancy? What cup size after pregnancy and nursing if you nursed? What are you now? What would you like to be? If cup size is not a consistent measurement, why do we ask? The answers to these questions give us a clearer understanding of how our patient sees her breasts. During our exam, measurements will precisely define the size of the patient's skin envelope.

Knowing what a patient **thinks she is** (by asking the questions) and knowing what she **really is** (from our measurements) helps us better understand the patient's perspective and her wishes.

***But we NEVER define the desired result by CUP SIZE alone.***

## Many women don't buy bras to fit their breasts ... a personal revelation from Dr. Tebbetts

During my first several years in plastic surgery, I was baffled by the array of bra types and sizes that patients applied to breasts that all looked very similar and that measured similar in size on exam. One of the more enlightening milestones of my plastic surgery career was the day I realized that women don't buy bras to fit their breasts. Most women buy bras to push their breast tissue where they think it looks best. Women don't necessarily buy bras that fit their breasts. They buy bras that the breast will fill. What do I mean?

The width of a breast (from side-to-side, Figure 4-1) increases with increasing cup size. But I was amazed that women who had measurements indicating a *D cup* width were often telling me they were a *B cup*. What they really meant was that they were wearing a B cup bra. Then one day I asked a patient to please put her bra on as I observed. The B cup bra did not fit the fold beneath the breast. The breast was wide, more like a D cup width. The bra she had picked was much narrower than the width of the breast. When the patient put it on, she leaned forward and tucked the outside part of the wider breast inward to fill the cup of the smaller and narrower B cup bra. A light went on! Then I understood! She picked the smaller B cup bra because the amount of breast tissue that she had would fill it! When she pushed the outside portion of the breast inward into the bra, it not only filled the bra but bulged at the top of the breast and toward the middle. More cleavage! From that day on, I have been able to put bra cup size in perspective and rely more on measurements to document the size of breasts.

## BREAST WIDTH AND CUP SIZE

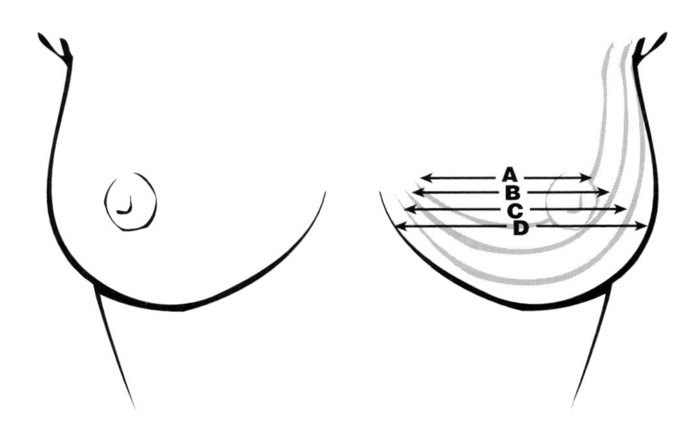


**The WIDER the breast,**
**the LARGER the cup size**

**Figure 4-1.**

Women buy a bra that they can **fill**.

Women buy bras to ***push breast tissue where they want it to go*** to create a specific appearance.

Women **don't necessarily buy bras that FIT** their breasts!

## Implant size in ccs

One measurement of the size of a breast implant is the volume (amount of filler) in the implant, measured in cubic centimeters (ccs). Do you know how much a cc is? How much is 300ccs? How many ccs are your breasts right now? How many ccs are in a B cup? How many ccs in a C cup? If you are thinking about trying to define what you want in terms of ccs, you should know the answers to all these questions. Fact is, some of these questions don't have an answer, at least not one correct answer. The answer to some of the questions is, "It depends."

Join a conversation with a group of women discussing their breast implants, and you might hear, "I have 300cc implants, and I'm a C cup." Another woman responds, "How can that be? I have 300cc implants, and I'm a D cup." They could both be correct. The message? A certain implant size in ccs does not guarantee a certain cup size. Why?

When teaching courses to surgeons, I have frequently asked the question, "How many ccs does it take to produce a C cup breast?" Invariably, one or more surgeons will respond with a specific number of ccs that will predictably produce a certain cup size breast, usually a less experienced surgeon. Also invariably, another surgeon will answer correctly by pointing out the following:

An augmented breast consists of the **skin envelope PLUS** the **implant PLUS** whatever **breast tissue** the woman had before the augmentation. Expressed as a formula for surgeons:

**Augmentation RESULT =**
**ENVELOPE + PARENCHYMA (breast tissue) + IMPLANT**

Now you can answer the question, "Why, if both women described above had 300cc implants, how could one have a C cup breast and the other a D cup breast?" The answer? The woman who ended up having a D cup breast after augmentation had more breast tissue *before* her augmentation compared to the woman who ended up with a C cup breast.

**A certain number of ccs in an implant does not make a certain cup size breast.**

*Be sure you **understand this concept**, and **be sure that your surgeon understands** it.*

The **final size of the breast** depends on the amount of **breast tissue the woman had prior to surgery PLUS** the **size of the implant** that was placed in the breast.

So a woman who has more breast tissue to begin with needs fewer ccs in an implant (smaller) to get to a C cup breast compared to another woman who had less breast tissue to begin with, and will need a larger implant to get to a C cup breast. If this concept is confusing, read it again until it makes sense.

Now that we know how *not* to define our desired breast size, how *do* we define it? At this stage, it's fine for you to specify what you want with the simple "want list" you made. Don't worry too much about specifics until you understand more about how breast size affects your tissues. Later, you and your surgeon can make more realistic estimates of what is achievable (and the tradeoffs) by thinking about your specific tissues. Do you have enough skin to create what you want? Do you have too much skin that will require more than what you want to fill it optimally? And a whole series of additional questions that will help answer the question, "Will your tissues allow you to have what you want? To what degree? And for how long?"

***Do you have what it takes (your tissues) to get what you want? And what do you have when you get it (the long-term result)?***

## How Much Is Enough?

How much breast is enough? The answer depends on two major factors: 1) Breast size in proportion to body size, and 2) the characteristics of each woman's breast skin and breast tissues. If balanced proportion is the goal, breast size should balance with other body proportions including height and hip measurements. Every woman's breast skin can only stretch and enlarge a certain amount without sustaining damage such as excessive stretching and thinning that allows the breast to sag or cause tearing of the skin undersurface that produces visible stretch marks.

From a practical, common sense perspective, a woman's breasts are "designed" to enlarge an amount that approximates the amount of enlargement that usually occurs with pregnancy. For most women, the breast usually enlarges an average of one to one and one-half cup sizes during pregnancy. Of course, the larger the breast *before* pregnancy, the greater the degree of enlargement *during* pregnancy. The larger the breast during pregnancy, the more the skin stretches to accommodate the enlarged breast tissue. After pregnancy, the breast tissue shrinks and falls to the bottom of the larger, stretched skin envelope. The result is a more sagging breast that is emptier in the upper breast. Extreme enlargement with pregnancy usually results in a very sagging breast with thin skin and visible stretch marks.

Similar changes occur following breast augmentation. The larger the implant, the larger the resulting breast. The larger the implant, the more the breast skin stretches, thins, and the more the breast will ultimately sag as a woman ages, losing upper fill.

**An augmented breast may not sag quite as much as an unaugmented breast of the same size, but the larger the implant, the more the breast will sag in the future as you age.**

## If a surgeon tells you that an augmented breast won't sag, locate another surgeon who understands tissue dynamics.

What is ideal fill for each woman's skin envelope? If a woman has had previous pregnancies, her skin envelope is already stretched. Envision a funnel and pitcher pouring liquid into a breast envelope (Figure 4-2, A). If the envelope has already been stretched, the fluid will initially fill the lower breast. As more fluid is added, at some point the breast appears full and natural, with a natural appearing upper breast slope (Figure 4-2, B). If more fluid is added, the upper breast begins to bulge outwardly as the skin envelope is overfilled.

Exactly the same principles apply to breast augmentation. To achieve an optimal aesthetic result, enough filler must be added (the size of the implant) to adequately fill the envelope (Figure 4-2, B). If a woman wants a very bulging upper breast, more filler (a larger implant) is required. But the larger the implant, the more the stretch, and the more the breast will sag in the future.

How much is enough? If the best long-term result is the goal, the answer is to fill the existing envelope to ideal fill and a natural breast contour (Figure 4-2, B). Any overfill past this point virtually guarantees that the breast will sag more in the future, increasing risks and decreasing the quality of the result (Figure 4-2, C). For women who have never been pregnant, the surgeon must estimate a normal amount of stretch that would occur with pregnancy, given each woman's breast tissue characteristics.

When you choose an implant that is too large for your skin to support, the implant can cause tissue changes that cannot be reversed and that can result in unsatisfactory consequences and additional surgery that are listed in Figure 4-2, C. Remember that your choice of breast size has long-term consequences.

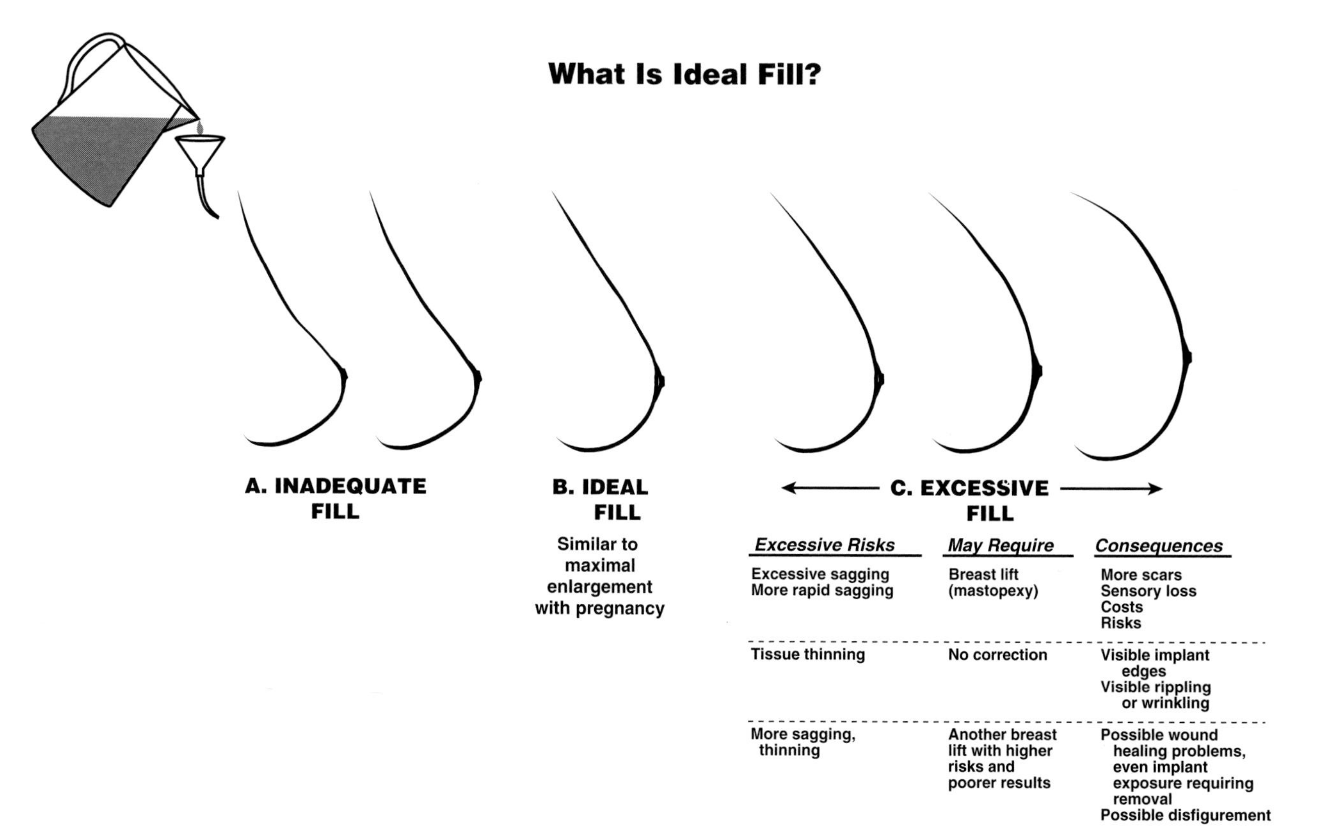


| Excessive Risks | May Require | Consequences |
|---|---|---|
| Excessive sagging<br>More rapid sagging | Breast lift (mastopexy) | More scars<br>Sensory loss<br>Costs<br>Risks |
| Tissue thinning | No correction | Visible implant edges<br>Visible rippling or wrinkling |
| More sagging, thinning | Another breast lift with higher risks and poorer results | Possible wound healing problems, even implant exposure requiring removal<br>Possible disfigurement |

Figure 4-2.

## WHAT DO YOU HAVE NOW?

**A surgeon can only work with the tissues that you bring the surgeon to work with.**

Look at your breasts in the mirror. Do they look exactly like any other woman's breasts that you've ever seen? No. Do they match side to side? Never. Do they look the same now as they looked five years ago? Probably not, if you look closely. No two women have exactly the same breast appearance because every woman's tissues and combination of tissues are different. The two breasts never match exactly because the tissues are never exactly the same in both breasts.

**No woman has two breasts that are the same, and no surgeon can create two breasts that are exactly the same.**

Your breasts don't look the same as they did five years ago because your tissues are five years older, and the characteristics of those tissues have changed. They will continue to change throughout your lifetime. I wish we could tell you they change for the better, but that "ain't so."

**Will what you have (your tissues) allow you to get what you want (your result)?**

Since a surgeon can only work with what you bring, whether you can get what you want depends on what you bring the surgeon — your individual tissues — to work with. Will your tissues allow you to get what you want? Do you have the optimal amount and type of skin to accept the implant that will create the breast you are ordering? If your tissues will accept the implant, how will your choices affect your breasts in the future? These are complex questions that don't necessarily have a single right answer. Begin by memorizing two inescapable truths, then tell every woman you know who is considering augmentation (and every surgeon you see who doesn't already know):

**The bigger the breast, the worse it will look over time (augmented or not)!**

*Think about the woman you knew at a younger age with large breasts. How do they look now?*

**Your tissues won't get better as you age; they will get worse!**

*Think about your grandmother's breasts or any woman's breasts after age 60.*

We aren't dealing with magic here. A little logic and common sense goes a long way. The bigger the breast you request (all other factors being equal), the bigger and heavier the implant, and the more that implant will stretch your tissues over time (Figure 4-3). Stretched breast skin sags. All this happens as you and your tissues are getting older and more stretchy on their own. You can't do anything about what you come with or how your breast envelope ages, but you certainly can affect how the implant may affect your tissues in the future by avoiding excessively large implants.

**The bigger the breast you request, the worse it will look over time.**

*Guaranteed. Slam dunk. For sure.*

*Repeat after me, aloud, ten times:*

***The bigger the implant I request, the worse it will look over time.***

Not only will it look worse, the bigger the implant you get now, the more likely you may pay in the future in additional operations and additional costs. You may, for example, require a breast lift (mastopexy) with additional scars, more risk of loss of sensation, and additional costs sooner if you select implants large enough to accelerate sagging. More about that later. For now, just recognize and acknowledge that:

**For the best long-term result, you might want to balance what you want with what your tissues will allow you to have.**

## Ageing in the Excessively Augmented Breast

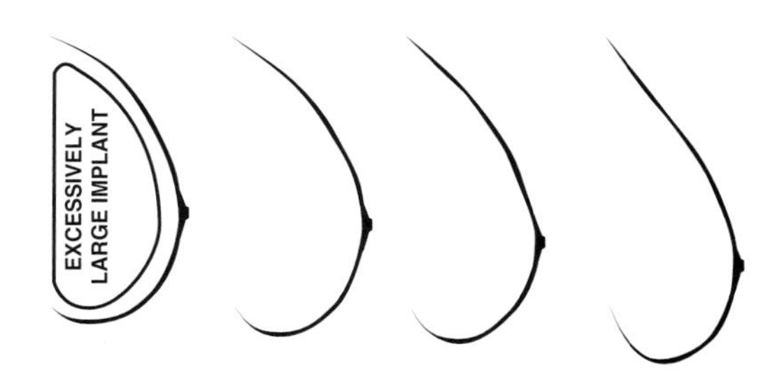


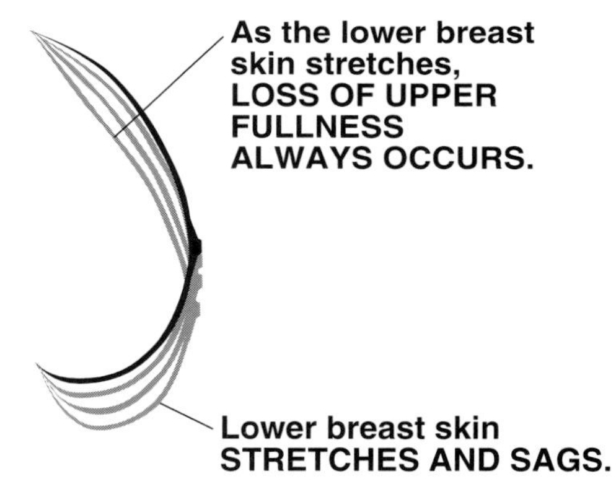


**The larger the implant, the more your tissue will stretch.**

**The more your tissues stretch, the more the breast will sag.**

**Risks of visible rippling, visible edges, feeling the implant, and reoperations increase.**

**Figure 4-3.**

*Your surgeon should help you understand the characteristics of your individual tissues and which options are realistic for you.*

**For the best long-term result, you might want to balance what you want with what your tissues can support over time.**

*Ask you surgeon specifically how the implants you select will affect your individual tissues over time, and take notes. This will make your surgeon aware that you are concerned about this and want the best result for the longest time.*

The real truth is that different patients' tissues react differently to the same implant over time. No surgeon can tell you exactly how your tissues will age, how soon you will sag, or when you may need a breast lift. But you should remember this: If a surgeon doesn't bring up the subject of your tissue characteristics and how your choice of implant might affect your long-term result, stop and think. Just what are the chances that you'll get the best long-term result from that surgeon?

## TWO GOLDEN RULES FOR GOOD RESULTS—SHORT TERM AND LONG TERM

For an **optimal result**, the surgeon must **adequately fill** the existing breast envelope.

**Any fill more than that required** for an optimal, aesthetic result **will detract from the long-term result**.

These principles will make more sense by applying them to two patient examples:

1) Sharon, a fictitious name but real patient,(Patient number 1, Figure 4-4) had a C cup breast before pregnancy and enlarged to DD during pregnancy. After pregnancy, her envelope remained stretched (as usually occurs), but her breast tissue

shrank and fell to the bottom of the envelope. She now has what appears to her a sagging breast, empty in the top and fuller and saggy at the bottom. Her breasts won't look good unless the stretched envelope is adequately filled. Imagine a funnel in the top of the breast. If we poured in liquid, the bottom of the breast would fill first. Pour more into the funnel, and the middle will fill next. The top fills last. At some point, with the patient sitting, the breast would look optimal, with adequate but not excessive upper fill. At that exact point, the amount of filler that we added to the breast is *precisely the amount required to produce an optimal result.* Exactly the same thing happens with breast implants. Too small, and you won't fill the top. Too large and the top will bulge, and the breast will sag more rapidly.

**The size of implant that will be required to fill a larger, stretched envelope will be greater than the size required to fill a smaller, less-stretched envelope.**

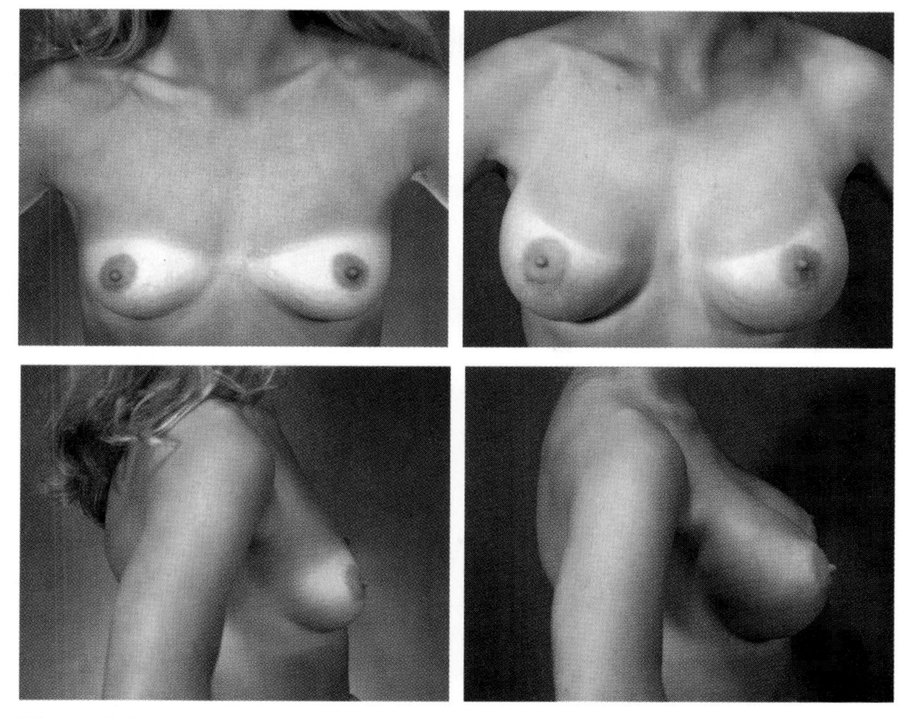

**Figure 4-4.**

2) Consider a different patient we'll call Janet (Patient number 2, Figure 4-5). Younger, no children, with an A cup breast. The skin is tight, has never been stretched by pregnancy, and there is very little breast tissue (parenchyma). Janet's envelope is totally different than Sharon's envelope. It is tight, with less room for an implant. The larger the implant placed, the more the skin will push against the lower implant, and the more the upper breast will bulge. The bulging will decrease over time as the skin of the lower breast stretches, but if the implant is too large for the amount of stretch that can occur, the breast will have permanent, excess upper bulging. If the implant is too large for the patient's skin characteristics, the lower breast skin will stretch excessively, and the breast will appear saggy or have a "bottomed out" appearance — both are bad. The implant that will produce an optimal long-term result for Janet will be smaller than the ideal implant for Sharon. Janet has smaller breasts to begin with and *skin that has never been stretched*. To apply the principles, use enough implant to fill the envelope, allowing for stretch, but not so much implant that excessive stretch and sagging will occur with time.

**The smaller and tighter (unstretched by pregnancies) the envelope, the less implant the envelope can accept and give an aesthetically optimal result and a good long-term result without problems.**

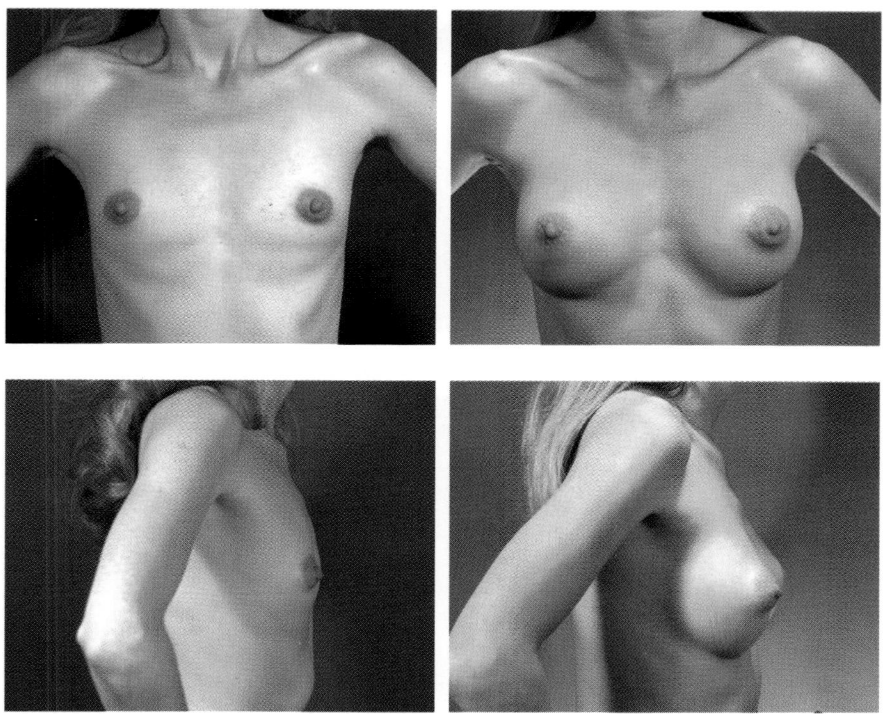

**Figure 4-5.**

No surgeon can totally predict what a patient's tissues will do over time, but every surgeon and patient should consider these issues when making implant choices. Even if Sharon and Janet were the same height, with the same torso proportions, and both wanted the same, optimal result, the implant required to produce that result would be different in the two patients. Why? *Because their tissues are different.*

**No implant will produce the same result in two different patients.**

Just because your best friend had a round, smooth, saline-filled, 300cc implant that produced a certain breast, rest assured that the same implant will not produce the same result in your breast because your tissues are different.

## ARE YOU WILLING TO LIVE WITH WHAT YOU'VE ORDERED?

Now we get to balance what you want with the tradeoffs of what you're willing to live with. What if you are Janet and you want Baywatch breasts? For those who were never treated to this prime example of video artistry, a Baywatch breast is *very large, very round, and very bulging at the top, even without clothing*. With your tight skin, can you get very large, round, bulging implants? You bet! If you can afford them, and you can describe them, you can find a surgeon who will fill your order — guaranteed. I mean you're guaranteed to be able find a surgeon who will fill the order, but the surgeon would have to be brain dead to guarantee the work.

Assume that now you've got them — the Baywatch breasts. Awesome! You love them, your significant other loves them, and most men must love them because they can't look in your eyes when they talk to you. You got 'em — now what have you got? What will predictably happen to the extremely large breast over time?

This really isn't a tough question; just think about what always happens to large breasts. The skin can't adequately support the weight of the breast tissue over time, so the breast sags. It's a little different with implants — they usually don't sag quite as much over time as a non-augmented breast the same size, but they still sag. The weight of the implant stretches and thins the skin. The thinner the skin, the more the breast sags. The weight of the implant pulls on the skin enough to create visible ripples around the edges of the breasts or in the upper part of the breast. If you need a reoperation for sagging or rippling, now what does the surgeon have to work with? Thinner, stretched skin. Poorer quality tissues. Operating on poorer quality tissues often brings poorer results and more potential problems. You ordered them. Now you have them. What have you got?

Does this mean that no woman should have larger breast implants? Not necessarily. Sometimes, larger implants are required to adequately fill a woman's existing breast envelope. Some women simply want to have larger breasts and implants, and they certainly have the right to have what they want. But they also should understand what will happen over time.

What's important is,
**regardless of personal choices and choices dictated by your tissue characteristics, you should be INFORMED and AWARE of the potential long-term implications of those choices BEFORE SURGERY.**

It's your job to see that this happens.

## REALISM AND THE PERFECT BREAST

Regardless of how much homework you do, how well-informed you become, and which choices you make, another inescapable truth is:

**PERFECTION IS NOT AN OPTION.**
**Surgeons can only produce improvement.**

Hopefully, you'll view the improvement as perfection compared to what you had before, but perfection doesn't exist in plastic surgery. Your breasts won't exactly match, you likely won't get every single thing you want, and even if you select a perfectionist surgeon, I guarantee you the surgeon won't be able to achieve perfection. Your tissues aren't perfect. Time isn't kind to tissues, and neither you nor your surgeon can stop the clock.

Go in with your eyes wide open. Do everything you can right, but be realistic about your expectations. Pin your surgeon down with questions that help you be realistic. Hopefully, your surgeon will do all this automatically, but, ultimately, it's your job to pick the surgeon who best meets these goals.

## THE PLEASURES AND PERILS OF WINDOW SHOPPING FOR BREASTS

Although I'm risking putting myself in a position I might not want to be in (and I should know better by now), I have observed that most women like to shop! If you needed a new dress, chances are you'd shop for it. If you were ordering a dress, you'd want to see a picture before placing the order. Deep down, you know that shopping for a dress isn't the same as shopping for a breast, but instinctively, you're likely to apply some of the same principles. As an informed consumer, you'd like to know what's available. You'd really like to know what your breasts are going to look like before you proceed with your augmentation. Pictures and images are common ways to address these issues. Three commonly used media are magazine pictures, pictures from a surgeon's before and after ("brag") book, and pictures on a computer imager.

### Magazine Pictures

**The only picture that truly represents breast characteristics is one totally without clothing, standing or lying down.**

Most pictures in magazines don't meet these criteria. If nude, the model is almost always posed in a position that best compliments her positives. Often the positioning interferes with (or contributes to) the appearance of the breast. At any rate, it doesn't allow an objective appraisal. If the model is wearing any clothing that touches the breasts (much less pushes the breasts to make them or the clothing look more appealing), you can't make objective judgements about the breast.

If you see breasts that you like, it's fine to take the pictures with you when you visit a surgeon. Pictures may help a surgeon understand what you like, and pictures may help you judge the surgeon:

**If a surgeon looks at a picture and says, "Sure, we can make that breast! No problem!"**

**RUN THE OTHER WAY!**

*There could be a real problem if your tissues don't match the tissues of the person in the picture (and they never do). Either the surgeon may not know, or the surgeon may not care. Exception: If the picture is a picture of a woman standing, nude, with tissues exactly the same as yours. Does she exist?*

**On the other hand, if the surgeon replies, "Let's look at your tissues and compare you as best we can to the person in the picture,"**

**BETTER!**

*Problem still is, the surgeon can't evaluate the tissues of the woman in the picture.*

**If the surgeon replies, "I'll use the pictures to help me understand what you'd like, and then I'll try to help you understand our best options and tradeoffs, given your tissues,**

**GREAT!**

### Surgeon "Before-and-After" Brag Books

We'll cover this subject later when we discuss surgeon consultations. Some basic rules that we'll mention again are:

**If you can find a patient in the book who looks almost exactly like you BEFORE her augmentation, it's possible that you MIGHT be able to look SOMEWHAT like her result AFTER your operation.**

*If you can't find someone who looks like you before her surgery, it's still fun to look.*

*The best lessons you can learn from any before-and-after book are:*

**If the surgeon doesn't have pictures to show you, consult other surgeons.**

**If every result looks good, consult other surgeons.**

**If the book does not contain a wide variety of breasts with some results better than others, consult other surgeons.**

**A surgeon's habits are reflected in the quality of the pictures as well as the quality of the results.**
*Look at the quality of the pictures! Are they standardized? Good quality? Is the background consistent in all the pictures?*

**If the surgeon or his personnel can't fully explain any question you ask about the pictures, consult other surgeons.**

## Computer Imagers and Images

Again, we'll cover this topic more later, but keep in mind for now that:

**Anyone, even a technician, can produce changes on a computer that no surgeon can produce with living tissue.**

**If the surgeon uses the imager to help you understand some points, fine.**

**If a technician or the surgeon uses the imager to sell you something that doesn't make sense or to sell you other non-breast operations, BEWARE.**

**If the surgeon morphs (changes the appearance of) your breasts on the computer and prints you a simulated before and after picture, don't look at it too much, and try not to fix the image in your mind. Your result definitely won't match the image exactly.**

**We are all human. Once we have seen a simulated result, we tend to expect that result, even if the computer screen is covered with disclaimers informing us that this is only a simulation.**

The computer can be a wonderful tool when used as a constructive tool to discuss options with you or provide you useful information. We use it a lot. When it's used primarily as a marketing tool to sell you an operation, you're likely not getting all that's best for you. To date, no one can precisely represent your tissue characteristics on a computer.

When it comes to images, shop all you want, but don't buy. Use pictures constructively, but base your buying on ***information*** and an ***evaluation of your tissues***.

## AND NOW...

Now that you have a feel for reconciling your desires with reality, let's move on to the next step — implants.

[CHAPTER FIVE]

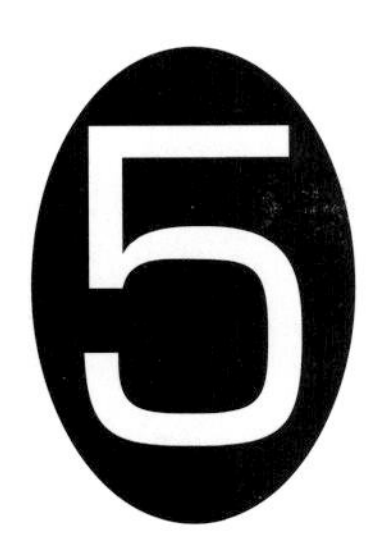


# BREAST IMPLANTS: The Devices and the Choices

***"The implant you choose is the implant you'll live with — understand the tradeoffs of different implants and choose carefully."***

Implant choices? There are many. Round shape, anatomic shape, underfilled, adequately filled, overfilled, smooth outer shell, textured outer shell, saline filled, silicone gel filled. Each of these choices is currently available somewhere, and each is a valid choice in certain situations. Each has benefits and tradeoffs. How do you choose? Start by learning about the alternatives! This chapter contains a lot of information — maybe more than you think you'd like to know! But the alternative — not knowing — could cost you significantly in the future. The only way to make the best decisions is to fully understand the many issues regarding implants.

**You can't know too much about implants — the issues and the choices.**

**Not knowing now could cost you** significantly in the future — **in quality** of results and **in complications** and **need for additional surgery!**

***The future price of poor decisions from lack of knowledge is too high for any patient to pay!***

## BREAST IMPLANTS ARE DEVICES ...

A breast implant is a device. Can you name any device that's perfect? Can you name any device that lasts forever? Can you name any sophisticated device that never requires maintenance? Probably not. So let's start out with three basic truths:

**Breast implants are NOT PERFECT.**

**Breast implants DON'T LAST FOREVER.**

**Breast implants may REQUIRE SOME MAINTENANCE.**

If you believe these three statements, you've taken a big step. If you accept that something's not perfect, you can begin learning about its imperfections and whether you're willing to accept them. If you accept that something won't last forever, you can begin to understand the factors that affect its longevity and make choices that help prolong its life. You can also decide whether you're willing to have maintenance if it becomes necessary.

***If you can't accept the imperfections of implants or if you're unwilling to have maintenance,***

**DON'T HAVE A BREAST AUGMENTATION.**

## IMPLANTS: WHAT DO I NEED TO KNOW?

This chapter is organized to meet the information needs of two different groups of women. If you want basic information about the currently available alternatives, and don't want to spend more time understanding all of the issues about implants, read the first half of the chapter. If you want more detailed information that focuses on the important issues that affect implant longevity and the tradeoffs between naturalness and longevity, read the entire chapter. Many of the most important issues about breast implants are not addressed in any other written information for the public. Although some of these issues may seem too detailed, dry, or boring, they affect your long-term result, risk of reoperations in your future, and risks of complications and problems.

## THE BASIC CHOICES

Figure 5-1 outlines the basic choices in breast implants currently available in the world in 1999. In the United States, implant filler choices are limited to saline, except in special studies under FDA supervision. Additional choices will almost certainly become available in the United States after FDA studies are completed, realistically in 2002 or later.

**Figure 5-1.**

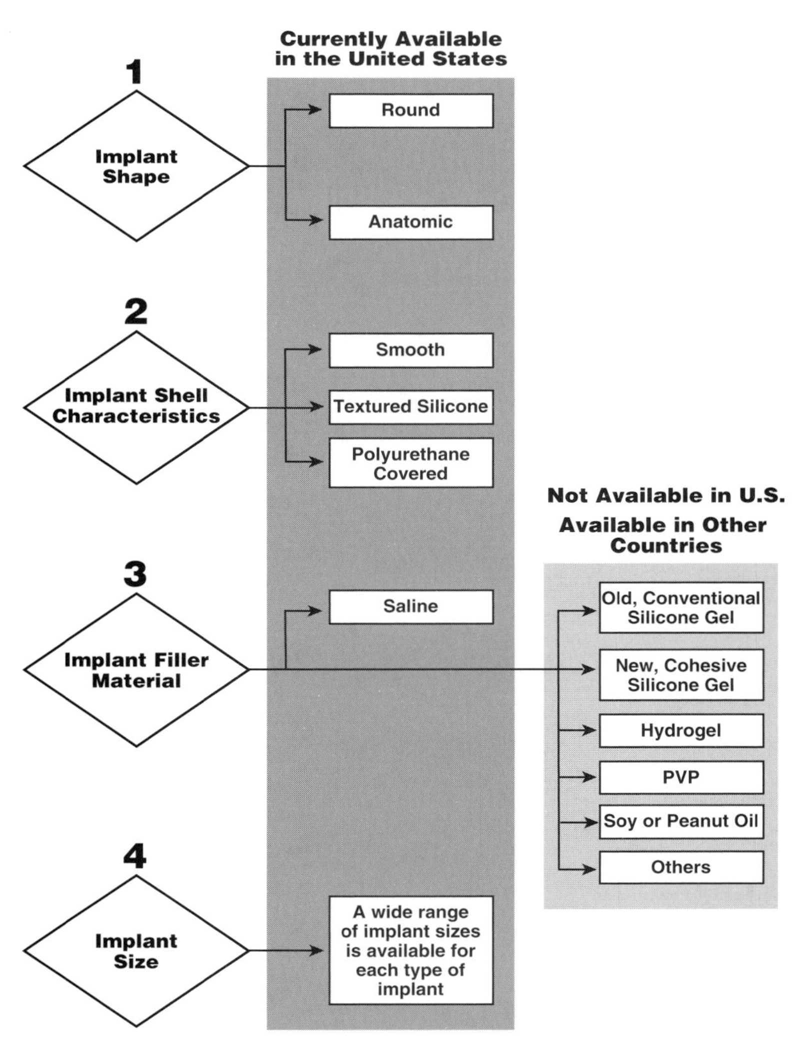

## IMPLANT SHAPE — ROUND OR ANATOMIC

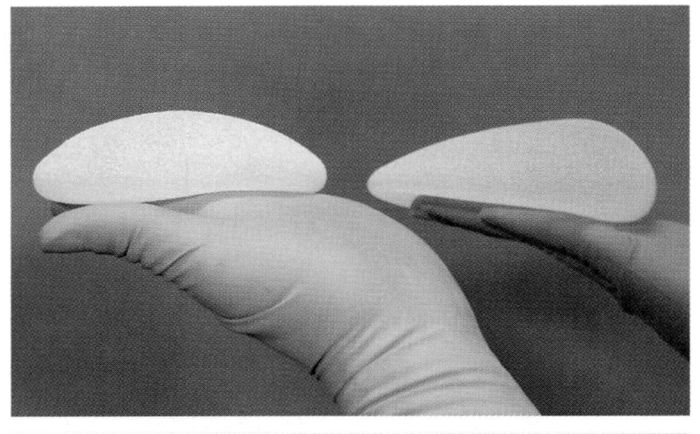

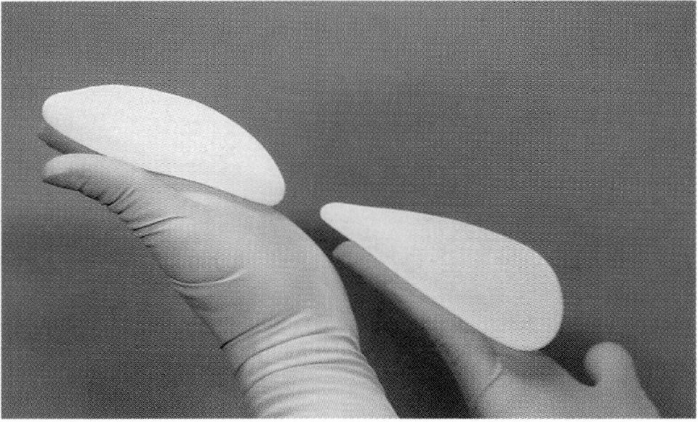

**Figure 5-2.**

### A round implant is round. An anatomic implant is shaped. Which looks more like a breast?

You can get a good result with either a round implant or an anatomic implant. Which is better for you? It depends on your answers to the following questions: Write down your answers, then continue reading.

**NO** **YES**

1. Do you want a result that looks more natural than excessively round and bulging in the upper breast?

| NO | YES | |
|---|---|---|
| ☐ | ☑ | 2. Do you want a full upper breast but not an overly bulging upper breast? |
| ☐ | ☑ | 3. Do you want an adequately filled implant with minimal risk of shell folding and risk of shell rupture? |
| ☐ | ☑ | 4. Do you want to maintain fullness in your upper breast (without a folded shell)? |
| ☐ | ☑ | 5. Do you have a surgeon who has experience with both types of implants? |

If your answer to all of the questions is ***"yes"***, you'll almost certainly want an **anatomic implant**.

### Round Implants

Round implants are designed on a round base, and when properly filled, create a more round appearance in the breast, a more globular appearance with a more bulging upper breast (Figure 5-3). Is it possible to create a natural appearance using a round implant? Yes, and Figure 5-4A is an example of a round implant creating a natural-looking breast—but there's a catch. What is it?

If an augmentation result looks natural (with a gradually sloping, full upper breast) and contains a **ROUND** implant, chances are overwhelming that the round implant is **UNDERFILLED** and the **SHELL IS FOLDED**.

***Shell folding risks premature shell failure and implant rupture.***

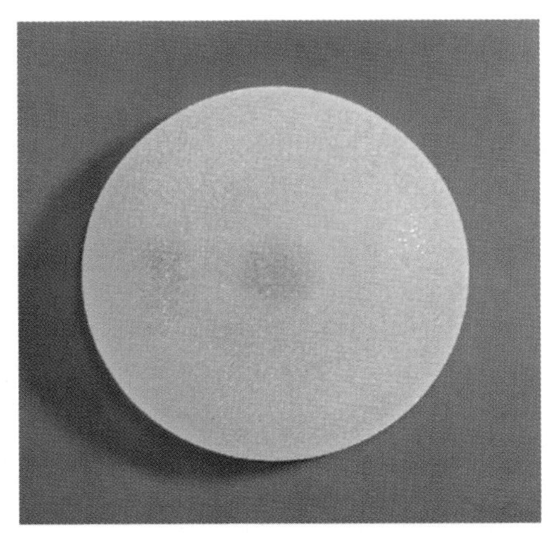

**Figure 5-3.**

If the round implant *were adequately filled to prevent upper shell collapse and folding, the upper breast would bulge more* and/or the breast would appear more globular (Figures 5-4B, 5-5B)—in virtually every instance. The only way the upper breast can look normal is if *the upper portion of the round implant collapses downward in the pocket* (Figures 5-4A, 5-5A). If the upper implant collapses, the implant shortens vertically and the shell collapses downward, reducing the bulging in the upper breast. Problem is, the shell is folded. Do you know what is likely to happen to a folded shell? It may wear out sooner. This phenomenon of upper shell collapse in a round implant explains what you might hear from some surgeons: "Round implants become anatomic in the pocket." No, round implants do not become anatomic. Round implants collapse because most are underfilled.

**Figure 5-4.**

## The Catch 22 with ROUND IMPLANTS — Solved by McGhan 468 and 410 Anatomic Implants With Adequate Fill

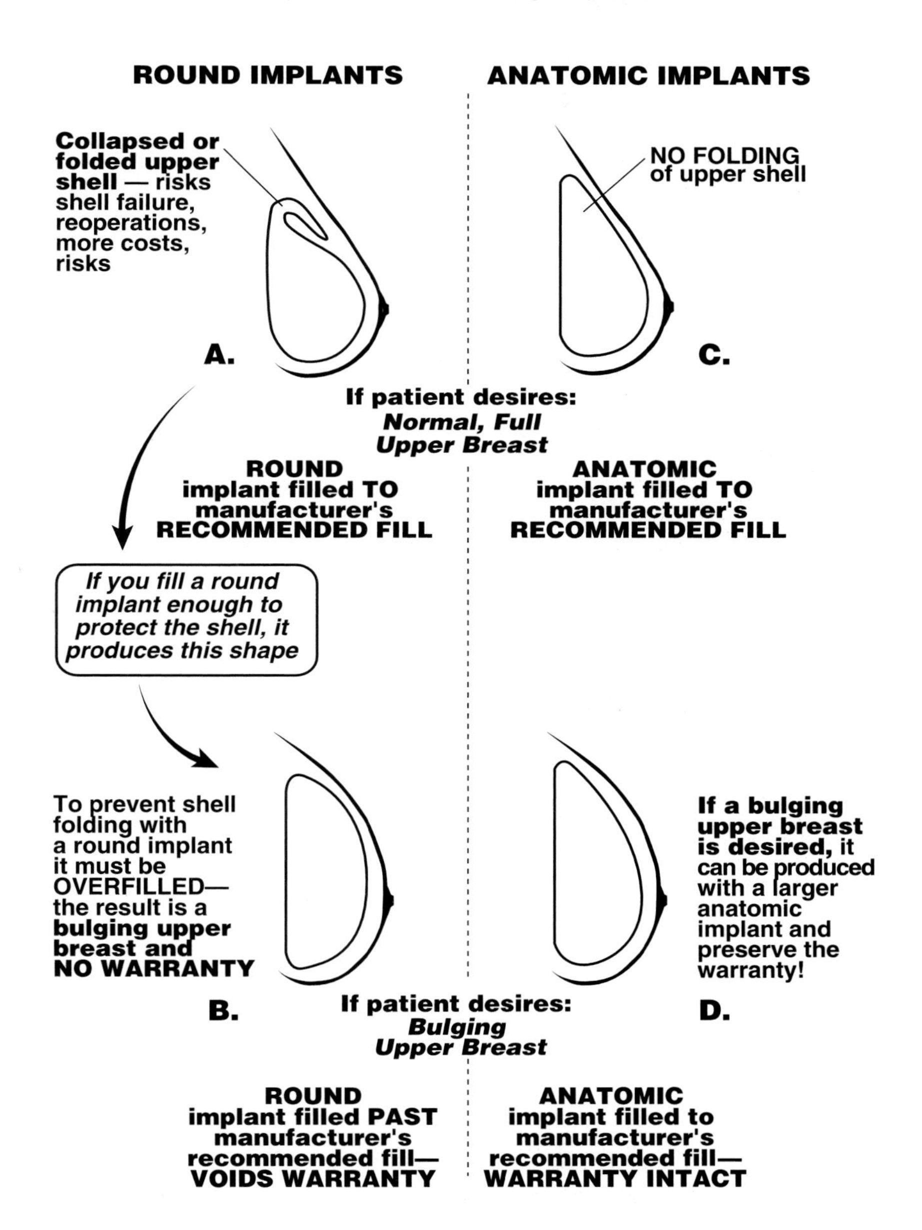

**Figure 5-5.**

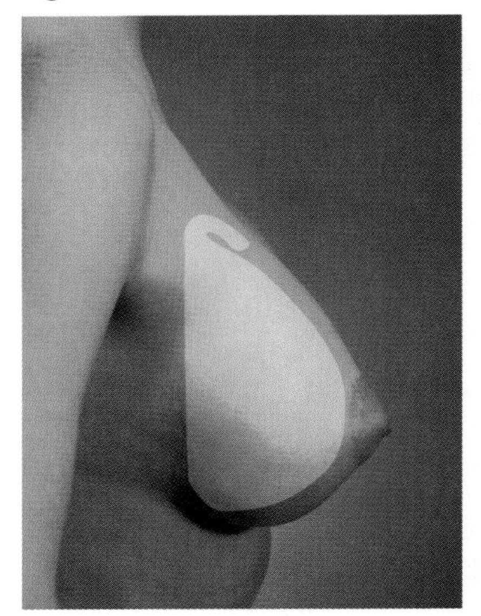

**A. The upper shell is collapsed and folded.**

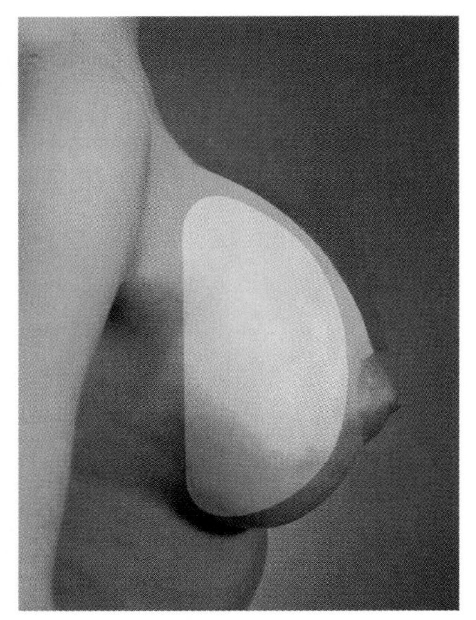

**B. If overfilled to protect the shell, a round implant produces more upper bulging.**

## Round Implants: The Catch 22

To produce a *natural appearing breast with a round implant,* a surgeon must *underfill* the round implant according to the tilt test (we know already that we can't trust *manufacturer's recommendations* alone to determine adequate fill). If the surgeon fills the round implant to manufacturer's recommendations, the implant shell will fold and collapse (Figures 5-4A, 5-5B). The breast may look natural, but the shell is folded. If the surgeon *overfills* past recommendations to prevent shell folding (Figures 5-4B, 5-5B), *the surgeon voids the implant warranty*. When our patients request a round implant, or when we think a round implant may be better (usually in a multiple reoperation case where it's difficult to control an anatomic implant), the patient must sign a permit indicating *only one* of the following choices:

1) *I want Dr. Tebbetts to fill my round implant to manufacturer's recommendations. I understand that this amount of fill may not prevent shell folding, and I accept that shell folding may cause my implant to wear out sooner.*

**OR**

*2) I want Dr. Tebbetts to fill my round implant more than manufacturer's recommendations until Dr. Tebbetts feels that the implant passes the tilt test and contains adequate filler to minimize risks of shell folding and shell collapse in the upper implant. I understand and accept that filling above the manufacturer's recommended fill voids the manufacturer's warranty, and I am responsible for all costs of implant replacement whenever it becomes necessary.*

With today's round implants, you must choose a **rippled, folded shell OR give up the manufacturer's warranty** if you overfill the implant!!!

*With current round implants from any manufacturer,* ***you can have only ONE of the two choices listed above, NOT BOTH.*** *Neither is perfect, so....you choose.*

If you request that your surgeon overfill your round implants, be sure to specify that you want the implants filled adequately to pass the tilt test. Many surgeons intuitively overfill past manufacturers' recommendations, but the amount of overfill is still inadequate for the implant to pass the tilt test. Later in this chapter, we'll explain the tilt test in detail.

**When overfilling past manufacturer's recommendations to protect the implant shell from folding, continue adding filler until the implant passes the tilt test.**

Some surgeons fill round implants a fixed *amount* over manufacturers' recommendations. Others fill a fixed *percentage* above manufacturers' recommendations. Neither is as foolproof as filling the implant to pass the tilt test.

**The larger a ROUND implant, the more fill above manufacturer's recommendations is required to prevent shell folding.**

In contrast, it is ***unnecessary to overfill McGhan anatomic implants past manufacturers' recommendations***, because at manufacturers' recommendations, McGhan anatomic implants for augmentation pass the tilt test!

***The fill volumes for McGhan anatomic implants were defined higher by the manufacturer to pass the tilt test. Round implants were not!***

The upper shell of round implants may not collapse and fold immediately after surgery (Figure 5-6A) because the tight skin envelope pushes back against the lower implant. However, over the first six months following surgery, the lower breast envelope stretches, allowing the filler to redistribute into the lower implant (Figure 5-6B). As the filler redistributes into the lower portion of an underfilled round implant, the upper shell collapses and folds, risking premature shell failure.

When round implants are overfilled to protect the shell (Figure 5-6C), the upper shell may not collapse and fold, but with current round implants, overfill voids the manufacturer's warranty (Figure 5-6D).

We are currently designing new round implants that will have adequate fill to protect the shell AND preserve the manufacturer's warranty. Call us for details and projected availability.

## ROUND Implants — What Happens Over Time?

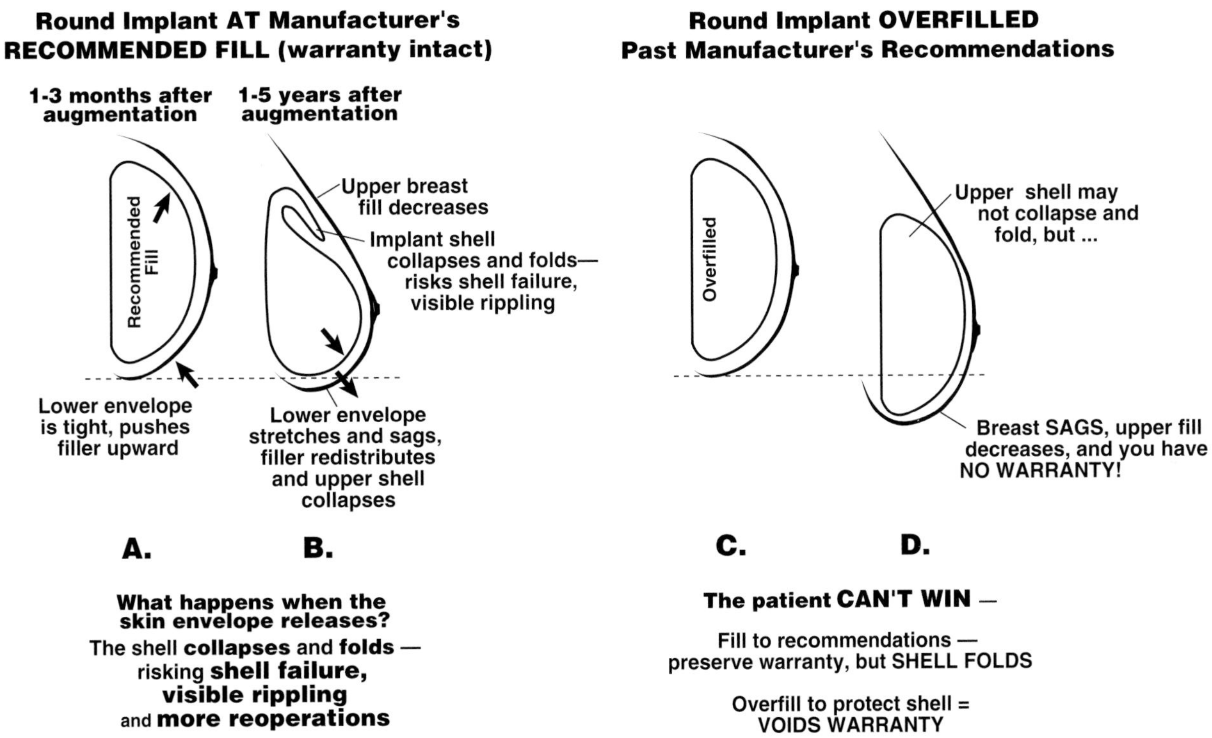

**Round Implant AT Manufacturer's RECOMMENDED FILL (warranty intact)**

**1-3 months after augmentation**

Recommended Fill

Lower envelope is tight, pushes filler upward

**A.**

**1-5 years after augmentation**

Upper breast fill decreases

Implant shell collapses and folds— risks shell failure, visible rippling

Lower envelope stretches and sags, filler redistributes and upper shell collapses

**B.**

**What happens when the skin envelope releases?**

The shell **collapses** and **folds** — risking **shell failure, visible rippling** and **more reoperations**

**Round Implant OVERFILLED Past Manufacturer's Recommendations**

Overfilled

**C.**

Upper shell may not collapse and fold, but ...

Breast SAGS, upper fill decreases, and you have NO WARRANTY!

**D.**

**The patient CAN'T WIN** —

Fill to recommendations — preserve warranty, but SHELL FOLDS

Overfill to protect shell = VOIDS WARRANTY

**Figure 5-6.**

## Anatomic Implants

Anatomically shaped implants are shaped like a natural breast (Figure 5-7A). Some surgeons refer to anatomic implants as "teardrop-shaped" implants. Either the surgeon hasn't looked closely at a teardrop (Figure 5-7B), or the surgeon hasn't looked closely at an anatomically shaped implant (Figure 5-7A). They don't look the same to me; do they to you? Ten years ago, I became very interested in anatomic implants after finding that I could not adequately fill round implants to protect the shell and still end up with a result that looked like a breast.

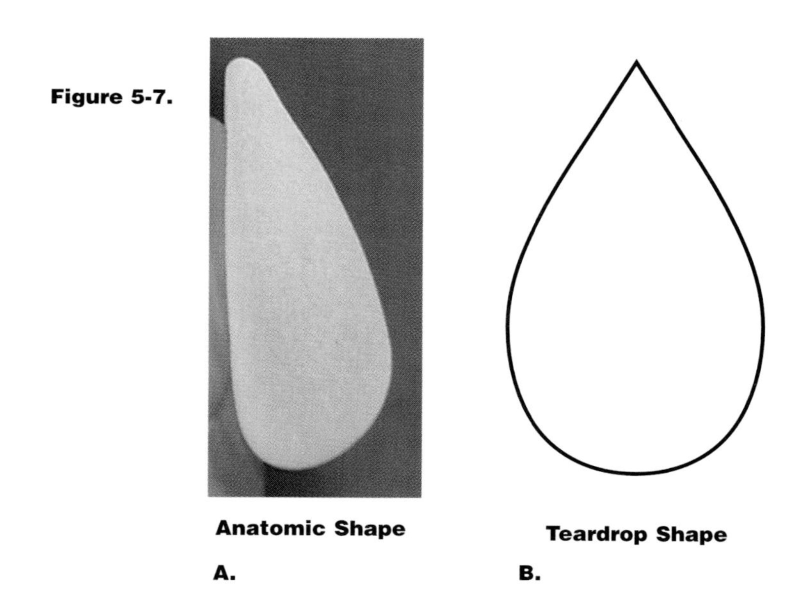

**Figure 5-7.**

**Anatomic Shape**

**A.**

**Teardrop Shape**

**B.**

**With an anatomically shaped implant, it is possible to adequately fill the implant to prevent shell collapse and folding and still produce an optimal aesthetic result** (Figure 5-4C).

***I was frustrated that I could never achieve shell protection and optimal aesthetics with any round implant.***

The message? For most first-time augmentation patients, anatomics seem **SAFER** (less risk of shell folding and early rupture) and **MORE EFFECTVE** (a more natural result with a full but not excessively bulging, upper breast).

The first anatomic implants that I experienced were silicone gel filled and covered with polyurethane foam. Tissues attached to the polyurethane foam and held the implant in proper position. They produced excellent aesthetic results and dramatically reduced risks of capsular contracture—excessive tightening of the lining around a breast implant that makes the breast excessively firm. Capsular contracture will be discussed in more detail later. But polyurethane-covered, silicone gel implants were not perfect (remember, no implant is perfect). The implants were underfilled and were designed on a round base with excessively tapered upper edges. Because the shells were thin and underfilled (we didn't know this back then), some of the shells failed, and the implants ruptured earlier than we liked (anytime is too early for us). We thought we could do better, so we began redesigning anatomic implants. We didn't try to redesign round implants, because if we filled any round implant enough to protect the shell, it was impossible to get the best possible aesthetic result.

What changes did we make with the new anatomic designs? We simply addressed the problems with the older designs. Instead of building the implant on a round base (breasts aren't round), we made the implant slightly taller than it is wide, like a full, natural breast. We replaced the excessively sharp upper edge that was sometimes noticeable with a more rounded upper edge. Most importantly, we filled the implant adequately to prevent upper shell collapse and folding by the tilt test.

## Anatomic, Silicone Gel-Filled Implants

Simultaneously, we were looking at possible alternate fillers to silicone gel. Two main objections existed at that time regarding silicone gel: 1) When the implant ruptured, the gel was "gooey" and could be displaced into the breast tissue or other tissues, and 2) tiny amounts of the gel material could escape through the implant shell (gel bleed). We have always been interested in alternate fillers, including saline, peanut oil, polyethelene glycol (antifreeze), and several other possible fillers. But every alternate filler that we have ever seen has at least as many, if not more, tradeoffs than silicone gel. While looking at alternate fillers, we thought, "Why not look simultaneously at silicone gel and try to correct its weaknesses (tradeoffs 1 and 2 above)?" After all, we have over 25 years of medical data on silicone gel. Accumulating a comparable amount of data on any newer filler would require another 25 years.

**Figure 5-8.**

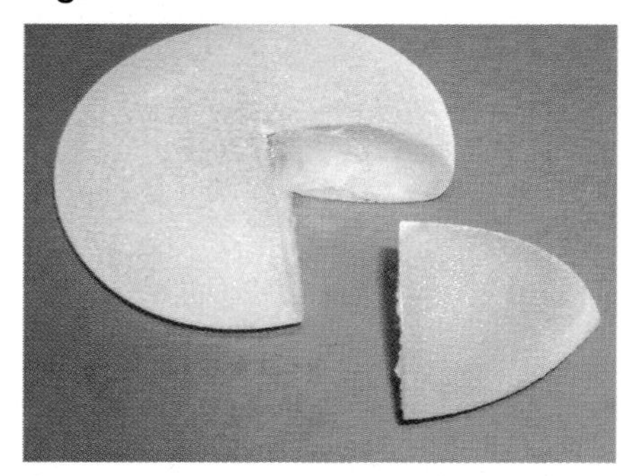

**A.**

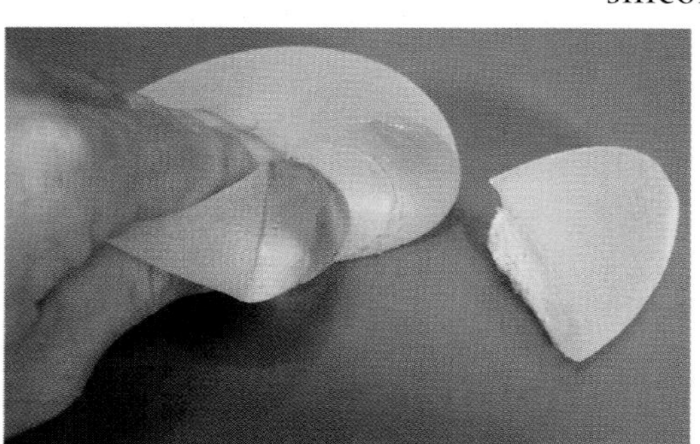

**B.**

Today's state-of-the-art anatomic implants are manufactured by McGhan Medical Corporation, the originator of modern anatomic implants and the world's largest manufacturer of anatomic implants. Instead of the older, "gooey" silicone gel, these new anatomic implants contain a newer, more cohesive silicone gel. This gel is so adherent to itself and the implant shell that you can cut a pie-shaped wedge out of the implant with scissors (Figure 5-8 A,B), and then squeeze the implant, and the gel won't migrate away from the implant.

**A major anatomic implant advance is a filler material (cohesive gel) that does not migrate following rupture of the implant shell.**

***Implant shell rupture can be caused by shell folding, a defect in manufacturing, surgical trauma, or trauma following surgery. All implant shells will eventually fail. A filler material that will not migrate after shell failure is an advantage.***

By putting an adequate amount of filler in the shell, the upper shell does not collapse or fold with the implant upright.

**Another major advance is adequate fill to prevent shell folding.**

This implant—the McGhan Style 410 Anatomic Cohesive Gel Implant—has now been in clinical use for over six years. More than 40,000 McGhan anatomic, cohesive gel implants have been used in countries other than the United States. Overall, aesthetic results have been excellent in a wide range of breast types.

The McGhan Style 410 cohesive gel anatomic implant makes **three significant advances:**
**1)** adequate fill to maximally protect the shell,
**2)** a filler that doesn't migrate, and
**3)** optimal aesthetic results.

Unfortunately, if you live in the United States and choose to have surgery here, this implant is not an option for you. The FDA currently bans the use of gel implants for augmentation (while allowing older, less advanced, underfilled, round gel implants in current studies that we will discuss later in this chapter). When the FDA ban on silicone gel-filled implants seemed imminent, we immediately began working toward a similar anatomic implant filled with saline.

## Anatomic Saline-Filled Implants

Today's state-of-the-art, anatomic *saline-filled* implants are also manufactured by McGhan Medical Corporation. To prevent shell folding with a saline-filled anatomic implant, we needed to add slightly more filler to the implant compared to a cohesive gel-filled implant. Adding more filler to protect the shell makes the implant slightly firmer, but protecting the shell is more important, in our opinion, than a tiny increase in firmness. Fill issues are discussed in more detail later in this chapter. Figure 5-9 is an anatomically-shaped, saline-filled McGhan Style 468 implant. Held upright during a tilt test (Figure 5-10), the implant upper shell does not collapse and fold. At the same time, the upper shell stays full (necessary to maintain fullness in the upper breast), the upper shell does not bulge excessively, and it's more natural. It is simply impossible to achieve all of these objectives with any currently manufactured round implant.

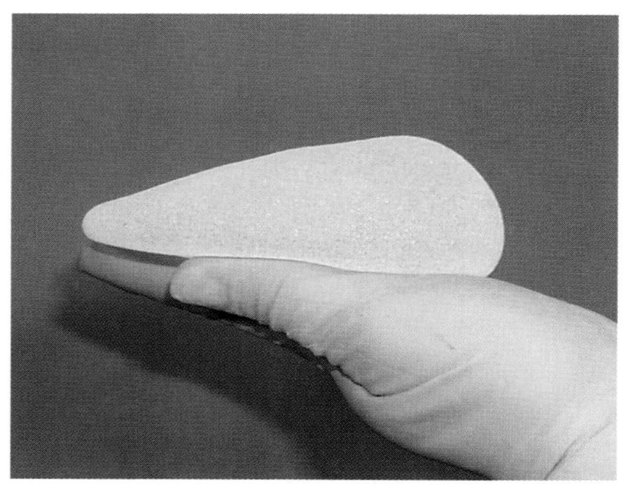

**Figure 5-9.**

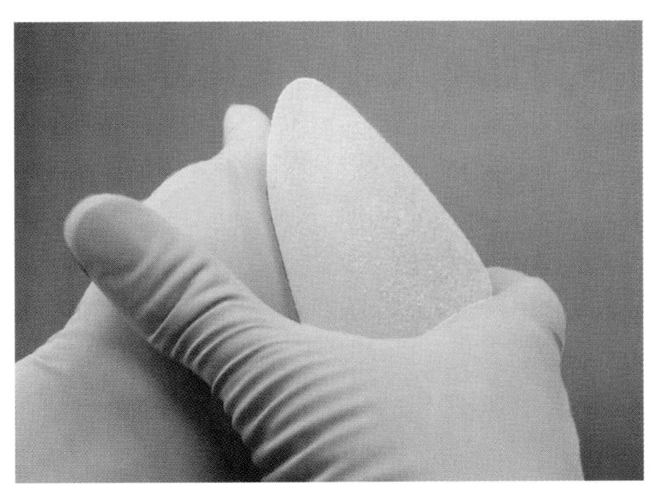

**Figure 5-10.**

When we defined fill volumes for McGhan anatomic saline implants, *I insisted that McGhan define the fill volumes high enough to prevent upper shell folding*. As a result, *if you select a McGhan saline-filled anatomic implant for augmentation, your surgeon does not need to overfill the implant above manufacturer's recommendations to prevent upper shell folding and prolong the life of the shell.* Before releasing anatomic implants, we set higher fill volumes compared to round implants. Because of its anatomic shape, we were able to put more filler in the implant without compromising the aesthetic result because of the shape of the implant! And, you can keep your warranty! **Gone is the Catch 22** of current round implants (Figure 5-4A,B) When filled to McGhan's recommended fill, anatomic style 468 saline and 410 silicone anatomic implants do not experience upper shell folding (Figure 5-4C).

*McGhan* ***anatomic*** *augmentation implants* ***do not need to be filled past manufacturer's recommendations*** *to prevent shell folding.*

**With McGhan Style 468 anatomic-shaped, saline implants, you get SHELL PROTECTION, and YOU KEEP YOUR WARRANTY — no choosing between the two! NO CATCH 22!**

*With round saline implants, you must overfill to prevent shell folding, and overfilling voids the warranty (*Figure 5-4A.B).

## Tradeoffs of Anatomic Gel and Saline Implants

As we've said, no implant is perfect. No implant shape is best for every patient. Anatomically-shaped implants demand more of the surgeon. The pocket the surgeon develops to receive the implant must be much more precise with an anatomic implant compared to the pocket for a round implant. With an anatomic, the pocket should "fit" the implant. Because full-height anatomic implants are taller than they are wide, if the pocket fits the implant in a side-to-side direction, the implant does not rotate or malposition unless the tissues stretch excessively.

**Some surgeons find the additional demands of anatomic implants too technically challenging or time consuming, so they don't offer their patients anatomic implants.**

However, many board certified plastic surgeons have rapidly developed the necessary skills to use anatomic implants with the help of the excellent educational materials and seminars provided by McGhan Medical Corporation.

In many cases that require reoperation, patients' tissues can become so thin and stretched (especially if they previously had large implants) that a surgeon cannot assure that the pocket will fit the implant. In *reoperations* (in contrast to first-time augmentations), until a surgeon has considerable experience with anatomic implants, the surgeon (and the patient) are probably better served using round implants, regardless of the tradeoffs. If a patient has very thin tissues and requests very large implants (in general, larger than 350cc), the weight of the implant will almost always stretch the patient's thin tissues and cause the implant pocket to enlarge. If the pocket enlarges substantially, an anatomic implant may rotate. Hence, *round* implants are probably a better option when *a very thin patient requests a very large implant*. You'll learn more about implant size and ccs later.

**Anatomic implants may not be the best option for reoperation cases until a surgeon has gained considerable experience.**

***Anatomic implants*** *are* ***ideal*** *for the majority of* ***first- time*** *augmentation patients.*

**Anatomic** implants may **not** be the best option for **thin patients** who request **excessively large implants** larger than 350cc.

All saline implants (not just anatomics) currently manufactured in the United States have a valve that is used to put filler (usually saline) in the implant. A valve is a device that is separate and additional to the implant, although it is incorporated into the implant. Any device has a failure rate, so adding any valve to any implant theoretically increases the failure rate of the implant. All saline implants (not just anatomics) need to be adequately filled to minimize risks of visible shell folding or rippling, audible sloshing, and shell folding that risks early rupture. A prefilled, round saline implant currently exists that does not have a valve, but this implant is manufactured by a company based outside the United States. The implant is underfilled by the tilt test (at my last testing in 1998), and the shell collapses with the implant upright.

## Importance of the Surgeon's Experience

If a surgeon has minimal or no experience with anatomic implants, the surgeon may not offer you this option, or the surgeon may offer the option, but discourage you with negative comments. Always ask your surgeon specifically how much experience the surgeon has with each type of implant. Ask to see pictures of results. Remember that you can't necessarily distinguish a round from an anatomic implant in a picture — a round implant can be underfilled and the result can look quite natural, but the shell is folded, even if you can't see shell folding or rippling. If a round implant looks natural following augmentation, chances are that the shell is folded.

My personal experience began with round implants. I used round implants exclusively for 10 years until anatomic implants became available. Today I have 20 years' experience with round implants and 10 years' experience with anatomic implants. I use both. I simply present patients all options and discuss those options with respect to each individual patient's tissues. The patient and I together choose the implant based on her wishes, her tissues, and the tradeoffs she is willing to accept (a TEAM DECISION).

A question that patients frequently ask a surgeon is, "How many augmentations have you done?" A better question (though difficult to ask in a tactful manner) is, "How many augmentations have you done WELL?" I personally know surgeons with smaller case numbers who consistently deliver better augmentation results than certain surgeons with much larger case numbers. Surgeons are like every other professional, with some more skilled than others. Some are more demanding of themselves than others. Numbers of cases are less important than the surgeon's self-critical pursuit of perfection.

## SMOOTH OR TEXTURED SHELL? IMPLANT SHELL CHARACTERISTICS

### It Won't Make Sense Unless You Know the History

Early generations of implants had *smooth* outer shells. *Textured* implant shells were developed to help reduce risks of capsular contracture. When any device is implanted in the human body, the body forms a lining or capsule around the device. This capsule forms around every implant in every patient, but the capsule can behave differently from patient to patient. All capsules tend to contract or tighten around any device. If the capsule around a breast implant tightens excessively, the capsule squeezes on the implant. This can make the implant feel too hard and can push it out of position, usually upward. The term capsular contracture describes a breast after augmentation that is excessively hard, often misshapen, and often displaced. A typical statement from a patient with a capsular contracture is, "My implants got hard." Actually, the implant itself does not become hard. If it were removed from the capsule that is squeezing on it, it would feel soft. The pressure of the capsule surrounding and squeezing on the implant causes the implant to feel hard in the breast. Cases of capsular contracture are illustrated in Chapter 16.

With older, smooth shell, silicone gel-filled implants, capsular contracture was very common. Rates vary in reported studies, but a 30 percent capsular contracture rate was probably common (one out of every three patients developed some degree of excessive breast firmness). With all *smooth* shell implants, surgeons learned to make the pocket to receive the implant very large, so that the capsule could theoretically contract a lot before it began squeezing on the implant. Motion exercises were commonly prescribed for patients with smooth implants. The theory was that moving the implant could keep the pocket open against the tendency of the capsule to contract. Good idea, but you usually can't overcome Mother Nature. The body's healing mechanisms were often more powerful than motion exercises. Despite motion exercises, capsular contracture was still very common with smooth shell implants. Patients hated capsular contracture. Surgeons hated capsular contracture. Both still hate capsular contracture. Patients with significant contractures required reoperations to soften the breast. If the capsule was removed, and smooth implants put back in, a large percentage developed recurrent contracture.

Enter *polyurethane*-covered implants. A polyurethane covering was cemented to the outer surface of the implant silicone shell. The reduction in capsular contracture rates was astounding. In my personal series of patients undergoing first-time (primary) augmentations, capsular contracture rates fell to less than 2 percent (2 out of 100). Incredible. But polyurethane-covered, silicone gel-filled implants became unavailable in the United States when gel-filled implants were banned by the FDA. Additionally, questions were raised with regard to one of the breakdown products of polyurethane (TDA) causing cancer in mice. Subsequent studies have shown that TDA levels in humans with these implants are so low that the risk of any carcinogenic effect is insignificant. When polyurethane implants became unavailable, surgeons wanted another alternative to smooth shells to reduce risks of capsular contracture. Implant manufacturers responded to the question, "If a rougher, polyurethane surface retarded capsular contracture, why not produce a silicone shell with a textured outer surface?"

**Textured silicone shell implants were developed as an alternative to smooth shell implants to reduce the risk of capsular contracture.**

You don't need to know all the scientific data with regard to capsular contracture or smooth versus textured shells. You just need a summary. The summary that follows is my current best judgement based on 20 years of experience:

**Textured surface implants have a lower risk of capsular contracture than smooth shelled implants.**

The difference between smooth and textured implant capsular contracture rates is more pronounced with **silicone** gel-filled implants than with **saline**-filled implants.

Other filler materials have not been adequately tested in large enough numbers with adequate followup to make a valid judgement regarding smooth versus textured shells.

### Textured or Smooth — How Do You Choose?

*Anatomic implants require a textured surface* to help maintain optimal positioning of the implant in the pocket.

***If you choose an ANATOMIC IMPLANT, it should be TEXTURED to help maintain implant position in the pocket.***

If you choose a *round* implant, the implant can be smooth or textured. If you choose a round implant in the United States today, you will most likely receive *saline*-filled, round implants. With saline-filled implants, the difference in capsular contracture rates between smooth and textured implants is not as significant compared to silicone gel-filled implants. But even if the capsular rate is only slightly lower, you might prefer a textured surface implant. If you choose a *gel*-filled, round implant (at the current time you would need to be enrolled in a study approved by the FDA), your risk of capsular contracture will be lower with a textured implant.

***If you choose a ROUND IMPLANT, and you want the least risk of capsular contracture, choose a TEXTURED SURFACE.***

Why would anyone choose a smooth-shelled implant today in a first-time augmentation? Smooth-shelled implants are a no-brainer for the surgeon. Make a pocket—drop it in. The implant always falls to the bottom of the pocket. Even if it is underfilled and the shell folds, it's often unnoticeable from the outside because the smooth implant with a collapsed shell falls downward, and shell folding is often hidden by the patient's breast tissue. Great! Easy and great! Even if the shell collapses and folds with underfilling, the patient doesn't see rippling or shell folding and complain. Wait a minute! Great for who? Maybe great for the surgeon who doesn't see or hear about rippling, but what about the patient with the folded shell? What's likely to happen to the folded shell with time? A folded shell can lead to shell stresses and potentially cause shell rupture. In many cases, because the implant falls to the bottom of the pocket, neither patient nor surgeon can see the folded shell by looking at the breast. If the shell folding were visible on examination, the surgeon could replace the implant before rupture occurred.

**Three good reasons to choose a ROUND, smooth shell implant:**

*1. You are having a reoperation, not a first-time augmentation.*

*2. Your surgeon has little or no experience with anatomic implants.*

*3. You are not concerned about the risk of capsular contracture.*

Some surgeons feel that textured shells are thicker and are, therefore, easier to feel after augmentation. The difference in shell thickness between smooth and textured implants is only a *few ten thousandths of an inch*! Easier to feel? Perhaps. But more often than not, the reason any implant is easier to feel is because the patient has very thin tissues! *If the tissues are thin, any implant shell is easier to feel, whether it is textured or smooth!* If you're likely to feel it anyway, why not try to reduce the risks of capsular contracture by selecting a textured shell?

## *Two* MYTHS *that are* NOT BASED ON FACTS:

**Textured surface implants have thicker shells and are more easily felt in the breast.**

*The thickness of your tissues over the implant is much more important than the minimal differences in shell thickness.*

**Smooth shell implants have less rippling than textured surface implants.**

*Rippling is the result of underfilling or traction, not the shell surface.*

You might also hear that rippling is more common with textured surface implants compared to smooth-shelled implants. NOT TRUE. Rippling results from either inadequate fill in an implant (*underfill rippling*) or an excessively large implant (smooth or textured) pulling downward on an excessively thin skin envelope (*traction rippling*). If a textured surface implant adheres to the tissues around the pocket, and if that same implant is underfilled, rippling may be more visible. But the problem that most often causes wrinkling is underfill, not the texturing on the shell!

## Implant Filler Materials — Silicone Versus Saline Versus Other Fillers

Before the FDA banned silicone gel-filled implants in the United States, over 90 percent of surgeons preferred and used silicone gel-filled implants over saline implants. If silicone gel-filled implants were widely available in the United States today, many experienced surgeons and many patients would probably choose silicone fill over saline. Why? Because silicone gel filler is more natural, it is more predictable, and it is safe.

**Saline-filled implants cause more stretch of the breast envelope compared to silicone gel-filled implants of comparable size and shape.**

*Therefore, predicting and controlling the result is more difficult for most surgeons with saline than with silicone-filled implants.*

The demand for silicone gel-filled implants is very high in the United States today. Many women travel outside the United States to obtain silicone gel-filled implants, sometimes compromising their care in the process. Women in the United States deserve a full range of options, provided the options are accompanied by a full range of information. How logical is it to approve silicone implants for reconstruction in women with breast cancer and not offer the same option to women for primary augmentation? Beats us! We're supposedly experts in the field, and we're at a loss to decipher this one!

Saline is harmless if an implant ruptures. So is silicone if it is properly used. Even saline implants have a silicone shell. Silicone is silicone is silicone! If silicone is so bad (and scientifically it is not), why is a silicone shell on a saline-filled implant okay? It makes no sense, but the decisions that determine which options are available to you are not currently based on science.

If you're concerned that you're not allowed a full range of options, tell your legislators. Tell the FDA. Tell them over and over. You'll need to shout louder than the minority of lobbyists and "patient advocate" groups who are paid by plaintiff lawyers to bend the ear of your legislators and the FDA.

## TODAY'S PICKS (THEY WILL CHANGE WITH TIME; I GUARANTEE IT.)

Our biases? We'll gladly share them with you.

### First-time Augmentations

If I were a woman having a *first-time augmentation* (or if my wife asked my best opinion for her choice of implants), I'd advise: If you want a near natural breast, choose anatomic, cohesive silicone gel implants if you can get them (if you live outside the United States or if you're willing to travel abroad and accept the tradeoffs). Saline textured anatomic implants are a very close second choice. If you are having a first-time augmentation by a surgeon who is experienced using anatomic implants, you won't notice a significant difference between a saline and a silicone gel-filled anatomic implant. Hundreds of thousands of first-time augmentation patients are very happy with anatomic-shaped, saline-filled implants.

## REOPERATIONS...

If you need a *reoperation*, something wasn't ideal the first time around, or your body is making things difficult! The first operation is the best chance for success. Augmentation surgery never gets easier the second, third, or fourth time around. Results are less predictable, tradeoffs are greater, and risks are higher with each reoperation.

**Don't expect any implant to necessarily solve a problem that requires a reoperation.**

*Implants usually don't solve problems.*

Don't waste your time looking for a "magic" implant to solve a problem. It doesn't exist. Look for an experienced surgeon, get second opinions, and, at some point, don't beat the dead horse (remember what you get — a beaten, dead horse).

Need a reoperation? Select a round implant, smooth or textured, unless you have a surgeon who is *very experienced with anatomic implants.* All current round gel implants are underfilled, so beware of shell folding and possible early shell rupture. Until the newer gels become available in the United States, I'd prefer a round, saline-filled implant adequately filled to protect the shell (forget the warranty or ask the manufacturer for an exception), and I'd accept a slightly firmer, more globular breast. Many patients and surgeons would disagree and select an underfilled, round, smooth-shelled gel implant, but I'd have to question their logic. Haven't we been down that road before? Did we learn anything from the breast implant crisis? Instead of making bad team decisions, why don't we focus our efforts on bringing all options to women of the United States?

### "Forget natural, even large and natural. I want really big, round breasts..."

If naturalness is not a major concern, and you want very large, round breasts (implants larger than 350-400cc), assuming you've accepted the tradeoffs and future consequences, I'd select a large, round, saline-filled, smooth implant (or textured implant with minimal texturing). Don't waste your money on anatomic implants (they're more expensive, about $350 more per pair). You're not after a natural look anyway, and with a round implant you avoid risks of anatomic implant malposition after your tissues stretch (and they will definitely stretch). Enjoy them while you can, save your money, and plan for a reoperation sometime in the future. You'll look awesome—for a while.

### "I don't want huge, but I want a full upper breast..."

If your main goal is beautiful fullness of the upper breast (but not necessarily huge breasts), don't be misled by those who tell you that a round implant produces more upper fullness in the upper breast than an anatomic implant. IT'S NOT TRUE. Remember that most round implants collapse unless they are overfilled. If they collapse vertically, they shorten. You lose upper fill. McGhan anatomic augmentation implants, when filled to manufacturer's recommendations, do not collapse, so they maintain their vertical height. Full-height anatomics are also taller than they are wide. With a properly selected anatomic implant, you have a better chance of getting and maintaining upper fill.

**An ANATOMIC IMPLANT can maintain fill in the upper breast better than a round implant because:**

***The upper pole of the anatomic implant doesn't collapse—it maintains its vertical height.***

***McGhan Style 410 and 468 anatomic implants are taller than they are wide.***

But remember—the larger the implant, whether round or anatomic—and the thinner your tissues, the more and faster your breast envelope will stretch. When the lower skin envelope stretches, the upper fill (regardless of implant shape) will decrease. No implant can overcome the effects of gravity on your tissues over time. With time, aging, and larger implants, you'll eventually lose some upper fullness in almost any case. Many patients and surgeons fall into the trap of thinking that a larger implant will *produce* and maintain upper fullness. A larger implant will almost always produce upper fullness, but it usually won't maintain that upper fullness over time because that same implant will inevitably stretch the lower skin envelope. With only a little bit of stretch, you'll lose the upper fullness. It isn't magic—the bigger the breast or the implant, the less likely it will maintain upper fullness over time.

## "WHAT'S NEW, AND WHEN CAN I GET IT...?"

### New Implant Designs

We've already discussed the latest implant designs that are currently available today—the McGhan Style 410 cohesive silicone gel-filled, textured, anatomic implants. But they're not available in the United States. The nearest and best alternative is the McGhan Style 468 textured, anatomic, saline-filled implant.

When will the cohesive silicone gel-filled implants be available in the United States for clinical use for first-time augmentations? Your guess is as good as mine. Sooner rather than later, I hope. But it depends on your demanding your options to your legislators and the FDA. If you don't, it could be five years or more.

In the rest of the world, we're currently working on expanding the size and dimension options of the Style 410 cohesive gel implant, more different sizes and dimensions of the same implant to better match a wider variety of breast variations. These new sizes and dimensions are already being manufactured and tested outside the United States (Figure 5-11).

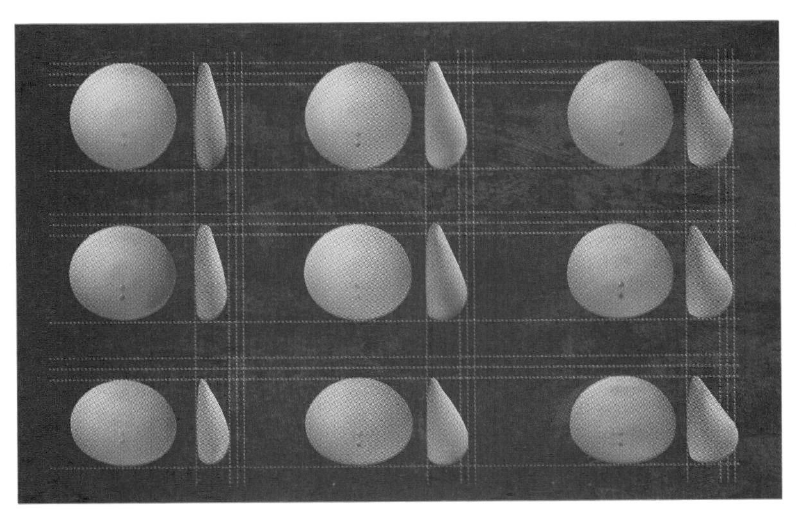

**Figure 5-11.**

## New Filler Materials

What about new filler materials? At the time of this writing, there is no radically new or better filler material that is likely to be available in the United States in the next two years. Peanut oil appeared promising from a mammogram standpoint, but the initial peanut oil implants had significant rippling problems, the filler material odor was objectionable to some patients and surgeons, and the manufacturer subsequently developed substantial financial problems, so the future of a peanut oil filled implant is uncertain at present. All other filler materials that I am aware of at this time are still in preliminary testing phases, and clinical availability is likely many years away. We've seen several "magic, new" implants with "magic, new" filler materials come and go in the past few years. Each one is advertised as the golden grail, but mysteriously, once it is used in a significant number of patients, suddenly it isn't so magical. Problems appear.

**When betting on new implant materials and fillers, don't place your bets until the product has at least a five-year track record.**

*History is replete with magic implant solutions that failed in the first two to three years of widespread use.*

After closely watching and participating in this field for the past 20 years, my opinion currently is:

**Don't discard silicone- and saline-filled implants (in that order) until there is a proven alternative that has at least five years of followup in a large number of patients.**

While you're thinking about what's new, remember what's important.

**Just because a breast implant design or filler is *NEW*, it's *NOT NECESSARILY BETTER*—no matter how promising it may seem.**

*If it's really good, it will stand the test of time.*

We continually learn. If you're the first to get a new device, or if you fall for premarketing that is not substantiated by long-term clinical experience, you may be the first, but your long-term result may not be the best. Think carefully before jumping on new bandwagons!

## IMPLANTS — WHAT'S BEST?

### If You Ask a Surgeon

When you ask a surgeon which type of implant is best, the surgeon will usually have an opinion based on that surgeon's experience. If the experiences were good, the surgeon likes the implant. Bad experiences, the surgeon doesn't like the implant. What if a surgeon never used a certain type of implant? The surgeon may, nevertheless, have an opinion. It's just not based on experience. If something bad occurs, surgeons sometimes blame the implant—sometimes justifiably, usually not justifiably. If a surgeon's opinions are based on experience, it's important to know what types of implants that surgeon has used. How many? Over what period of time? How long did the surgeon follow the patients to really know the long-term results?

**The best opinion about implants is an opinion based on experience.**

*If a surgeon has minimal or no experience with a certain type of implant, the surgeon should preface any opinion with, "I've never used that implant, but here's what I think of it."*

You'll rarely hear a surgeon admit lack of experience with any type of implant. Most surgeons will give you an opinion without specifying their experience, so it's your job to ask. Would you let someone operate on you if they said, "I've never done that operation, but would you like for me to try it on you?" Probably not. Do patients accept the first implant suggestion from a surgeon without knowing their options? Every day. You certainly want to listen carefully to your surgeon's recommendations, but you deserve to know all of your options before making choices. ***Become informed.***

**If a surgeon has experience with only one type of implant, that's likely the implant the surgeon will recommend.**

*Hopefully. It's scary to think about the alternative.*

**The more experience a surgeon has with a variety of implant types, the more options the surgeon can offer you, and the better the surgeon can put those options into a realistic perspective for you.**

## If You Ask a Patient Who Has Had a Breast Augmentation...

**Most patients who have had an augmentation will tell you that the type of implant they have is best. Otherwise, why would they have it?**

*When a patient tells you her type of implant is best, ask why. Find out how much she really knows.*

Ask what types of implant options she considered. Ask which implant options her surgeon offered. Ask why she and her surgeon chose her current implant. Even though the implant she has is "best," ask her to explain its tradeoffs, because every implant has tradeoffs.

**The more a previous patient knows, the more in-depth information you'll get. But don't be disappointed if you don't get much.**

*Many patients are never offered options. Many patients don't learn about options on their own.*

Does that mean that they have a bad result, or that they are unhappy with their result? Absolutely not. If you can be happy without knowing, is it really necessary to know a lot about implant choices and the tradeoffs inherent to any implant? Only if you want to know. Only if you want to make the best choices. You can hope to be lucky, or you can become knowledgeable. We're assuming you want to know.

If a patient has a bad experience with a certain type of implant, is it the implant's fault? Possibly, but usually not. Many factors can affect the result — patient tissue, patient choices, surgeon skill, surgeon experience, and healing factors—just to name a few. The implant is easy to blame, but it's often not the only cause of problems. So, when you ask your friends their opinions about implants, weigh the opinions, considering their knowledge and your knowledge. The issues aren't simple. Neither are the answers.

### Our Personal Opinion About What's Best...

Every surgeon and staff have biases when it comes to implants. We're no exception. Our biases are based on 20 years of experience performing augmentations using virtually every type of implant that has been available in the United States since 1977. Based on this experience, we have some very strong beliefs:

**A breast implant should be as SAFE as possible.**

A breast implant **should last** as long as possible.

***NO SINGLE TYPE*** *of breast implant*
***IS BEST*** *for every patient.*

***Every patient deserves information and choices.***

**WHAT'S BEST FOR YOU** depends on 1) what you want, 2) what your tissues will allow you to have, and 3) which set of benefits and tradeoffs you are willing to accept.

Most of these statements are common sense. Safety should be a paramount concern when you are considering placing a device inside your body for an extended period of time. We know that breast implants are medically safe. How can we make them safer? By making them last longer. The longer any implant lasts (before the shell wears out), the fewer times any woman will need a reoperation. The fewer reoperations, the fewer risks, tradeoffs, potential complications, and costs. Make sense? You bet! So our personal, Number 1 concern is maximizing the longevity of breast implants. To the extent that we can prolong the life of your implant, you are less likely to need reoperations with risks, tradeoffs, possible complications, and costs.

## IMPLANT LONGEVITY — THE MOST IMPORTANT ISSUE AND THE FACTORS THAT AFFECT IT

**The longer an implant lasts, the fewer reoperations you will need during your lifetime.**

*Reoperations involve additional risks (more than the initial operation), costs, recovery time, and the results are less predictable.*

Over the past 10 years, we have made implant longevity our primary concern. We have done this by making implant design changes, improving surgical techniques, and educating surgeons and patients about issues that affect implant longevity. Implant designs and materials will continue to change, but regardless of the design or material, the longer any implant lasts, the better for the patient. That's why we will continue to focus on implant longevity. That's why we want you to understand the issues, so that you can make informed decisions.

### Naturalness Versus Durability

Notice I said naturalness *versus* durability. With currently available materials that we are using and researching, I can assure you that:

**There are definite tradeoffs between naturalness and durability when it comes to breast implants.**

**If you want your implant to last longer, you'll need to accept some tradeoffs in naturalness.**

**The only natural breast is a natural breast. Natural breasts don't contain a breast implant. If you want a totally natural breast, don't have an augmentation.**

***What is natural?*** It depends on who you ask, and when you ask. Is "natural" the firm, perky, full breast in a typical 18-year-old woman, or is "natural" the less full, softer, slightly saggier breast of that same woman after three children when she is 40 years old? If this woman chooses to have an augmentation when she is 40 to refill her upper breast and improve the sagging, her implanted breasts will be firmer. They will feel more like the breasts she had when she was 18, before pregnancies. So are they unnatural? Compared to what? Yes, they're unnatural compared to softer, saggier, and empty at the top. But are they acceptably natural to her? You'd have to ask, but I'd bet the answer is yes. This scenario illustrates common changes that occur in many women's breasts with pregnancy and aging and points out that:

***Naturalness is relative. It depends on what a woman*** **HAS,** ***what a woman*** **WANTS,** ***and what a woman is*** **WILLING TO ACCEPT** ***in tradeoffs.***

## What Makes an Implant Feel More Natural or Less Natural?

**How natural an implant feels is determined by THREE main factors:**

1) The ***thickness of the implant shell***

2) The ***thickness of your tissues*** that cover the implant

3) The ***amount of filler material*** in the implant.

The *thinner* the outer shell of an implant, the less you can feel the implant in the breast. From the standpoint of naturalness, a thinner implant shell is better. But with current implant shell materials, *thinner is weaker*. Thinner is less durable. Most implants manufactured today have *thicker* shells compared to the shells of implants made 20 years ago. The 20-year-old implants may be more natural, but they're less durable. Today's implants generally have thicker shells to increase durability and, hopefully, increase shell and implant longevity. Notice, I said, "Hopefully."

Many factors affect the life of an implant shell, not just the thickness of the shell, but a thicker shell is a first step to make your implant last longer.

How thick is thick? You'll possibly hear different implant companies touting that their shells are thicker or less thick, depending on how you and your surgeon feel about naturalness versus durability. Surgeons don't like to hear patients complain about being able to feel their implants, so many surgeons will select or recommend implants with thinner shells. Question is, did your surgeon discuss *all of the issues* with you that affect naturalness? Did your surgeon ask *which you would rather have, an implant that feels more natural, or an implant that lasts longer?* These are important questions, important issues to resolve before choosing an implant!

The thickness of an implant shell is not the only factor that affects whether you may be able to feel your implants. The thickness and characteristics of your tissues are at least as important. Since you can't change your tissues, you should clearly understand the limitations and tradeoffs your tissues will impose:

***If you are thin and you can feel your ribs beneath your breast with your fingertip, you will probably be able to feel the edges or shell of any state-of-the-art implant in the world today, regardless of its shell thickness.***

***If you have thin tissues, you have thin tissues. You can't change that. Your surgeon can't change that.***

***The thinner you are, the more likely you'll feel some portion of your implants after your augmentation.***

***Since you can't change your thin tissues (gaining weight won't change them enough), if feeling your implant is unacceptable to you, don't have an augmentation.***

*Feeling* some portion of your implant is one thing—usually no more of an issue than feeling your ribs. *Seeing* the edges of the implant is a bigger problem to most patients. If you are thin, there are specific surgical options such as placing the implant behind muscle (more about that in Chapter 6) that can often help prevent your seeing an implant edge. But no technique or pocket location can consistently overcome thin tissues and guarantee that you won't be able to feel some portion of the implant.

Thin is in. Many women spend considerable time, effort, and money to get thin and stay thin. In our practice, a large percentage of patients are thin. Thin patients are just as happy with their augmentations as patients with thicker tissues. We almost never hear a thin patient complain about feeling her implants. Why? Partly, because we did everything surgically possible to cover the implant. Largely, because we discussed the issues and the patient made the choices and accepted the tradeoffs before her surgery!

## Why Is the Amount of Filler in Your Implant Important?

The amount of filler material in your implant (regardless of the type of filler, saline or silicone) is critically important and is an issue that is frequently overlooked by patients and some surgeons:

***The amount of filler in an implant largely determines whether the shell of that implant folds or collapses when the implant is in your breast.***

***If any implant shell (using today's materials) collapses or folds, this causes stresses on the shell that can make the shell wear out sooner.***

***If an implant shell folds, it increases your risks of feeling or seeing rippling in your breast.***

Assume for a moment that you are holding an empty implant shell. The size doesn't matter. The shell material doesn't matter. Even the filler material you're going to put in the implant doesn't matter. As you gradually add filler to the implant (like filling a balloon with liquid), the shell expands. When only a small amount of filler is added, the implant feels soft, but the shell is floppy. If you tilt the implant upright, the shell collapses and folds. The more filler you add, the more the shell expands, and the less likely the shell will fold when you tilt the implant upright.

With any implant and any filler material, the following occur:

The **more filler** you place in the implant, the **less risk of shell folding**.

The **more filler** you place in the implant, **the firmer the implant** — slightly firmer is a tradeoff for durability.

**Exceeding the capacity** of an implant shell **can cause distortions** of the shell.

Let's illustrate these points by actually filling an implant shell. The round, saline implant shell is empty and collapsed in Figure 5-12. The manufacturer recommends placing 300cc-330cc of saline (salt water) into this shell as an optimal amount of fill. In Figure 5-13, we have added 250cc of saline. Looks pretty good on the table, right? But when we place the implant in our hand and support (not pushing) the lower implant with the other hand and tilt it upright (Figure 5-14), what happens? The upper shell collapses and folds. Shell folding can cause visible rippling in your breast and can cause the implant shell to rupture.

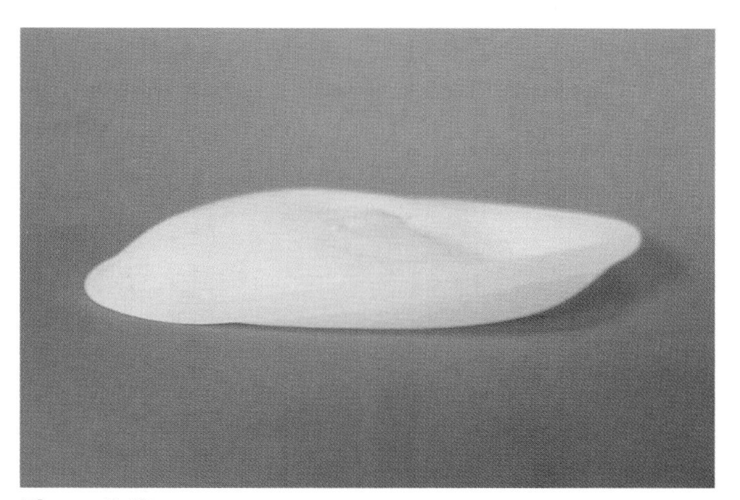

**Figure 5-12.**

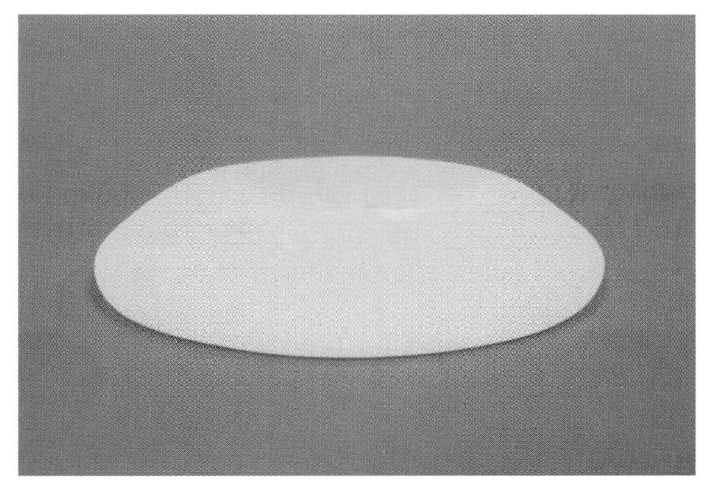

**Figure 5-13.**

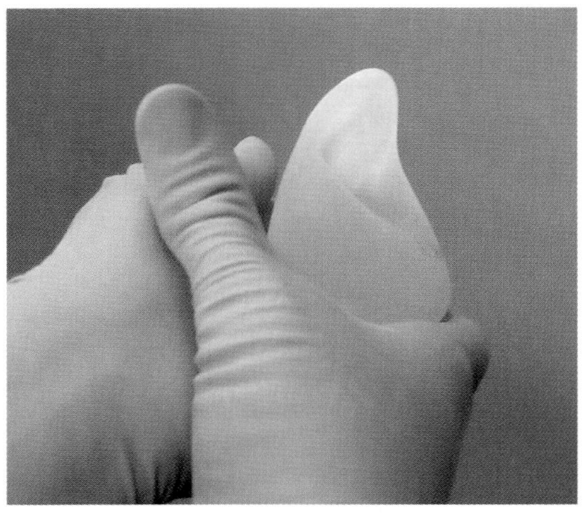

**Figure 5-14.**

**Any folding or collapse of an implant shell should worry you if you want the shell to last as long as possible.**

So let's add saline up to the manufacturer's recommendations and see what happens. Even after we reach the 330cc the manufacturer recommends (Figure 5-15), the shell still folds when we perform the tilt test! So let's see how much saline it takes to prevent the shell from folding when upright. We continue adding saline in small amounts until the shell first experiences no collapse or folding when upright (Figure 5-16). How much total saline was necessary to eliminate folding with the implant upright? 360cc! So why doesn't the manufacturer recommend more fill to prevent shell folding? An excellent question! To demonstrate that excessive overfilling creates problems, we continue adding saline until we create distortion and scalloping of the shell (figure 5-17) at 390cc, so it's obvious that, at some point, excessive fill creates problems.

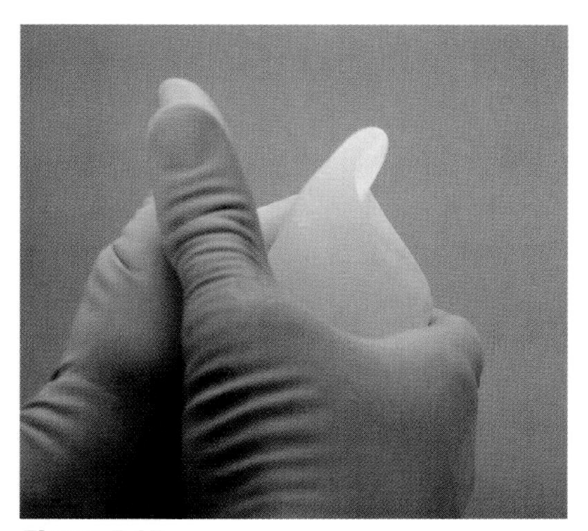

**Figure 5-15.**

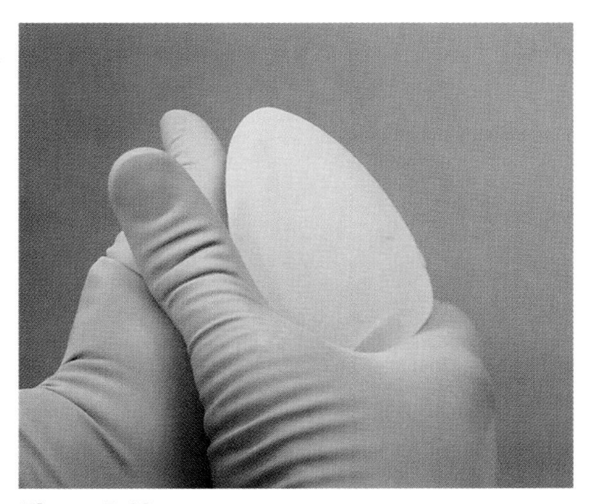

**Figure 5-16.**

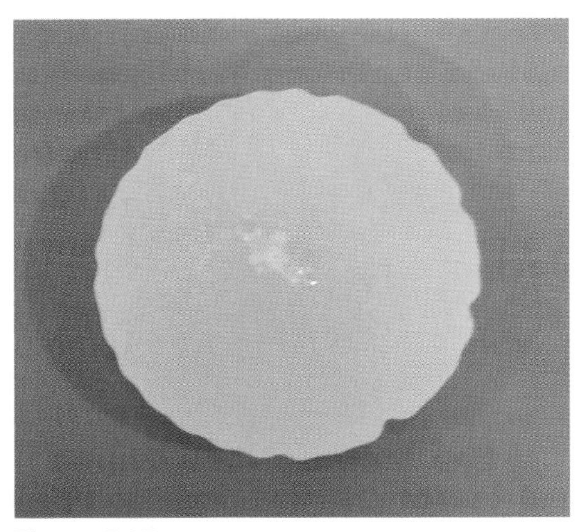

**Figure 5-17.**

## Optimal Fill Volumes and Implant Shape (Round or Anatomic)—How Do They Relate?

### All of today's ROUND implants are underfilled if filled to manufacturer's recommendations.

*With virtually all of today's round implants, regardless of the filler material or the size of the implant, shell collapse and folding occur if the implant is filled to the manufacturer's recommendations!*

Can't happen, shouldn't happen, you say? Most surgeons instinctively acknowledge this fact. Having experienced problems with patients having visible rippling and wrinkling with saline implants filled to manufacturer's recommendations, most surgeons overfill saline implants past manufacturer's recommendations to prevent patients having these problems. Problem solved? Not quite! Overfilling voids the manufacturer's warranty on the implant! Sound like a Catch 22? It is! If a surgeon fills the implant enough to prevent shell folding and protect the shell, no warranty! If the surgeon fills to manufacturer's recommendations to protect the warranty, the patient has a greater risk of experiencing visible rippling or premature implant rupture! So why don't the manufacturers just define fill volumes higher for round implants?

Manufacturers have not defined fill volumes higher for *round* implants, possibly because:

**Manufacturers believe that surgeons won't use and, therefore, won't buy round implants with more fill because the surgeon feels that the implant is too firm.**

*Historically, manufacturers respond to the pressures of their market like most successful companies.*

**Surgeons feel that firmer implants (even a tiny bit firmer), are unacceptable to patients.**

*Often they make this assumption without ever having used a significant number of firmer implants or asking patients which they would prefer, a slightly firmer breast or a reoperation sooner?*

**When round implants are filled adequately to prevent shell folding, they look very round, and the upper breast can look excessively bulging, even having a sharp, bulging stepoff.**

*Although some patients request an unnatural, excessively bulging upper breast, most don't.*

***These principles apply to***
**ALL ROUND IMPLANTS, REGARDLESS OF THE FILLER MATERIAL *in the implant.***

Older, round, silicone gel-filled implants were definitely softer than today's implants. But none of them could pass the tilt test. They were softer because they were underfilled. Perhaps some older implants ruptured sooner because they were underfilled and had folded shells. No way to know, no way to prove the point retrospectively. But enough of a question that I'd think we should consider simple ways to increase shell longevity—like just filling the shell adequately! Even today, the issue is not adequately addressed by many manufacturers and surgeons.

**Anatomic-shaped implants are more like a natural breast, fuller at the bottom, full and tapering at the top.**

**Because of the tapering upper pole, an *anatomic implant* can be *filled adequately to prevent shell folding* — without producing an unnatural appearing upper breast.**

**McGhan Medical has defined the fill volumes of their anatomic implants higher at the outset—so there is no need for the surgeon to overfill the implant to protect the shell!**

### What Can You Do to Influence Surgeons and Manufacturers to Protect the Shell of Your Implant?

If you want the shell of your implants to be protected by assuring adequate fill, and if you'd like to avoid visible wrinkling and rippling after your augmentation, we suggest that you:

**Require that any implant placed in your body pass the tilt test before it is implanted— regardless of the type, shape, or filler material.**

*Ask your surgeon to perform the test.*

This basic, simple test doesn't answer every possible question about factors that affect implant shell life. But the tilt test is something you or your surgeon can easily do, it's logical, and it's probably better than any other test currently available that can be applied in or out of the operating room! How do you do it? If your surgeon is unfamiliar with the tilt test, refer them to the following reference: Tebbetts, J.B. What is adequate fill? Implications in breast implant surgery. *Plast.Reconstr.Surg*. 97: 1451, 1996.

## What About New Implants and the FDA?



As a patient, you'll hear about every new "wonder implant" that might ever hit the market. In fact, you'll hear about it long before it's a reality, long before it's adequately tested (that's called *premarketing*). An excellent example is the highly touted peanut oil-filled implant. Another example is the prefilled saline implant—no valve on the implant. There will be countless more. Companies want you to be ready for new when it comes; they *want you to want it* even *before* it comes.

Did any of the ads for peanut oil implants ever mention shell wrinkling or rippling? In at least five academic presentations by surgeons using peanut oil implants, I saw large, prominent folds in the shells in patients' mammograms following augmentation. Did any surgeon mention the folded shell? No, they were emphasizing how well x-rays could pass through the implant. Improving mammograms is important, but so is adequate fill to protect the shell.

With another, prefilled saline implant manufactured in France and sold in the United States, I have heard the company tout the softness of its implant compared to other implants. When I performed a tilt test on the implant, guess what? It didn't pass; the shell folded significantly. Yes, it's a bit softer, because it's underfilled by the tilt test. Any company can produce a softer implant—just underfill it! But remember, an underfilled implant may cost you a reoperation!

Want more food for thought? The FDA, after telling women that silicone implants were potentially dangerous and removing them from use for augmentation in the United States (now proved scientifically not the case), is now allowing studies using *the same gel implants that they said were so bad in the first place.* Surgeons and patients, glad to have more options, are participating in the studies. Will any of these implants pass the tilt test? I encourage you to try it! So why would the FDA allow studies on underfilled implants? Ask them. Perhaps the FDA is not aware of the fill issue, or perhaps the FDA doesn't consider it important. *Why would manufacturers want to study the same implants that got them into litigation a few years back?* The only plausible answer is that manufacturers must sell implants to be able to provide implants to American women. American women need (and deserve) more options than saline implants for augmentation, and they deserve adequately filled implants to maximize the life of the implant shell and prevent reoperations.

But why regress? Why not pro—gress? Why study an old design, underfilled silicone gel implant of the type that the FDA banned initially, especially when newer, more advanced options are available! Why not study new, *cohesive* gel implants with a new filler material that are available in most of the rest of the world, used in over 40,000 patients, implants that *will* pass the tilt test. *And*, you can cut a pie-shaped wedge out of this implant with scissors, squeeze the implant, and the gel won't migrate (Figure 5-8)! We designed these cohesive gel, anatomic implants because we believe that they are safer, will last longer, and they are the implants I would unquestionably recommend over all other implants I've ever used (and I've used almost every type). Are cohesive gel implants perfect? No! Nor is any implant perfect! Is it best for every patient? No! But it is a step forward compared to most other implants. Now we're working on the next generation after cohesive gel, but if you're an American woman, you can't even get the current generation of the McGhan Style 410 cohesive gel implant in the United States! We will continue to be committed to the design and development of newer, better implants for our patients. Our goal is to be able to provide patients with implants that will last a lifetime. We're not there yet.

Is the amount of filler in an implant important? We believe it is very important! Should we adequately fill all implants, regardless of the design or filler material, to prevent shell collapse and folding. No doubt in our minds! Otherwise, every woman who receives an underfilled implant may require a reoperation sooner than she would were it adequately filled. More reoperations mean more risks and more costs.

**Which would you prefer — SOFTER, more natural with a FOLDED shell, or slightly FIRMER with a PROTECTED shell and LESS CHANCE OF REOPERATION?**

*You choose. It's your body.*

## WHO MAKES AND GUARANTEES MY IMPLANTS?

This is a critical question that many patients never ask! Why does it matter? Because you may be placing a device manufactured by a company in your body for many years. How good is the design? How good are the manufacturing processes? How good is the quality control? What happens if you have a problem? Who is there to support you? Does the company have the majority of its financial assets in the United States where its commitment is backed up by its money and large support staffs? All are questions that you should consider before selecting an implant, or before allowing your surgeon to select an implant for you.

### United States Companies

At the present time, two major companies manufacture breast implants in the United States — McGhan Medical Corporation and Mentor Corporation. Both are first-class companies committed to first-class patient care and state-of-the-art products. Both stand behind their products with strong guarantees, strong patient support, and commitments to research that advances the safety and efficacy of their products. Both companies are available when you need them, providing excellent service to patients and surgeons. We work with McGhan Medical Corporation, but we have the utmost respect for both companies, and we use implants manufactured by both.

### Foreign Companies

Foreign-based companies sell breast implants in the United States. Amazingly, the FDA allows foreign companies to sell breast implant products in the United States based on foreign data that may or may not conform to the standards that the FDA demands domestically of Mentor and McGhan. Does that mean that the products are not up to standards? Not necessarily. But a foreign-based company is often not subject to the same pressures, risks, and demands of a United States-based company. If the majority of a company's assets (capital) are located outside the United States, you could have a substantially more difficult time recovering money from that company if you had a problem with its product.

Ask the following questions of any company, foreign or domestic:

How long have you been in business?

Are you a publicly traded company in the United States?

Are most of your assets in the United States? Ask for documentation.

How long have you been selling breast implants in the United States?

How much money have you spent on breast implant research and development? Ask for documentation.

What are the terms of your guarantee on your breast implants? Do you cover all of my expenses for my lifetime with respect to implant replacement and surgery in the event of implant failure? Listen carefully to the answers, and ask for written documentation.

How many salespeople and support staff do you have in the United States? Where are they located? Ask for documentation.

**The company that manufactures your breast implants doesn't matter until you need to replace its implants.**

**It's easier to assure that you'll have a company's support when you need it *BEFORE* you put its product in your body.**

**Look into the company that manufactures your implants before you have an augmentation, or don't complain later.**

## "WHEN IS AN IMPLANT DOOMED TO DISAPPOINT ME?"

Any implant will disappoint you if you expect it to do something that an implant can't do?

An implant is likely to disappoint you if...

*You are very thin and expect that you won't feel some portion of your implant.*

*You have extremely saggy breasts and think an implant alone will solve the problem (it may, more about that later, but it may not—it depends on several factors).*

*You select excessively large implants that your tissues can't support over time.*

*You don't realize that your tissues won't get better with time, and select your implants accordingly.*

## THE NEXT STEP

Now that you're knowledgeable about implants, let's examine different surgical options.

[CHAPTER SIX]

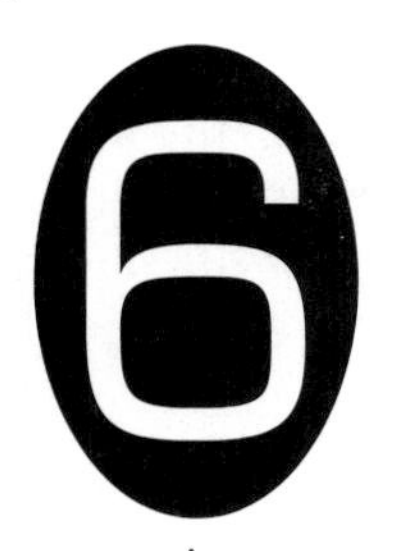

# SURGICAL OPTIONS:

# Over/Under Muscle, Implant Shape and Size, Incision Location

***"No set of surgical options or implant options is perfect for every patient—every option has tradeoffs."***

Many different surgical options exist in breast augmentation. To be able to offer you options, a surgeon must be familiar with different approaches and implants and have the experience and skill to apply those options confidently.

**NO specific set of surgical options is BEST for every patient.**

*If you are offered only one set of options, consult other surgeons.*

**Every patient tends to think that the options they chose are also the best options for someone else.**

*That isn't true because **no two women are exactly alike.** Your tissues are definitely different!*

**NO SURGICAL OPTION IS PERFECT. No surgical option is without tradeoffs.**

*The question is whether you know the relative benefits and tradeoffs and pick the options that best **maximize the benefits and minimize the tradeoffs.***

**If you choose surgical options without thinking about your tissues, you'll need to blame something or someone for the consequences.**

*You'll probably blame the implant or the surgeon, when it's really **YOU** who's largely responsible.*

## LOCATION OF THE POCKET FOR THE IMPLANT

### Over or Under Muscle?

The simple answer is: If you are extremely thin (and we'll show you how to measure later), you may need to put the implant behind muscle to assure adequate tissue cover over the implant. If you don't, you run more risks of seeing the edges of your implant. But there is much more to making the decision!

Breast implants are usually placed in one of **two locations**:

**1)** Behind your breast tissue but *in front* of your pectoralis muscle — **retromammary placement** (Figure 6-1), or

**2)** Partially *behind* your pectoralis muscle — **partial retropectoral placement** (Figure 6-2).

**Retromammary Placement**

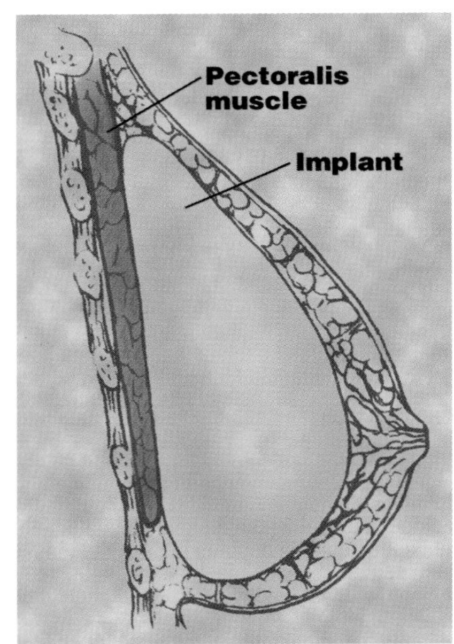


**Figure 6-1.**

**Partial Retropectoral Placement**

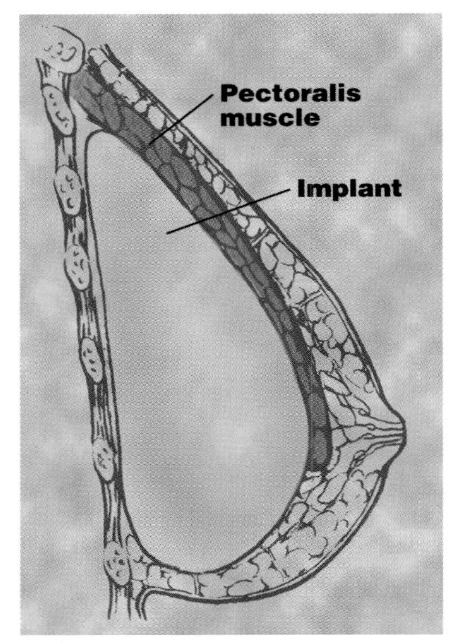


**Figure 6-2.**

When silicone gel-filled implants were available and widely used in the United States, surgeons began placing implants partially behind the pectoralis muscle because *silicone gel implants* had a lower risk of capsular contracture (excessive firmness) when they were placed partially behind the pectoralis. With *today's saline-filled implants,* the risk of capsular contracture is about the same whether the implant is placed in front of the muscle or behind the muscle. So, what difference does it make, and how do you choose? The choice is based on the thickness of your tissues — how much thickness you have to cover your implants.

## What Muscle, and Where Is It?

Let's review our anatomy from the Introduction! Figure 6-3 shows a cross-sectional side view of the upper body. Let's look at the layers of tissue beginning with the skin over the breast. Beneath the skin is a layer of fat—variable from patient to patient. The skin and fat layer make up what we call the "skin envelope" of the breast. The skin envelope covers the breast tissue, the next deeper layer. Beneath the breast tissue is the pectoralis major muscle that lies on top of your ribs. Implants can be placed behind the breast tissue but in front of the pectoralis (retromammary), or they can be placed behind the breast tissue and behind the pectoralis muscle (partial retropectoral). To understand why we use the term "partial" retropectoral, let's look at a front view of the anatomy.

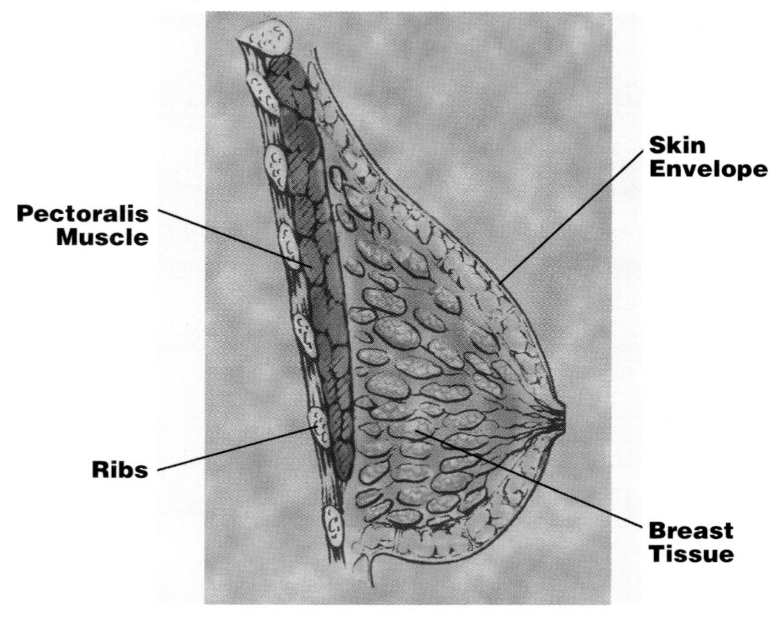


**Figure 6-3.**

The pectoralis muscle lies beneath the upper half or upper third of the breast (Figure 6-4). When an implant is placed in f*ront of the muscle*, the implant is covered in the lower portion by breast tissue and in the upper portion by only skin and fat (Figure 6-5). When an implant is placed *behind* the pectoralis major muscle, the upper portion of the implant is covered by muscle, but the lower portion (especially the lower, outside portion) of the implant is still covered by breast tissue (Figure 6-6). Hence, the term "partial" retropectoral—the implant is only partially behind muscle in the upper breast. In the lower breast, the implant is not totally covered by muscle.

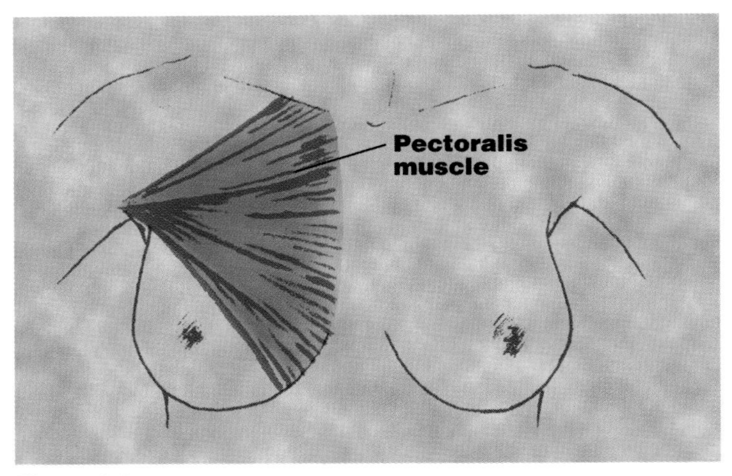


**Figure 6-4.**

**Partial retropectoral placement** *means that the upper portion of the implant is partially covered by the pectoralis major muscle.*

**Retromammary Placement**

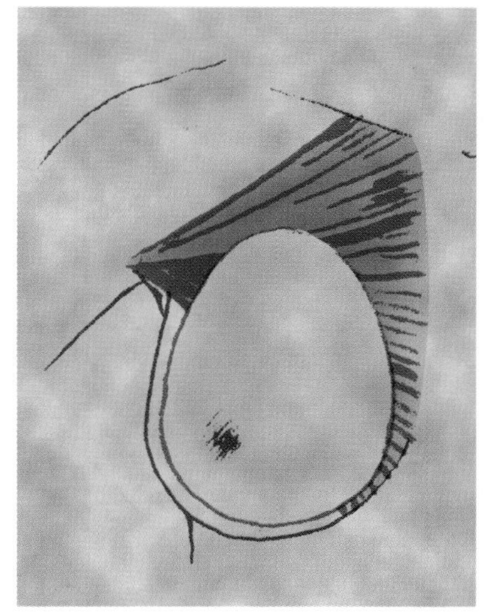

**Figure 6-5.**

**Partial Retropectoral Placement**

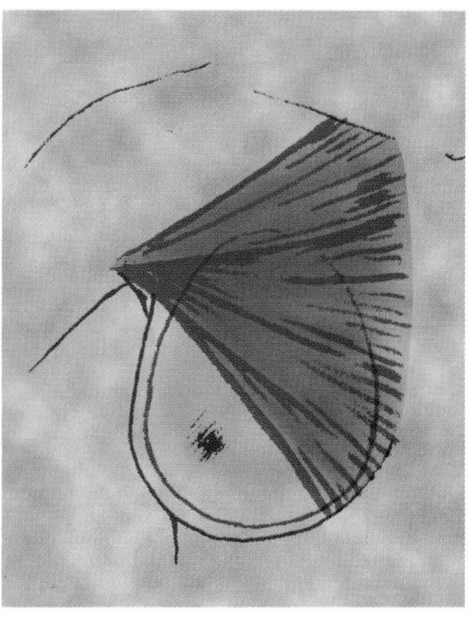

**Figure 6-6.**

Below and to the side of the pectoralis muscle is the serratus muscle. Although this muscle can be lifted to provide total muscle coverage of an implant, this option is best reserved for difficult reconstruction cases, *not* for augmentation. When an implant is totally covered by muscle (total submuscular), the shape of the lower breast is seldom as good and never predictable. The fold beneath the breast (the inframammary fold) is flatter and doesn't stretch as predictably with time. The additional pressure of the serratus muscle on an implant can also cause upward displacement of the implant, requiring reoperation. These tradeoffs generally mean that:

***Although sometimes possible, total muscle coverage is rarely the best option for a first-time augmentation.***

Rare exceptions exist where total muscle cover may be a good choice, but only in very, very thin patients who will accept all of the tradeoffs listed above.

## Retromammary (Behind Breast Tissue Only) Placement — Benefits and Tradeoffs

The goal of augmentation is to produce the best breast. The implant helps produce the best breast by putting pressure on the overlying breast tissue and skin envelope to fill and shape the breast.

**The closer the implant is to the tissues it is trying to shape, the more accurate and predictable the result.**

**An implant placed in FRONT of the muscle (behind breast tissue, retromammary) will always more PREDICTABLY CONTROL BREAST SHAPE.**

*If a surgeon tells you otherwise, I would respectfully disagree and ask how much experience the surgeon has with both types of placement.*

**A more perfect aesthetic result is usually possible when an implant is placed in the retromammary position.**

*That doesn't mean that every implant should be placed retromammary.*

From a practical standpoint, what are the advantages of retromammary (behind breast only) placement?

### Advantages of Retromammary Placement

**More precise control of cleavage —** the distance between your breasts

**More precise control of upper breast fill —** especially upper fill toward the middle of your chest

**Less chance of muscle pressure pushing your implants to the side over time,** widening the distance between your breasts

**Less chance of distorting your breast shape** when you tighten (contract) your pectoralis muscle

With all these advantages, why in the world would you ever put an implant behind muscle? There's one overwhelming reason—to provide adequate soft tissue coverage over the implant so you don't see the edges of the implant.

If you are *thin* and you place your implants *only behind breast tissue,* you will have a greater risk of *feeling or seeing an edge of the implant.* How thin is thin? How do you determine when "thin" is "too thin"? In a moment, we'll tell you. Another issue with placing implants only behind breast tissue and not behind muscle has to do with mammograms. More about that later. For starters, memorize this one:

**One of the most important principles in breast augmentation is providing ADEQUATE SOFT TISSUE COVER OVER AN IMPLANT.**

**If you are very thin, adequate tissue cover is more important than all of the advantages of retromammary placement combined and is always the FIRST PRIORITY!**

**The main tradeoffs of retromammary placement are:**

1) This location may not provide adequate soft tissue cover to prevent your seeing the edges of your implant if you are exceedingly thin, and
2) This location may make your mammograms more difficult (more about this later).

### Partial Retropectoral (Behind Pectoralis Muscle) Placement—Benefits and Tradeoffs

### Advantages of retropectoral Placement

You already know the main advantage of putting an implant partially behind muscle—to prevent seeing an edge of the implant.

**The major advantage of placing an implant behind muscle is to PREVENT IMPLANT EDGE VISIBILITY.**

*This does not mean that you may not feel portions of the implant, especially in the fold under the breast and the outside portion of the breast.*

**A second stated advantage of subpectoral placement is BETTER REDUCTION OF RISKS OF CAPSULAR CONTRACTURE compared to retromammary placement.**

*This difference is more marked with silicone gel implants than with saline implants. With saline implants, risks are about the same.*

**Better mammograms?**

*Maybe, but a soft breast that can be pulled away from the chest for mammography is also important.*

A third stated advantage of retropectoral placement is that some radiologists believe that placing the implant behind muscle improves mammogram interpretation. Although this concept is well-established in the medical literature, it's not an absolute (remember, most medical "facts" are shades of gray). One of the most important requirements for getting a good mammogram is that the breasts are soft (no capsular contracture). If the breasts are soft, it's easier for the technician to pull the breast tissue forward (away from the implant) to get a better picture. Other factors can significantly affect mammograms: The skill of the technician performing the mammogram, the skill of the person interpreting the mammogram, and the consistency and characteristics of your breast tissue — just to name a few. Also, mammograms are not perfect, with or without implants. Earlier, we told you that a significant number of breast cancers may not show up on a mammogram. A mammogram is not the only way to assess a breast. Your personal exam and your physician's exam are equally as important. Remember, every implant interferes with mammograms to some degree. If you have a strong family history of breast cancer (mother and grandmother), don't have a breast augmentation. Ask your surgeon about mammogram issues with implants; then make your own decisions.

## Tradeoffs of Retropectoral Placement

When an implant is placed behind the pectoralis muscle, the following tradeoffs can occur. They may occur to different degrees in different patients, but you should be willing to accept them, if necessary, in exchange for minimizing risks of upper implant edge visibility and possibly better mammography. The pressure of the pectoralis muscle overlying the implant causes the following:

### Distortion of breast shape when you tighten (contract) your pectoralis muscle

*This varies tremendously from patient to patient and is not predictable.*

### Shifting of the implants to the side over time, widening the distance between the breasts

*This also varies tremendously but is usually worse the thinner your tissues, the thicker your pectoralis, and/or the larger your implant.*

### Less control of upper breast fill, especially upper and toward the middle

*The pressure of the pectoralis on the upper implant reduces control of fill in these areas.*

### More stretch of the lower breast tissues over time

*Usually not a big issue, but the muscle puts pressure on the upper implant, transmitting more pressure to the lower envelope.*

### Increased risk of upward displacement of the implant

*This is related to the surgical techniques used. With optimal surgical technique, it is rare unless capsular contracture occurs and closes the lower pocket, pushing the implant upward.*

With all of these tradeoffs, why would anyone put an implant under muscle? Because the *Number 1* issue should be *adequate soft tissue coverage, regardless of the tradeoffs.* Without adequate soft tissue coverage, you may see or feel edges of your implants, you'll hate it, and you'll probably require a reoperation to correct it. More surgery, more costs, more down time — all bad. Make good team decisions at the beginning!

## Feeling or Seeing an Implant Edge

If you place an implant under the pectoralis muscle, you have done all that is possible to prevent seeing the upper edge of the implant. What about feeling the implant? The muscle only covers the upper and middle portions of the implant, not the lower and outside portions. In the lower and outside portions of the breast, if you are very thin and can feel your ribs with your finger, you will almost certainly be able to feel the edge or shell of your implant, especially in the fold under the breast or at the outside of the breast. You can't see the area under the fold of the breast (when standing), no matter how thin you are, so seeing an implant edge under the breast isn't much of an issue.

At the outside part of the breast, if your skin envelope is extremely thin, you may be able to see an implant edge in certain body positions — no matter what implant — no matter how much skill a surgeon may possess! Why? Because you can't change your tissues, and the only tissues covering the implant at the sides (laterally) are skin and fat. If skin and fat are thin, you may see or feel an edge of the implant! No way around it! If the surgeon tries to cover the lower, outer areas with muscle, you'll have other tradeoffs described previously.

## ABOVE OR BELOW MUSCLE — WHAT IS THE DECISION BASED ON?

**Decide to put your implants above or partially beneath muscle based on:**

### The thickness of your skin and fat layer above your breast tissue

*If you are thin (and we'll tell you how to measure it) and don't want to see the upper edge of your implants, put them behind the pectoralis muscle!*

### Your assessment of the relative benefits and tradeoffs of placing implants above or below muscle

*Nothing is perfect. You'll have to accept some tradeoffs with either location.*

How thin is thin? That's a tough question to answer! At what degree of thinness do risks of seeing an implant edge become significant? An even tougher question! The answers to these *should not be made based on subjective opinions* (yours or your surgeons'), but should rely on *objective measurements.*

We use a simple, quantifiable *pinch test* to determine whether soft tissue coverage will be adequate with retromammary placement, or whether the tissues are so thin that retropectoral placement is a better option.You can do it yourself if you have a caliper. Isolate the breast tissue (parenchyma) by pinching to pull the breast tissue down and forward. Above the breast tissue, firmly pinch the skin and underlying fat, and measure the thickness with a caliper (Figure 6-7). If the thickness is *greater than two centimeters (cm.),* your tissues are thick enough that retromammary placement is an option, with minimal risks of seeing an implant edge. On the other hand, if the pinch thickness is two cm. or less, you should definitely place your implants in the partial retropectoral position!

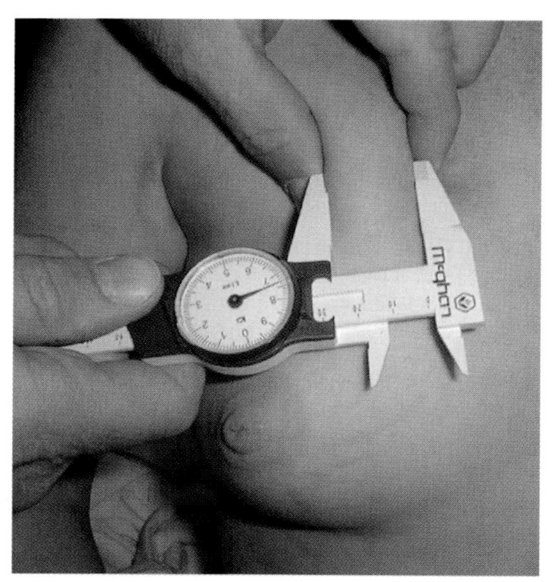

**Figure 6-7.**

**If the pinch thickness of your tissues above your breast tissue is less than two cm., RETROMAMMARY placement of an implant is NOT the best option for most patients.**

*If you put your implant under inadequate soft tissue cover, don't be surprised and don't complain when implant edges are visible.*

***Don't try to cheat on this!*** It truly isn't worth it! Regardless of the tradeoffs of partial retropectoral placement, they're far better than facing the possible consequences of placing your implants under inadequate soft tissue cover: Visible edges, visible traction rippling or wrinkling, visible implant shell — and the list goes on. If you are thin, measure your pinch thickness. If you measure less than two cm. on the pinch test, and a surgeon recommends retromammary placement, ask why? Also ask the surgeon about the risks listed above.

**One more time for emphasis:**

1) **If you are extremely THIN (less than two cm. pinch thickness above your breast), you should put the implant BEHIND MUSCLE to assure adequate tissue cover over the implant.** *If you don't, you run more risks of seeing the edges of your implant and risk other long-term problems.*

2) **If you have adequate thickness of tissues (more than 2 cm. pinch thickness above your breast), weigh the advantages and tradeoffs listed above and choose above or below the muscle based on your preferences and your surgeon's recommendations.**

### Myths About Muscle...

You may hear some popular myths about muscle, so let's mention them:

**Myth 1**
**Under muscle prevents capsular contracture.**

Not true. You can definitely develop a capsular contracture whether your implants are above or below muscle. Only with silicone gel implants does over or under muscle make a significant difference.

**Myth 2**
**Under muscle supports the implant better.**

Not true. The theory here is that the attachments of the pectoralis muscle to the ribs (near the fold beneath the breast) act as a sling to support the implant. In fact, when these attachments are all left intact, they tend to cause two problems: Upward implant displacement (a high riding implant with excessive upper bulge), and more lateral (to the side) displacement of the implants, widening the gap between the breasts!

### Myth 3
### Over muscle is never good.

Not true. In fact, *provided you have adequate soft tissue cover,* over muscle allows your surgeon better control of breast shape and fill.

### Myth 4
### Under muscle is never good.

Not true. If the pinch thickness of your tissues (above your breast tissue) is *less than two cm., under muscle is always better.*

## INCISION LOCATIONS

Figure 6-8 illustrates four commonly used incision locations for augmentation.

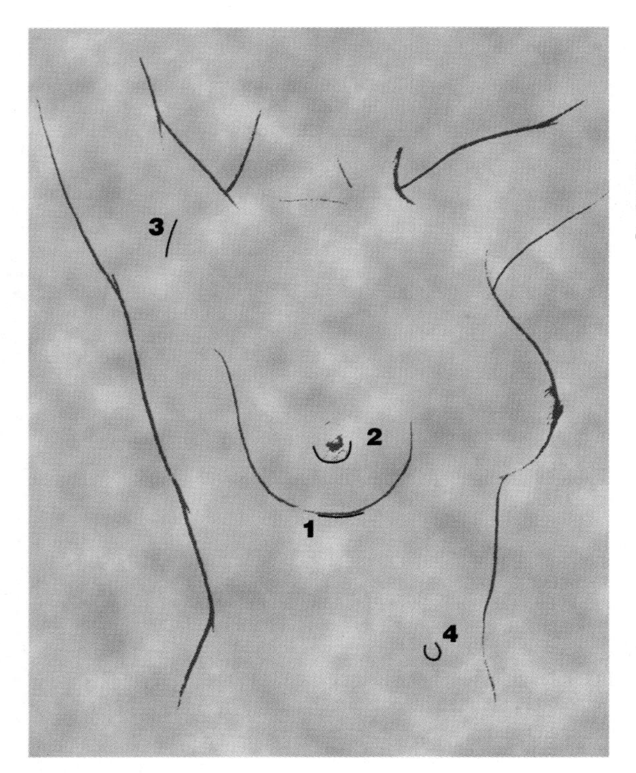


**INCISIONS**

**1 - Inframammary**
**2 - Periareolar**
**3 - Axillary**
**4 - Umbilical**

**Figure 6-8.**

Based on 20 years of experience with all incision locations, I am convinced of the following:

**Most patients worry far more about incision location before the surgery than they care after the surgery (provided they have a good result).**

**If an incision is on you, you will notice it!**

**If you have a beautiful breast, neither you nor anyone else will care where the incision is located.**

**Every patient thinks that the incision location she has is best.**

**Incision location is a common way that surgeons use to market their augmentation practice.**

*If a surgeon touts the "X incision" as unquestionably the best, and states, "I am the expert at the "X incision," run the other way.* ***No incision is best****, and the likely message is that the surgeon doesn't know how to do it any other way.*

**If a surgeon is EXPERIENCED with ALL incision locations, the surgeon will offer you ALL OPTIONS.**

**If you hear negative comments about an incision location from another patient or surgeon, it's usually because neither has much experience with that incision location.**

**No incision location is always best. Each location has advantages and tradeoffs.**

Every woman's breasts, at some time in her life, are likely to acquire a blemish — a stretch mark or a biopsy scar. A well-executed incision scar is usually no more noticeable than these other blemishes, and if the breast is beautiful, who notices? Who cares?

Just because your friend had a certain incision doesn't mean that incision location is best for you. In most cases, it doesn't matter. A few, very rare breast deformities are best addressed through a certain incision, and when these deformities occur, we don't hesitate to tell a patient, "With this specific breast deformity, a specific incision location gives us better control over your operation, and, hopefully, we'll get a better result." But *in over 90 percent of patients that we see, we offer the patient a choice of incision locations.* If a surgeon is experienced in all incisional approaches, the surgeon is less likely to recommend one location over another. Instead, the surgeon will give you a full range of options.

Don't form an opinion about incision location until you know about all the alternatives! *Incision location is one of the* ***LEAST*** *important decisions you'll make in augmentation.* Each incision location has relative advantages and tradeoffs.

## What About Scars?

We've said it once, and we'll say it again. No scar location is necessarily always better than another. Let's examine some myths about scars:

### Myth 1
### For patients with minimal or no breast tissue, a scar under the breast isn't a good choice.

Not necessarily. Assuming an augmentation is well done, that patient will develop a good crease beneath the breast. If the scar is properly positioned exactly in the crease, it will be minimally noticeable.

We've heard from more than one patient, "My boyfriend (a medical student on a medical fact finding mission, I'm sure ) said that he saw a scar on a topless dancer that was up on the breast, and it was terrible. I don't want that incision." The facts? More topless dancers have inframammary incisions than any other incision. The reason the scar was more noticeable was that it was improperly located. If the scar is placed too high above the fold, it's in an area where it is maximally stretched by the pressure of the implant. If it were kept exactly in the fold, there's less stretch, and the scar would be narrower. A popular misconception I've heard from surgeons is that inframammary scars should be placed above the fold "so that it won't show when she raises her arms in a bikini." Fact is, less than 1 percent of a woman's life is spent in a bikini. Fact is, a good scar exactly in the fold is far better than a widened scar that occurred because it was placed above the fold. If a surgeon is experienced in all incision locations, you can just choose! If you don't like one, choose another!

### Myth 2
### One incision location is less noticeable than another.

Not true. It depends on the patient's body position, who is looking, how long after the surgery (whether the scar is mature and faded), and the quality of the scar (largely dependent on each patient's healing tendencies). What is always less noticeable is a better quality scar, regardless of its location.

### Myth 3
### A shorter scar is always better than a longer scar.

Not true. The *quality* of a scar is much more important than its length. A short, ugly scar is always more noticeable than a slightly longer, thin, faded scar. Experience has taught many surgeons that when you make an incision too short to minimize scar length, you often stretch that incision and "beat up" the incision edges excessively during surgery. The scar does not heal as well, often stays redder longer and becomes wider. The result is a shorter scar, but also an uglier scar. A better quality scar, even if it is slightly longer, is far better than a short, ugly scar.

### Myth 4
### If you can put the incision off the breast in the armpit or the belly button, it's always better.

Not true. We'll cover specific advantages and tradeoffs of each incision location later in this chapter, but there are definite tradeoffs for both the axillary (armpit) and umbilical (belly button) approaches that may not appeal to some patients. Fact is, after surgery, scar location usually becomes a non-issue if the patient has an excellent result.

### Myth 5
### One scar location or another always preserves breast sensation better.

Not true. We formerly believed the axillary (armpit) incision preserved sensation better than other approaches, but after many more years' experience, we don't think that is necessarily true. The factors that most affect sensation are 1) Surgical technique—the more the surgeon directly visualizes the anatomy and the less bleeding, the less risk of nerve compromise, and 2) the size of the implant—the larger the implant, the more stretch it places on nerves, and the greater the chance you'll lose more sensation.

### Myth 6
### Surgeons pick scar locations because they think one is best.

Not necessarily true. Surgeons usually pick scar locations based on their experience. If they have a lot of experience with different scar locations, they'll offer you all options and discuss the tradeoffs. If they've only done augmentations one way (or even the majority one way), that's the scar location they're most likely going to push (hopefully).

## THE INFRAMAMMARY INCISION

Located in the fold beneath the breast, the inframammary incision is the most widely used incision in augmentation. The reasons? It gives the surgeon excellent access for augmentation in a wide range of breast types, offers better control of the operation in many instances, and is a "gold standard" that most surgeons learned during their residency training. More women have had augmentation through an inframammary incision than all other incision locations combined.

**The greatest advantage of an incision beneath the breast is the degree of control it allows the surgeon in a wide range of breast types.**

*More augmentation patients have had this incision location than all other incision locations combined!*

**The greatest tradeoff of an inframammary incision is the presence of a scar in the fold beneath the breast.**

The tradeoff of the inframammary incision is the scar beneath the breast. Properly placed in a patient with normal healing, after the scar matures, the scar is less noticeable than the imprint of your bra on your skin when you remove your bra. A very small percentage of patients form less than optimal scars (more about that later). If you have formed very heavy scars on your chest area in the past (that did not improve with time), you may want to consider another incision location. No test can predict the quality of scar you will form. But for the vast majority of patients (well over 90 percent) , the inframammary scar location is an excellent choice.

## THE PERIAREOLAR INCISION

This incision is placed around the edge (or just within) the areola, the pigmented skin surrounding the nipple. In most instances, the skin around the areola is thinner than the skin in the fold beneath the breast. There is some evidence that, all other things equal, thinner skin forms better scars than thicker skin. Some surgeons tout a periareolar (around the nipple-areola) scar as less visible than a scar beneath the breast. Is that true? Not necessarily. It depends on the quality of the scars in the two places, and that's not totally predictable.

**The greatest advantage of an incision around the areola is that it's located in thinner skin that usually heals well.**

**The greatest tradeoffs of a periareolar incisions are increased exposure of the implant to bacteria normally found in the breast, and, if you develop a bad scar, a scar located in the most visible location on the breast.**

A periareolar scar is located on the most visible area of the breast. As long as the scar is good—great. But if it's not so good, and we don't know who may form a bad scar, it's not so great. It's true that the skin of the areola area usually heals well, but if it does not, the less than optimal scar is noticeable every time you look at the nipple or areola.

Another stated advantage of the periareolar incision is that it's easier for the surgeon to reach all parts of the breast from a central incision. Truth is, a skilled surgeon can reach all parts of the breast under direct vision *by all incisions* (with the exception of the belly button incision where a portion of the dissection is usually "blind").

Tradeoffs of the periareolar approach? If you have a very small areola, incision length can be inadequate without extending the incision onto breast skin which forms less optimal scars. When you cut skin, you cut nerves. When you cut nerves, most grow back, but not all, and not predictably. You might think that an incision around the areola would always make patients lose more sensation compared to other incisions, but it doesn't! Why not? We don't know! Probably because sensory loss is very unpredictable and may be more related to how the surgery is done (more about that later), or the size of the implant (the larger, the more stretch on nerves and potential sensory loss).

Every woman's breast tissue contains bacteria. These bacteria live on the skin of healthy women and enter the breast through the nipple. They don't usually cause infection because the body is accustomed to their being in the breast. But put a large, foreign object, your breast implant, in the area, and the bacteria can sometimes produce problems. When an implant is inserted through a periareolar incision, the breast implant is more directly exposed to breast tissue than with other approaches. With more exposure to bacteria, you might think that infection rates would definitely be higher with this approach, but increased infection risk has not been scientifically documented. Even if an implant doesn't get infected, bacteria around the implant are probably a major factor contributing to capsular contracture, so you might expect a higher risk of capsular contracture with a periareolar incision. Again, not scientifically confirmed.

If you happen to form bad scars (and this can happen, regardless of your history of scars), the areola would not be an ideal place to have a bad scar. Bad scars are very rare in any location, but to date, we have no way of reliably predicting which patients will develop bad scars.

## THE AXILLARY INCISION

Placed in the deepest area of the armpit, the axillary incision is probably the least conspicuous of all augmentation incisions. Proper incision placement is critical. If placed in the highest portion of the armpit hollow, the scar is unnoticeable in virtually any body position. Even with arms fully raised, and even before the scar fades, losing its pink color, the incision looks like a normal crease. Once the scar is mature, it is almost impossible to detect in most patients, even with the arms raised. Another stated advantage of the axillary approach is better preservation of sensation in the breast. Actually, sensory preservation is quite variable and is more likely related to the type of dissection performed and the size of the implant.

**The greatest advantage of an incision in the armpit is that its location makes it the least visible of all scars for augmentation.**

**The greatest tradeoff of axillary incisions is that a surgeon must be experienced, and the operation time is usually slightly longer if the surgeon uses state-of-the-art techniques.**

With older axillary techniques, after making the incision in the armpit, the surgeon used various types of blunt instruments to "blindly" create a pocket for the implant. The development of an instrument called an endoscope (Figure 6-9) allows surgeons to see inside the body on a television screen to more precisely control the operation. With the advent of modern endoscopic instrumentation, surgeons can see to precisely create the pocket for the implant instead of bluntly, blindly tearing tissues. This minimizes bleeding, maximizes accuracy, and shortens recovery. The longer operation time required for endoscopically assisted axillary augmentation is more than compensated by increased accuracy and control. A slightly longer operating time can mean more costs, but should not increase any risks associated with the operation. Ask your surgeon.

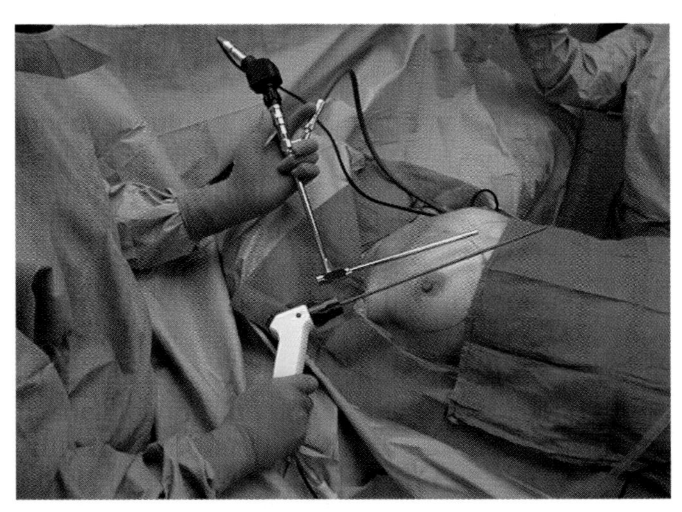

**Figure 6-9.**

The axillary approach using endoscopic instrumentation is technically more demanding of the surgeon compared to periareolar and inframammary approaches and is difficult for some surgeons to learn. If you are considering an axillary approach, be sure that your surgeon is experienced in endoscopic techniques and that the surgeon minimizes blunt, blind dissection.

## THE UMBILICAL INCISION

Umbilicus is the medical term for your belly button. The incision for the umbilical approach is placed in and around the belly button. I use the terms "in" and "around" because, to some degree, the location of the incision depends on the size of the belly button. Most women's belly buttons are small, and the incision required is one inch or more in length. The surgeon may not make the initial incision one inch, but the instruments required for the operation usually stretch the incision, and portions of the incision can sometimes extend outside the boundaries of the belly button.

The main advantage of the belly button incision is that it is located off the breast. The belly button incision sounds very acceptable to many women because they are familiar with other endoscopic procedures in the abdomen that use similar incisions, such as ligation of the fallopian tubes (tubal ligation). Actually, the incision required to insert a breast implant through the umbilicus is much larger than that required for many abdominal procedures.

**The main advantage of an incision in and around the belly button is that the incision is located off the breast.**

**The main disadvantages of the umbilical incision compared to other incisions are:**

*It offers the surgeon the **least control** of all incisional locations and the least predictable results.*

*It is **located further from the breast**, and normal tissues in the upper abdomen are disturbed to get to the breast.*

*Access to the breast is created by* ***bluntly pushing*** *a* ***one-inch-diameter tube*** *from the umbilicus to each breast through the tissues of the upper abdomen.*

*The pocket for the implant is developed by inserting an uninflated implant, blowing it up, then* ***pushing it vigorously*** *side to side to* ***tear a pocket*** *to receive the implant.* ***The surgeon cannot see inside the pocket*** *to create the most precise pocket with the least bleeding.*

*When the pocket is created by any method other than direct vision,* ***the pocket is less accurate, bleeding is increased, and control is less****.*

*Most surgeons who use the umbilical approach do not offer implant placement behind muscle.* ***If you are thin, behind muscle is better long term****.*

So why would anyone want to use this approach? It sounds good, unless you really look at it objectively. Does this mean that you can't get a good result through this incision? No. It just means you should be able to expect an even better result in the same patient through an axillary approach. The armpit incision satisfies the advantage of moving the incision off the breast. The armpit incision is much closer to the breast, so much less normal tissue is traumatized getting to the breast, and the risk of depressions or troughs in the abdomen from bluntly pushing a large tube through the fat are avoided. From the armpit, the entire pocket can be created *precisely* and *bloodlessly* under *direct vision* for a more accurate, more controlled pocket with less bleeding. Your surgeon can also easily place the implant above or below muscle via the armpit, depending on your tissue needs.

Why would any surgeon want to use the umbilical approach? The umbilical approach allows some surgeons to differentiate themselves from other surgeons by advertising: "I can do it, and they don't. Come to me." The umbilical approach can be appealing from a marketing perspective, but I challenge any surgeon to debate me in a scientific forum on the logic of why it is really better. We have many patients who are interested in umbilical augmentation— until they hear the facts. Having performed umbilical augmentations, I can categorically state that there is no comparison with other approaches if precision and control are objectives. In fairness, I hope that one day the umbilical approach will be able to offer the same level of control as other approaches and avoid unnecessarily traumatizing a normal area of the body (the abdomen) to get to the breast. When it can, I'll be happy to endorse the approach—we can always use more options—provided they make sense.

## IMPLANT SHAPE AND IMPLANT SIZE

Much of the information you need about implant selection and size is included in Chapter 5. Some of the information is worth repeating, and you'll need some new information that relates implant choices to the surgical choices previously discussed in this chapter.

### The Implant Selection Process

A few guiding principles first:

**Implant selection** is ideally a team **decision** between you and your surgeon.

Assuring **adequate soft tissue cover** (selecting the pocket location, above or below muscle) is **more important** than **implant selection.**

When selecting implant **shape** (round or anatomic), think about the **potential risk of shell folding** and how that could affect the **life** of your implants.

When selecting **implant size,** the **larger** the implant, the **more tradeoffs and risks** you'll encounter, especially long-term.

## Incision location is LESS important than implant selection.

Don't worry too much right now about selecting your implant. Wait until you visit with surgeons and determine which surgeon best understands what you want and can best explain in detail your tissue characteristics and how they will affect your augmentation. Listen carefully to your surgeon's implant recommendations and the reasons. Then make your decision.

### Implant, Pocket Location, Implant, and Incision: Combinations That Are Available

The following table shows you that almost any implant can be put in almost any pocket location through almost any incision— provided you select an experienced, qualified surgeon. This table shows you the options that are currently available. A "yes" means that this is an accepted combination that has been scientifically confirmed and presented. A "no" means that although someone may be doing it, the jury is not in yet.

| Implant Shape | Implant can : be placed Retromammary (over muscle) | Implant can be placed: Partial retropectoral (under muscle) | Implants can be placed over or under muscle through all incisions |
|---|---|---|---|
| **ROUND** | | | |
| Smooth | Yes | Yes | Yes |
| Textured | Yes | Yes | Yes |
| **ANATOMIC** | | | |
| Textured | Yes | Yes | No - Anatomic implants cannot be accurately placed through an umbilical incision at this time, and implants cannot be readily placed under muscle through the umbilical incision. |

If anyone tells you that a combination labeled "yes" is not available, keep searching. I assure you that the options are there for you if you find a surgeon with experience in all approaches.

## HOW THE SURGEON CREATES THE POCKET FOR YOUR IMPLANT

You'll undoubtedly hear discussions about surgical techniques in your quest for the best breast. Most patients are not qualified to judge the details of surgical techniques. That's what you're paying your surgeon to do. But some basics are worth knowing.

**There's a difference between doing things because they're EASIER and doing them because they are BETTER.**

**Surgeons are human. Some surgeons do things because they are easier,** *and may even convince themselves that they're better. It's possible to achieve* **easier and better**.

**In surgery, better is usually more difficult until you LEARN MORE—then BETTER IS EASIER.**

**Nothing is easy in surgery. Everything is difficult until you learn to do it well—then everything's easier.**

**If I (as a surgeon) don't know any better, I simply don't know any better. That doesn't mean that better doesn't exist or can't exist.**

Surgical techniques evolve, and most get better with time. There's always something new. The new things that are really better survive the test of time. Do all "better" surgical techniques become widely accepted? I wish it were true, but not necessarily! When better things are more difficult, it almost always takes much longer for them to become widely accepted, sometimes until a new generation of surgeons comes along.

A good example is techniques used to create the pocket to receive a breast implant. Traditionally in surgery, sharp instruments, scalpels or scissors, were used to cut tissues. Problem is, when tissues are cut with sharp instruments, they bleed. Blood covers and stains adjacent tissues and obscures details that allow a surgeon to be more accurate. Blood loss, even if it is not life threatening, is messy, wastes time, and compromises accuracy.

If a technique is easier or faster, I guarantee it will find its way into many surgeons' bag of tricks. Blunt dissection, a technique used to create the pocket for the implant, is an example. Basically, a blunt dissector is an 18" round rod about the diameter of a ball point pen that is bent into a curve at one end (Figure 6-10). This instrument is used to tear, rather than precisely cut tissues. After the surgeon inserts the instrument, the remainder of the pocket dissection is "blind." The surgeon is not looking inside the tissues as the instrument sweeps from side to side, tearing and separating tissues to create the pocket. During my residency training 21 years ago, I was taught to use blunt dissection to create a pocket for a breast implant. It works, and it's fast, but it's also very traumatic to tissues and causes a lot of bleeding. Surely, there had to be a better way! I started searching, and I found the electrocautery.

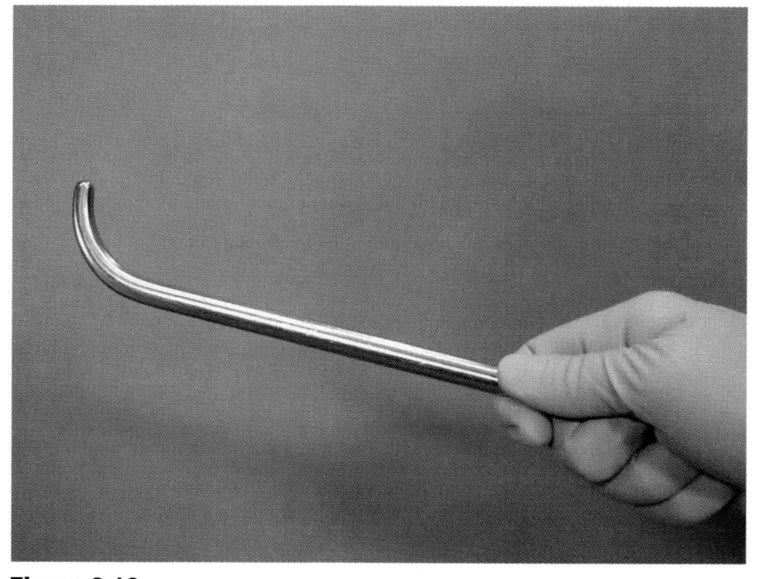

**Figure 6-10.**

Electrocautery instruments use electrical current to cut tissue, and to stop (coagulate)bleeding vessels(Figure 6-11). With electrocautery dissection, tissue cutting and blood vessel coagulation occur simultaneously! Incredible benefits! Dramatically less bleeding! The surgeon can see. The surgeon can be more accurate and spends less time stopping bleeding. Sound great? You bet! So everybody uses it to create pockets for implants, right? Wrong. A lot of surgeons still use blunt dissection.

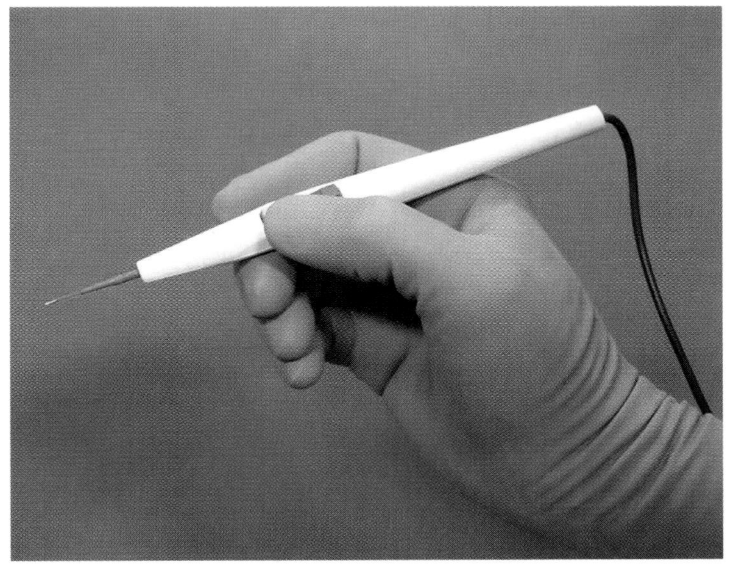

**Figure 6-11.**

**BLUNT dissection techniques for creating the implant pocket cause MORE TISSUE injury, TEAR TISSUES, create MORE BLEEDING, and result in a LONGER RECOVERY time compared to state-of-the-art electrocautery dissection techniques.**

During the seven years that I used blunt dissection, most of my patients (especially when the implant was placed beneath muscle) could not return to normal physical activities for 10-14 days. Today, the vast majority of our patients (even submuscular augmentations) return to normal activities in *less than three days!*

Why? ***No more blunt dissection!*** Today, regardless of the incision location (and we offer all of them), regardless of over or under muscle, we never use blunt dissection.

Compared to electrocautery dissection, creating a pocket by blunt dissection injures tissues more than precise electrocautery dissection, prolongs recovery, and carries a higher risk of complications.

Having used all types of dissection, I can't bring myself today to sharp dissect or blunt dissect a pocket! Thank goodness for progress! You are the benefactor. Think of the difference between a ***two-week*** recovery and potentially, a ***two-day*** recovery! No surgeon can guarantee every patient a two-day recovery, but avoiding blunt dissection can dramatically shorten recovery times!

## THE NEXT STEP...

Now you know about different surgical options. The next step is learning about the *problems* that can occur in breast augmentation, regardless of the options you choose.

[CHAPTER SEVEN]

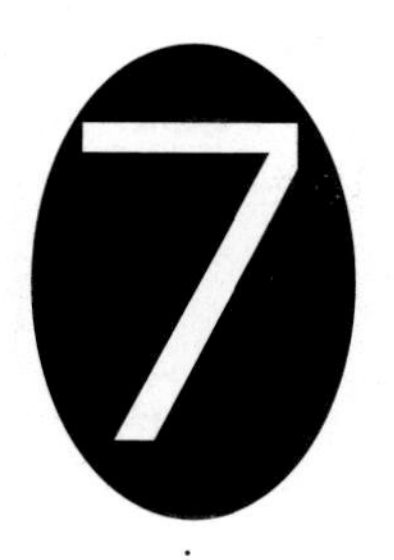


# NOTHING IS PERFECT: Tradeoffs, Problems and Risks

***"Every choice in augmentation has tradeoffs. Risks can be reduced by making the best choice based on good team decisions."***

Don't fool yourself. Nothing in life is perfect; nothing is without tradeoffs. Augmentation is no different. You can't choose a set of options for breast augmentation that doesn't come with a package of tradeoffs. Tradeoffs are compromises that you accept when you select an implant, a pocket location, an incision location, or any other option in augmentation. You *will* accept tradeoffs, whether you know it or not. The more you know about tradeoffs of each option, the better choices you can make.

In our practice, any *surprise* that occurs in augmentation is a *problem*. When educating patients prior to surgery, we tell them, "If it's a surprise, it's a problem!" We don't want surprises. We certainly don't want problems.

**The better we help you understand what to expect before surgery, the more you know, the FEWER SURPRISES— and the FEWER PROBLEMS.**

When you decide to have an augmentation, you are deciding to take risks. Every medical procedure requires that you take certain risks to potentially gain certain benefits. Every cosmetic surgical procedure is totally elective. You choose it. You don't require it. There is no medical reason that requires you to have it. For any procedure that you *want*, but don't really *need*, the potential benefits should far outweigh any potential risks. To decide whether a set of risks is reasonable and justifiable, you must first know what the risks are and how likely it is that those risks will occur.

## TRADEOFFS

The following table lists tradeoffs that are associated with common options available in augmentation. This list is not comprehensive — other tradeoffs can occur. The purpose of this overview is to emphasize that:

**No option or set of options in augmentation is without tradeoffs.**

The potential benefits of each of these options are described in Chapters 5 and 6 for comparison with the tradeoffs.

| OPTION | POTENTIAL TRADEOFFS |
|---|---|
| **1. Implant shape** | |
| ***a. Round implant*** | Less natural appearance<br>Increased risk of shell folding if filled to manufacturer's recommendations<br>If overfilled to prevent shell folding, voids manufacturer's warranty |
| ***b. Anatomic implant*** | More expensive<br>More demanding of the surgeon<br>Can rotate or malposition if pocket is not accurate or if tissues stretch excessively |
| **2. Implant shell surface** | |
| ***a. Smooth shell surface implant*** | Higher risk of capsular contracture, especially with silicone gel filled implants<br>Does not develop tissue adherence to reduce risks of capsular contracture<br>Does not develop tissue adherence to control implant position<br>Does not develop tissue adherence to help support weight of implant<br>Implant always falls to bottom of pocket created for the implant<br>Implant may shift more to the side when lying down |
| ***b. Textured shell surface implant*** | Some surgeons believe that a slightly thicker shell is easier to feel in very thin patients (shell thickness only varies a few ten thousandths of an inch from smooth to textured, and a thicker shell may be more durable)<br>Some surgeons believe that small particles of silicone can shed from textured surfaces (never demonstrated in a large study of augmentation patients)<br>Textured surfaces vary from manufacturer to manufacturer |
| **3. Implant pocket location** | |
| ***a. Retromammary pocket (behind breast tissue, not behind muscle)*** | Possibly more exposure to bacteria in the breast tissue (but no scientific study proves a higher infection rate)<br>Possibly higher risk of capsular contracture with silicone gel filled implants (no higher risk with saline implants) |
| ***b. Partial retropectoral pocket (behind the pectoralis muscle)*** | Distortion of breast shape with muscle contraction<br>Less control of upper breast fill (especially upper toward the middle)<br>Tendency of implants to shift to sides over time, widening distance between the breasts (worse in thinner patients or with larger implants or with thicker pec muscles)<br>Longer recovery when muscle is manipulated |

| OPTION | POTENTIAL TRADEOFFS |
|---|---|
| **4. Implant pocket creation technique** | |
| ***a. Sharp dissection to create the pocket*** | More bleeding, obscures anatomy detail during surgery<br>More bruising after surgery<br>More risk of fluid or blood collection around implant |
| ***b. Blunt dissection to create the pocket*** | More traumatic to tissues<br>More bruising<br>More pain<br>Longer recovery |
| ***c. Electrocautery dissection to create the pocket*** | Can cause tissue charring if electrocautery is improperly set<br>Requires specific technical skills of the surgeon<br>Requires special instrumentation |
| **5. Incision location** | |
| ***a. Inframammary incision location (under the breast)*** | Scar located under the breast<br>Scar more visible lying down compared to axillary (armpit)<br>If not positioned optimally, can locate higher on underside of breast where it can stretch and widen. |
| ***b. Periareolar incision location (around the areola)*** | Scar located around the areola<br>If suboptimal healing, scar is on the most visible portion of the breast<br>May interfere more with nipple sensation (though not scientifically proved)<br>May expose implant to more bacteria in breast tissue (not scientifically proved) |
| ***c. Axillary incision location (in the armpit)*** | Technically more demanding of surgeon<br>If improperly positioned, scar can be visible without raising the arms (scar is least visible of all scars in all body positions when properly located)<br>Requires special instrumentation to perform optimally |
| ***d. Umbilical incision location (in and around the belly button)*** | Visible scar in and around belly button<br>Least accurate control of all approaches<br>Injures abdominal fat tissues to gain access to the breasts<br>Risk of visible troughs on abdomen, abdominal bruising after surgery<br>Pocket dissection is blind, no direct visualization during pocket dissection<br>Access is farthest from breast<br>Creates pocket by manually tearing tissues using an inflated device |

**Tradeoffs always depend on the details of each specific case.**

**The characteristics of your tissues can significantly affect the tradeoffs.**

**The experience of your surgeon with different options can significantly affect the tradeoffs.**

**After a surgeon examines you, be sure to ask about specific tradeoffs and how they relate to your specific tissues and the surgeon's experience with different options.**

## PROBLEMS

If it's a **SURPRISE**, it's a **PROBLEM**.

There are two kinds of surprises:

***A surprise can be SOMETHING YOU DON'T KNOW ABOUT that confuses or frightens you,***

**OR**

***A surprise can be a MEDICAL COMPLICATION that causes untoward medical events.***

The first type of surprise, something you don't know about that confuses or frightens you, is potentially preventable. The second, a medical complication, can occur despite all best efforts by you and your surgeon.

### Problems (Surprises) That Result From Things You Don't Know

Most people deal with the unknown problems better if they know what's coming. When you have an augmentation, your body will do predictable (and sometimes unpredictable) things in response to your surgery during the healing process.

**The more you know about what to expect and what is normal, the less confused or frightened you will be when it occurs.**

***It's a TEAM job to assure that you know what to expect after your surgery.***

**It's the responsibility of your surgeon and your surgeon's staff to provide information for you.**

## IT'S YOUR RESPONSIBILITY TO USE IT!

If you don't receive comprehensive information from your surgeon, you can't very well read and digest it! The amount and quality of written and verbal information that you receive from surgeons is an excellent way to evaluate different surgeons. If you receive good information and you don't read and digest it, you aren't doing your job, and you are making your life more difficult during recovery. You can't possibly remember every detail about what to expect. That's why most surgeons will give you specific, written information to use as a reference. Keep it; use it. Despite good reference material, things can occur that reading an explanation just doesn't solve. Call your surgeon or the surgeon's staff. Helping you is their part of the team job.

Before your augmentation, be sure that all of your questions are answered. If you are the least bit unclear about anything, ask! Take notes, and spend time going over them. The more you know, the more comfortable you'll be, the fewer surprises you'll have, and the fewer problems.

### Problems (Surprises) That Result From Medical Complications

The other type of problems that can occur fall into the category of medical risks — untoward events that can occur following any type of surgery. These problems can be very significant, and you should understand and consider all medical risks very thoroughly before deciding to have breast augmentation surgery.

## RISKS ASSOCIATED WITH BREAST AUGMENTATION — THE BASICS

**Every breast augmentation operation carries inherent risks.**

**Medical complications are not totally preventable by you or your surgeon.**

**Do not have an augmentation unless you thoroughly understand and accept the potential risks and tradeoffs of the procedure.**

When you are first learning about risks, be sure that you thoroughly understand exactly what the risk involves. Secondly, ask how often each risk occurs. A risk can sound terrible, but if it only occurs once in every 100,000 cases, it's logical to be *informed* but not excessively *worried* about that particular risk. In other words, try to put all risks into perspective. How bad is it, what are the possible consequences, and how often does it occur? In this chapter, you'll learn the basics, but **always ask your surgeon three basic questions:**

***Exactly what does the risk involve?***

***What are the possible consequences?***

***How often does the risk or problem actually occur?***

The risk of your developing a specific problem or complication is usually expressed as a percentage. For example, the risk of your developing a hematoma (collection of blood inside the pocket, around the implant) may be 2 percent. That means that this problem occurs in approximately two out of every 100 patients. When you are trying to decide whether to have an augmentation based on risk factors, it's logical to always consider the worst-case scenario. Always ask if the quoted risk factor is *an average figure reported in the medical literature* (these are averages that are derived from large scientific studies). Risk figures derived from large scientific studies more closely represent a possible worst case scenario compared to figures based on a surgeon's personal experience.

Let's consider an example from our practice. Over the past 20 years, I am aware of only three patients who experienced bleeding following augmentation that required additional surgery (hematomas) out of more than 3,000 cases. However, in all of my literature and discussions with patients, I quote the risk of hematoma as one or two in every 100 cases, 1 percent or 2 percent. My personal rate of hematomas is much lower, but every patient should base her decision about whether to have surgery on the higher number, and assume that she has at least a 1 percent or 2 percent risk of developing a hematoma after augmentation.

## DETAILS OF BREAST AUGMENTATION RISKS—FROM THE FDA

In 1997, the FDA released a statement that details augmentation risks that the agency thinks are important. The entire text of FDA information for patients regarding augmentation is available from the FDA's web site at http://www.fda.gov.

For each category of risk, the text from **the FDA statement is labeled "FDA," and is printed in bold type**. Our comments regarding that same risk follow, and are labeled "JT" and are printed in regular type.

**FDA: SURGICAL RISKS OF IMPLANTS**
**In addition to the risks of anesthesia and surgery in general, following are some of the complications that may**

**result from any surgical procedure that places a foreign object (including a breast implant) in the body. It is not known how frequently these occur.**

JT- Although the FDA states that "It is not known how frequently these occur," most surgeons can give you an estimate based on published scientific studies, with references to the medical literature if you desire.

*FDA- Hematoma:* **A hematoma is a collection of blood or a blood clot from a leak in a blood vessel that may form within hours after surgery in the pocket where the implant has been placed. If this happens, swelling, pain, and bruising may result. Large hematomas may have to be drained surgically for proper healing. Surgical drainage may cause scarring, which is minimal in most women.**

JT- A reasonable guideline is that hematomas occur in about one or two cases out of 100 (1-2 percent). Large hematomas should *always* be drained, and you may have a drain tube in place for several days. The risk of capsular contracture (excessive tightening of the capsule around the implant producing an excessively hard breast, sometimes misshapen) is *substantially* higher following a hematoma. If you have any history of abnormal bleeding, you MUST advise your surgeon. Avoid all medications that contain aspirin for at least three weeks before and after surgery, and ask your surgeon for a list of other medications to avoid— medications that could impair normal blood clotting.

*FDA- Infection:* **requires immediate medical attention if it occurs. If you notice signs of infection such as pain, redness, swelling, tenderness or fever, call your surgeon immediately. If the infection does not subside promptly with the appropriate treatment, removal of the implant may be necessary. (If that happens, a new device can usually be implanted after the infection has completely cleared.)**

JT- The usual risk of infection is less than one in 100 cases. We take an even harder stand about infection compared to the FDA.

In our practice, we advise every patient *before* augmentation that if they develop an infection, we recommend removing *both* implants, and we do not ever recommend replacing either implant. Although this is a very hard position for both patient and surgeon, it definitively solves the problem, forever. Any attempt to salvage an infected breast implant is tenuous at best. No matter how long you wait after removing an infected implant, there is a significant risk of reinfection if you attempt to replace the implant, regardless of treatment techniques used. Even if a replaced implant does not become reinfected, there is a substantial risk of capsular contracture in the previously infected breast. Reinfection or capsular contracture both require additional surgery with additional risks, potential complications, costs, time off work, and possible permanent deformity. Not worth it! Take them out and leave them out! Fortunately, infection is very rare, but if it occurs, implant removal is the best option.

## FDA: OTHER IMPLANT-RELATED RISKS

**In addition to the surgical risks discussed above, other risks are associated specifically with breast implants. The surgeon should discuss these with you way in advance of surgery.**

**If possible, a month before the surgery, ask your surgeon and anesthesiologist or anesthetist for full information on the risks associated with breast implants, including: the patient package insert for your specific type of implant(s), the patient information sheet for women considering saline-filled implants and a copy of the informed consent form usually given to the patient prior to surgery for either saline or silicone implants.**

**The adverse effects from breast implants fall into two categories. The first consists of known risks that are clearly associated with these devices. The second consists of problems that have not been scientifically shown to be associated with breast implants but have been reported by some women who have them.**

JT- We couldn't agree more. Read the surgeon's information materials, the manufacturer's package insert and informational materials, and all consent forms. If you have any questions at all, ask for answers well in advance of your surgery. Consider the information very carefully before you proceed.

**FDA: KNOWN IMPLANT-RELATED RISKS**

*FDA- Rupture, deflation, and leakage:*
**Breast implants are not lifetime devices and cannot be expected to last forever. Some implants deflate (or rupture) in the first few months after being implanted and some deflate after several years; yet others are intact 10 or more years after the surgery.**

JT- We've already told you that no device lasts forever, especially breast implants. Many factors affect the life of a breast implant. The implants that are available today are technologically the best implants in history, but their life span is not predictable. Assume the worst—if you needed to replace an implant in the first few months after surgery, is it worth it? Both McGhan Medical and Mentor currently guarantee their implants. See their informational literature for details.

Rupture means that the outer shell of the implant disrupts in a major way—allowing most or all of the filler material in the implant to leave the implant. If you have a saline implant, the breast usually decreases significantly in size, making rupture easy to recognize. Since saline implants are inflatable, the term "deflation" is used synonymously with rupture — the shell disrupts. Remember that your body forms a capsule around every implant. If your capsule is intact, with saline implants the body absorbs the saline. With silicone implants, provided you did not have a closed capsulotomy (squeezing on the implant and capsule to break the capsule), and provided the capsule is intact, most or all of the silicone remains inside the capsule and is removed when the implant is replaced. With older silicone gel-filled implants, even if a closed capsulotomy was not performed, it is possible for silicone gel to escape from the capsule into the breast or adjacent tissues, but in my personal experience, escape of significant amounts of silicone through an intact capsule is exceedingly rare.

Leakage refers to escape of smaller amounts of filler from an implant without gross disruption of the implant shell. Leakage is a very poorly defined term. If a saline implant "leaks," it usually deflates, partially or totally. All silicone gel implants experience some "leakage" — trace amounts of silicone can escape the shell of the implant. This phenomenon is called "gel bleed." The key questions are: How much escapes? What is the result? With gel bleed, only trace amounts of silicone escape. What is the result? The answer depends on whom you ask. Silicone is contained in many cosmetic products that women use every day. Many antacid preparations contain simethicone. Silicone has been used for decades in a variety of implantable devices from lenses in the eye to shunts in the brain. And even needles and syringes used every day in most fields of medicine are lubricated with ***liquid silicone!***

**FDA-** ***Saline implants*****:**
**Saline implants may be more vulnerable to damage and deflation than gel-filled implants. When a saline implant deflates, it usually happens quickly. Surgery is then required to remove the ruptured implant and replace it, if desired. Since salt water is naturally present in the body, the body will absorb the leaked saline solution from the implant instead of reacting to it as foreign matter.**

**It is clear that the rupture rate for saline implants varies and seems to be dependent on many factors, including manufacturing quality standards and length of time since manufacture, etc.**

**It is not known when deflation is most likely to happen. The implant may break due to injury to the breast or normal aging of the implant, releasing the salt water filling. Because of the uncertainty about the actual rupture rate of saline breast implants, FDA has advised the manufacturers that they must conduct a study of the frequency of rupture in**

**women with saline breast implants for a period of at least 10 years. This study must be included in the applications to continue marketing (Premarket Approval Applications, or PMAs). This study, to be completed in 1996 or 1997, is part of the companies' 1994 agreement with FDA on the studies they will conduct in order for their saline-filled breast implants to stay on the market.**

JT - Saline-filled implants are not inherently "weak." I've actually filled implants, placed them on a hard floor, and stood on them to demonstrate the strength of the shell (and I'm a big guy). Any inflatable implant contains a valve. Every additional device added to the shell of an implant has a failure rate. Although we can't prove all the answers, the life span of saline implants is probably shorter than comparable silicone gel-filled implants for several reasons: A less cohesive filler that does not buffer movement forces transmitted to the shell, *underfill* (see Chapter 5), and the presence of a valve (an additional device). So many factors can affect the life of an implant that it will be difficult or impossible to ever precisely estimate implant life, regardless of what type of study is done. The bottom line is: If you're not willing to undergo replacement, regardless of when it becomes necessary, don't have an augmentation.

**FDA-** ***Silicone gel implants*****:**
**When silicone gel implants rupture, some women may notice decreased breast size, nodules, uneven appearance of the breasts, pain or tenderness, tingling, swelling, numbness, burning, or changes in sensation. Other women may experience a rupture and not notice any differences. If the problems are severe, the implants may have to be removed. If you are considering the removal of an implant and the implantation of another one, be sure to discuss the benefits and risks with your doctor.**

**The rate at which silicone gel-filled implants rupture -- and thus their durability -- remains unknown. However,**

**using different methods for detection, published studies suggest between 5 and 51 percent of women experience rupture, an enormous range. A 1992 study by Destouet et al. analyzed the screening mammograms of 350 women with breast implants who had their implants for 1 to 27 years and had no symptoms. The study suggested that 5 percent of them had experienced "silent rupture" of their implants, although the mammogram readings were not confirmed by surgical removal of the implant. Robinson et al. studied 300 women who had their implants for 1 to 25 years and had their implants removed for a variety of reasons. They found visible signs of ruptures in 51 percent of the women. Severe silicone leakage -- silicone outside the implant without visible tears or holes -- was seen in another 20 percent. Robinson et al. also noted that the probability of rupture increases as the implant ages.**

**Mammograms do not necessarily detect ruptures. New information indicates that magnetic resonance imaging (MRI) may be used for evaluating patients with suspected rupture, deflation or leakage. Discuss this and other options with your doctor.**

**In addition to the length of time the implant has been in the body, the chance of rupture also increases with injury to the breast. Closed capsulotomy, a technique used to break capsular contracture by squeezing the breast, has been implicated as a possible cause of rupture.**

JT - The consequences of silicone gel implant rupture can vary widely depending on many factors. A key factor is whether the lining (capsule) surrounding the implant is intact. Provided another surgeon has not forcibly squeezed a hard breast to disrupt the capsule (a procedure called *closed capsulotomy*), I personally find it very *easy* to remove all visible gel from within the capsule and replace the implant. If the capsule and implant were broken while squeezing the breast to break a capsule, there is a greater risk of manually forcing silicone gel into adjacent tissues. When silicone gel remains in adjacent tissues, the body can form firm nodules (granulomas) around the gel.

Detecting a ruptured breast implant is similar in some ways to detecting breast cancer—there's no test that is 100 percent accurate. Even expensive MRI's are not totally accurate. The only sure way to know is to open the incision and take a look at the implant. Despite the nuisance and slight risks, it will answer the question—definitively. Not knowing is the worst solution. If you don't want to open it and take a look, just how worried are you? If you're really worried, perhaps the best solution is to remove and not replace your implants.

## FDA- OTHER KNOWN RISKS (FOR ALL BREAST IMPLANTS):

***FDA- Capsular contracture*** **is a tightening of scar tissue around the implant. It can sometimes cause pain, hardening of the breast, or changes in breast appearance. Although it seems to occur to some extent in most women with breast implants, there is no reliable data on how often this happens. If the changes are severe, more surgery may be needed to correct or remove the implants.**

JT - A capsule or tissue lining forms around every device implanted in the human body. Capsular contracture is not a medical complication—it's a normal body response to a foreign body—but there is too much of that response in some women! In most women, the capsule surrounds the implant but does not squeeze excessively on the implant, even if the capsule contracts a bit. Problems occur when the capsule contracts or tightens excessively, squeezing on the implant, making it feel hard, and sometimes pushing it out of position, distorting breast shape. The implant itself doesn't become hard. If you removed it from within the capsule, it is still soft. The breast *feels* hard because the capsule is squeezing on the implant. With current *saline* filled implants, the risk of capsular contracture is roughly 3-5 percent.

Our preferred correction of capsular contracture is to completely remove the existing capsule surgically and replace the implant. Most surgeons would suggest a textured surface implant, especially if replacing a silicone gel implant.

With respect to capsular contracture, we take a much stronger stand than many surgeons. Because we have no test to predict which patient will develop capsular contracture, and we don't know definitive causes or methods of predictably preventing it, we always worry about it. Fortunately, today's implant technology has substantially reduced the risks of capsular contracture. Most patients who develop capsular contracture will develop it in the first year following surgery, but a small percentage can develop it much later. My advice to patients today prior to surgery is this: "If you develop significant capsular contracture, we will go back to the operating room, remove as much of the capsule as possible, and replace your implant. If you develop a second capsule, I will recommend that you remove your implants and not replace them. I can't force you to do this, but your body is giving us a message—you are a capsule former. Since we don't know how to predictably prevent another capsule in patients who tend to form capsules, removing your implants reduces or removes all the risks, costs, and tradeoffs of additional operations in the future. If you're not willing to agree to this good team decision up front, I'd rather refer you to another surgeon."

While technology has made giant strides, a small percentage of patients will form capsules and continue forming capsules despite everything we know today. It's better to remove implants than repeatedly reoperate —I can't begin to tell you the number of problem cases that result from repeated reoperations. Patients almost never want to part with their implants, and surgeons try to please their patients. Sometimes bad team decisions result, and the consequences are rarely satisfactory. Repeated operations are one of the most common causes of severe problems.

***FDA- Calcium deposits*** **may form in surrounding tissue and may cause pain and hardening of the scar tissue. In some cases, these deposits may need to be surgically removed.**

JT - In my experience, this is a rare problem and usually occurs around silicone gel implants more than 10 years old. Most calcium deposits that I have seen are immediately adjacent to, or contained as part of, the capsule surrounding the implant. Most are very easily removed with the capsule. Calcium deposits can, however, form in any scar tissue anywhere in the body, so theoretically, they could certainly form in areas of the breast that have been treated surgically.

***FDA- Changes in nipple or breast sensation* may result from the surgery. These changes may be temporary or permanent. They may affect sexual response and the response of the nipple during breast feeding. A woman whose nipple is removed as part of her mastectomy will not have the ability to nurse.**

JT - What do we tell patients? "If you are like most patients, you will lose some sensation, and you will get some back. It's possible to lose all sensation, but this is exceedingly unusual. If you can't cope with that, don't have an augmentation. The larger the implant we use, the larger the pocket we have to make, the more nerves we have to cut or stretch, and the more sensation you're likely to lose." If you consider your breasts abnormal or unattractive before augmentation, that could also affect your sexual response.

***FDA- Interference with mammogram readings* can occur with breast implants. The presence of the implants requires a special mammography technique and increases the technical difficulty of taking and reading mammograms. This interference may delay or hinder the early detection of breast cancer by "hiding" suspicious lesions. Women with implants should always inform the radiologist and mammography technologists about the implants when scheduling the appointment for mammography and before mammography is performed. This is to make sure that the mammography technologists use the special technique for women with implants and that they take extra care when compressing the breasts to avoid rupturing the implant. Several factors affect the success of special mammography techniques in imaging the breast tissue in women with breast implants. The procedure involves pushing the implant back and gently pulling the breast tissue into view. Therefore, the location of the implant, the degree of capsular contracture, the size of the breast tissue compared to the implant and**

**other factors may affect how well the breast tissue can be imaged. Also, a radiologist may find it difficult to distinguish calcium deposits in the scar tissue around the implant from a breast tumor when he or she is interpreting the mammogram. Occasionally, it is necessary to remove and examine a small amount of tissue (biopsy) to see whether or not it is cancerous. This can frequently be done without removing the implant.**

JT - To my knowledge, there are no definitive scientific studies that prove that breast implants hinder the early detection of breast cancer by mammography. The FDA uses the word "may" in their statement. Many factors affect the accuracy of mammograms and the accuracy of breast cancer diagnosis. Breast implants are one of those factors, no doubt. If you are not willing to sacrifice some degree of mammogram accuracy, don't have a breast augmentation!

***FDA- Shifting of the implant:*** **Sometimes an implant may shift from its original position, giving the breasts an unnatural look and possibly causing pain and discomfort. An implant may become visible at the surface of the breast as a result of the device pushing through the layers of skin. Further surgery is needed to correct this problem. Placing the implant beneath the muscle may help to minimize this problem.**

**Other problems with appearance could include incorrect implant size, visible scars, uneven appearance, and wrinkling of the implant.**

JT - All of these things can happen. If an implant shifts from its original position AND causes pain and discomfort, the usual cause is capsular contracture. Implant "shifts" can also occur from skin stretch due to an excessively large implant under excessively thin tissues. Visible implant edges indicate inadequate soft tissue coverage over the implant, best prevented by measuring soft tissue thickness before surgery and making decisions on pocket location (over or under muscle) based on those measurements. An excessively large implant in a patient with thin tissues is a setup for implant visibility. The implant further stretches and thins already thin tissue, and the implant becomes visible. Once the problem of a visible implant occurs, it's exceedingly difficult to correct. Better to make the *right team* decisions before the first operation.

Incorrect implant size is a difficult issue that requires very careful, compulsive communication between you and your surgeon before your augmentation. A large percentage of augmentation patients, if questioned more than a year following surgery, state that they would like to be larger. Some surgeons, recognizing this predilection, rationalize, "Why not just make them bigger to begin with?" Decisions about breast size should be team decisions between patient and surgeon, based as much as possible on measurements that are quantifiable, not on subjective cup size. No method currently exists to precisely predict breast size. If you are not totally comfortable that your surgeon understands your "wants," don't proceed with augmentation. At the same time, be sure that you are honest with yourself and your surgeon about your true desires. Always remember: The larger the implant, the worse the result and the higher the risks long-term as ageing occurs.

Visible scars, unequal appearance, and wrinkling and rippling are subjects that are addressed in detail in other chapters. Reiterating a few key principles: All scars are visible to some degree, especially if they are on you. No one can predict the quality of a scar. If you have a beautiful breast, it's unlikely anyone will look at the scar. All breasts are unequal. No woman has two breasts that are the same, and no surgeon can create two breasts that are the same. Don't expect it. Wrinkling and rippling are most often due to either an underfilled implant or an excessively large implant in a patient with thin tissues.

## DEALING WITH PROBLEMS

**The best way to deal with a problem is to deal with it—NOW!**

All patients and all surgeons hate problems. But when they occur, it's best to deal with them, and the sooner the better. Often it's a good idea to get another opinion to make everyone more comfortable and assemble as much brainpower and experience as possible.

**There isn't a surgeon alive who wants an unhappy patient. Keep your lines of communication open!**

**No surgeon can solve a problem unless the surgeon is aware that a problem exists! Most of the best surgeons will encourage you to seek another opinion — don't hesitate to ask!**

Try to keep the team together. Honesty is important. Communicate with your surgeon. Confront the problem, discuss the alternatives, get other opinions if necessary, and then make joint decisions. If, for any reason, you aren't comfortable with your surgeon or vice versa, try to stay friends and seek additional help. You'll almost always benefit from a non-adversarial approach. I haven't seen many lawyers solve complicated medical problems!

One principle is worth repeating: If you have any problem twice, or if you have the same problem twice, remove your implants or don't complain later. If problems occur, seek additional information or other medical opinions, and use common sense!

***You are partially responsible for what happens to you.***

**If problems occur, remember there are worse things than removing and not replacing implants!**

## THE NEXT STEP...

By now, you've digested a lot of information. You're informed about implants, different surgical options, and potential problems. The last step before consulting a surgeon is learning about recovery and the factors that affect recovery, so you can ask the right questions and make the right decisions.

[CHAPTER EIGHT]

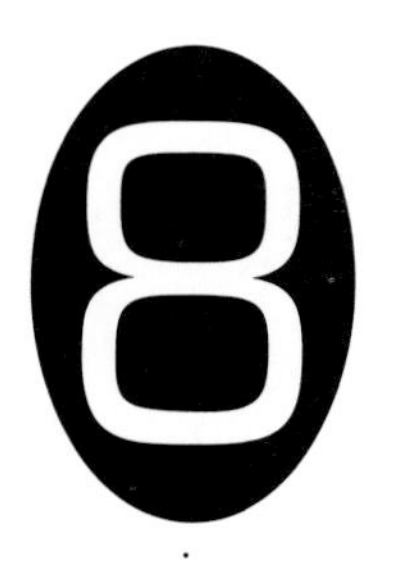

# RECOVERY: Learn About It Before Surgery!

***"Learning about your recovery can tell you a lot about a surgeon. A more skilled surgeon usually offers you a simpler and faster recovery."***

Learn about recovery *before surgery*? You must be kidding! Why not just worry about that when the time comes? Because...

**Learning about recovery can tell you a lot about your augmentation operation—before you have it!**

**Your experiences during recovery are a direct consequence of what happens during your surgery.**

***The less traumatic your surgical procedure, the easier and faster your recovery.***

**You won't see what your surgeon will do in the operating room, but you can gain insight by asking about your recovery.**

Would you like to have an easier and faster recovery? Would you prefer less time away from your normal activities? Less time off work? Less bruising? No drain tubes coming out of your body? No tight bandages or special bras? All of these things are possible, but only if you choose the right surgeon! In fact, all of these are routine in some augmentation practices. But not in all augmentation practices! The only way you'll know is to ***ask about recovery before your augmentation!***

## WHAT'S TO RECOVER FROM?

### Tissue Trauma

Any operation causes some degree of injury (trauma) to your tissues. The more precise and delicate the surgery, the less trauma, but *some tissue trauma is unavoidable.* Your body responds to tissue trauma in predictable ways — pain, swelling, bruising, and stiffness after surgery.

**The greater the amount of trauma to your tissues, the more discomfort and other symptoms you'll have after surgery.**

**The greater the trauma, the longer it takes your body to heal and the longer it takes for you to feel normal and return to normal activities.**

To put an implant in your breast, the surgeon creates a pocket to receive the implant. The pocket can be behind breast tissue (retromammary), or behind breast tissue and behind muscle (partial retropectoral). If it's just behind breast tissue, the surgeon lifts the breast tissue off the pectoralis muscle to create the pocket. If you are thin and need more soft tissue coverage, you need additional muscle cover over the implant, and the surgeon needs to lift the pectoralis muscle and create a pocket behind the muscle. When muscle is manipulated, you can expect more discomfort, swelling, and a longer recovery. How much longer? It depends on your tissues, and it depends on how the pocket is created at surgery.

**Recovering from a pocket created behind breast tissue is easier than recovering from a pocket created behind muscle.**

*Why? There is less tissue trauma.*

**If you are thin and need muscle cover (or need it for other reasons), it is more important to have muscle cover than to avoid slightly more tissue trauma.**

*You and your surgeon must decide based on your tissues.*

**The more tissue trauma caused by your surgery, the longer and more difficult your recovery.**

**Ask about recovery and compare what surgeons tell you! Longer recovery times usually imply more tissue trauma at surgery.**

## Tissue Stretch — Another Form of Tissue Trauma

Your implant will stretch your tissues and also stretch nerves in and around your breast. The larger the implant, or the tighter your tissues, the more pressure the implant exerts on your tissues. This pressure subsides over time (weeks to months) as your tissues stretch to accommodate your implant. But pressure of an implant (especially a larger implant in tighter tissues) can produce more discomfort, more stretch on nerves in the breast, and more temporary or permanent loss of sensation. The message? Some tissue stretch injury is unavoidable, but

**Excessively large implants in excessively tight tissues can produce excessive stretch trauma that can cause more discomfort and temporary or permanent sensory loss.**

*Consider your tissues when selecting implant size.*

Tissue stretch can produce temporary numbness, tingling, pin prick sensations, and other weird feelings during the first few weeks of recovery. These sensations are a normal part of recovery. Sensation varies tremendously from patient to patient and is not predictable. If you select a large implant that stresses your tissues excessively, expect more sensory loss, and a longer time for sensation to return to near normal.

### Bruising and Swelling — What Causes It?

**Bruising is bleeding within your tissues.**

**Bruising and swelling are caused by tissue trauma.**

**The more tissue trauma, the more bruising and swelling.**

**The more bruising and swelling, the longer your recovery.**

**The more bruising and swelling, the longer before you'll return to normal activities.**

**You can judge a lot about your upcoming surgery by asking:**
***"Will I have bruising? For how long? What about swelling? When can I return to normal activities?"***

## TISSUE TRAUMA AND SURGICAL TECHNIQUE

In Chapter 6, you learned about different surgical techniques, different methods that surgeons use to create the pockets for your implants. The technique a surgeon uses to create the pocket can significantly affect how much tissue injury occurs, and, hence, can significantly affect your recovery.

**BLUNT DISSECTION techniques cause SUBSTANTIALLY MORE TRAUMA compared to electrocautery dissection techniques.**

**Sharp dissection techniques cause substantially more bleeding compared to electrocautery techniques.**

**Ask your surgeon specifically what technique will be used to create the pockets for your implants. If it's not electrocautery dissection, expect more bruising, swelling, and a longer recovery time.**

## TUBES COMING OUT OF YOUR BODY

No matter how tiny a tube, when you see it coming out through a puncture in your skin, it looks the size of a fire hose. You won't like it. You'll be told that it's necessary to remove fluid from around your implant, and that if you don't have it, your chances of collecting blood (hematoma), fluid (seroma), and chances of capsular contracture are increased. True? Not necessarily.

It is true that *if* substantial bleeding and tissue injury occur at the time of surgery, you body will release more blood and fluid into the pocket around the implant, and that it's better to remove the fluid with a drain than to leave it there. But *it's also true that*:

**In first-time augmentations (as opposed to reoperation cases), techniques exist that make drain tubes unnecessary in the vast majority of patients.**

Ask if you'll need drains. If the answer is yes, does that mean that the surgeon isn't good or isn't doing a good job? No. Does it mean that the surgeon is doing something wrong? No. You should consider many factors in choosing a surgeon, but this is one of those factors. Why does the surgeon need drains when other surgeons don't? Get answers from different surgeons, and then you decide.

## ANESTHESIA AND RECOVERY TIME

It's nice to have anesthesia when you're having surgery! Having anesthesia means that you will receive drugs. The longer the operation, the longer the anesthesia, and the more drugs you'll receive. When the drugs are discontinued following surgery, your body must break down (metabolize) the drugs before you will feel normal. Anesthetic drugs often cause some hangover. Hangover can be good—if it eases your discomfort immediately after surgery. But once you're feeling better, hangover that lasts longer is a nuisance because you don't feel normal as quickly.

Some people are prone to develop nausea following anesthesia. Even the best anti-nausea drugs don't totally prevent nausea in some patients. However, the fewer narcotic drugs you get, the less chance of your developing nausea. The shorter the anesthesia and the less tissue trauma during surgery, the less narcotic drugs you'll need.

**The longer your anesthesia and the more tissue trauma, the more drugs you'll need, the longer you'll be required to remain at the surgery facility, and the longer time before you'll feel normal.**

**Ask about surgery time, anesthesia time, time in the recovery room, and how long until you'll return home the day of surgery.**

*All of these factors will tell you a lot about how much anesthesia you'll receive and when you can expect to feel normal.*

**The shorter your surgery and the less tissue trauma, the fewer drugs you'll need, the less chance of nausea and hangover, and the more rapidly you'll return to normal.**

*I know I'm repeating, but I want to be sure you've got the picture!*

## General Anesthesia Versus Local Anesthesia With Sedation — What's Best?

**When considering anesthesia, what's BEST is what is SAFEST and allows your surgeon the greatest degree of CONTROL during your operation.**

Many people don't love the idea of being "put to sleep." It just has a bad ring to it! Everyone has heard about disasters that have occurred with anesthesia. All the disasters are reported, but you never hear about the hundreds of thousands of anesthetics daily that go without a hitch! So it's normal to think: The less anesthesia the better. If I can have this surgery without being "put to sleep," that's better. Right? **Wrong!**

When problems occur with anesthesia, most fall into two general categories:

1) You have a totally unpredictable reaction to a routine anesthetic drug (an idiosyncratic drug reaction), or
2) You regurgitate while you are asleep or heavily sedated, and instead of hurling the material out of your mouth, you suck stomach acid down your windpipe into your lungs. Your lungs react violently, and reflexes usually cause your heart to react by developing abnormal heart rhythms — a very bad combination.

Both of these potentially dangerous events are exceedingly rare, but they can occur. The first, an idiosyncratic drug reaction, cannot be predicted or totally prevented. If it occurs, it's treatable. The second event (aspiration), however, is *almost totally preventable* by inserting a small tube with a balloon into your windpipe after you're asleep. When the balloon is inflated, you can regurgitate all you want. The stomach acid can't get past the balloon and down your windpipe! The only price you pay is that your throat may be a little raspy from the tube for several hours after surgery.

The problem is, you won't enjoy having an endotracheal tube (the tube with a balloon in your windpipe) unless you're asleep. If you have *local* anesthesia, you are not asleep. Even more drugs along with the local anesthesia will heavily sedate you, but technically you're still not asleep. Mainly, you're not asleep enough to tolerate an endotracheal tube. If you have local anesthesia injected, it deadens the tissues, but you'll need additional drugs to stay comfortable. If you get uncomfortable during surgery, your surgeon may need to stop while anesthesia gives you more drugs. That slows things down. Remember, longer anesthesia, more drugs, and more nausea result in a longer recovery! Does local anesthesia work? Usually, but those additional drugs that keep you comfortable can also interfere with your gag reflexes. If you regurgitate, you may be too sedated to gag and hurl, and the stomach acid can go down your windpipe because you don't have an endotracheal tube in place.

**Local anesthesia with sedation (you're not asleep) usually does not allow you to have an endotracheal tube to protect you from aspiration.**

**General anesthesia (you are asleep) with an endotracheal tube in place better protects you against aspiration.**

**General anesthsia is more predictable at keeping you asleep and comfortable, you are less likely to remember events of your surgery, and your surgeon has more control.**

Some surgery facilities are not equipped to administer general anesthesia. You certainly don't want to have any anesthesia unless a facility and its personnel are equipped and optimally trained. Before surgery, ask your surgeon the following:

**What type of anesthesia will I have?**

**Which is safer, local or general?**

**Which offers better control, local or general?**

*Under local anesthesia with sedation, how am I protected against aspiration?*

**Can you offer me both options and let me choose?**

### Popular Misconceptions About Anesthesia, and the Facts

A popular misconception that general anesthesia causes more nausea than local anesthesia is not necessarily true. Nausea relates more to the *type and quantity* of drugs you're given, and *how* they are given. Some medical personnel administer anesthesia better than others. Ask your surgeon who will be giving the anesthesia. Is this someone the surgeon works with regularly? How regularly?

A second misconception is that general anesthesia requires giving you more drugs than local anesthesia. Again, not necessarily true. By having you asleep and your surgeon having optimal control, your surgery can proceed more smoothly in a shorter time. General anesthesia can require *fewer drugs* because of *more control* and a *shorter surgery time*. Again, it depends on who is doing it and how they do it!

A third misconception is that it takes longer to recover from general anesthesia. Again, not true. Recovery depends on the amount of drugs you received during and after surgery. The longer the operation, the more drugs you'll receive. Well-done general anesthesia involves a shorter recovery than many local anesthesia with sedation cases. If a surgeon does not have access to top-notch general anesthesia, local with sedation can be a better option.

You have a choice of surgeons and a choice of surgical facilities. No surgeon or facility can offer you risk-free anesthesia. It doesn't exist. But one of the major risks (aspiration) is almost totally preventable with general anesthesia. It's up to you to ask the right questions and make the best team decisions.

## BANDAGES, BINDERS, AND SPECIAL BRAS

Another aspect of recovery that can tell you a lot about your surgery is the use of special bandages, binders, and special bras.

**Devices don't produce optimal results. Optimal surgery produces optimal results.**

**The more you rely on external devices to produce a result, the less predictable the result.**

**The biggest problem with devices is that you have to use and tolerate them.**

**How much do you like wearing things that are tight, uncomfortable, or a nuisance?**

**What do you often do with things you don't enjoy wearing? Take them off!**

**So when a surgeon depends on a device that you can wear or not wear, the result is not as predictable.**

Does that mean that all external devices are a bad deal? Not necessarily. If a surgeon feels that a device is necessary after surgery, the surgeon usually has a reason. Ask for the reason. If other surgeons don't feel a device is necessary, ask why not!

## Bandages

Survey several surgeons, and you'll find that bandages vary from none to mummy-like, near-total body wraps! Why? Often because a surgeon was trained to use a certain type of bandage for augmentation and has used it ever since! During my residency training, I was taught that it was necessary to firmly wrap every augmentation patient with an elastic bandage that covered everything from the neck to the waist. The reason given was that the elastic wrap would put pressure on the breasts to reduce risks of bleeding and provide support to keep the patient comfortable. Sounded logical to me, so I did it. Patients tolerated it for a couple of days because they thought it was necessary. But when I asked them how it felt, they all said, "Horrible. It's tight, rolls up, is hot, itches, and I can't take a bath and wash my hair!" My patients have taught me that they would much rather be able to bathe and wash their hair.

Bandages to stop bleeding? Why not just do the surgery in a way that you don't have bleeding in the first place? How you do the operation is what determines the amount of bleeding! Not a bandage, not a wrap, not anything else! So I improved the way I do the operation and did away with bandages completely. No bandages on any patient for the past 10 years! Any bleeding?

One case out of more than 1,000 augmentations! Bleeding can occur after surgery — no matter what technique is used. But...

**Bandages don't prevent bleeding as well as specific surgical techniques do.**

**Bandages are a nuisance that prevent you from showering and washing your hair.**

**Bandages are largely unnecessary, provided certain surgical techniques are used.**

Bandages to improve patient comfort? Ever been wrapped in an elastic bandage for a couple of days? Ever had adhesive tape pulled off? Ever been unable to bathe or wash your hair for a day or two? In some operations, bandages are necessary. Following augmentation, they are not, provided specific surgical techniques are used.

### Binder Devices, Straps

Quite an array of binder devices exist, mostly touted as essential aids to keep an implant in place or to push it somewhere — upward, downward, inward, outward. Surgeons utilize these devices in a variety of ways for a variety of reasons, usually due to a bad experience with implants "going" somewhere that neither the surgeon nor the patient likes.

Implants largely "go" where implants are put at surgery. If the pocket to receive the implant is substantially larger than the implant, the implant can move. When implants are put "under the muscle," you'll hear from some surgeons and patients that the implants "tend to ride up." Behold, an opportunity for a device, some type of strap or binder across the upper breast to "hold" them down.

The reason implants tend to "ride up" is usually due to one of three causes:

1) Excessive tissue forces are pushing on the lower implant,

2) The implant was positioned too high at surgery, or
3) The implant chosen was too large for the patient's tissues.

The most common reason for excessive tissue pressure on the lower implant is that the implant is too large for the patient's tissues. When too much implant is placed into too tight a pocket, the pocket pushes back, especially in the lower breast, and the implant is pushed upward. Under muscle, the pocket tends to be even tighter, especially if specific techniques aren't used to release pressure of the lower muscle on the implant. If you're thinking about a larger implant and have tight tissues, a binder or strap may make some sense, but...

**Specific surgical techniques — accurate, precise pocket development and control — are more effective than binder devices at controlling implant position.**

**When you and your surgeon select an implant that is excessively large for your tissue characteristics, the risk of implant displacement increases.**

How long are you willing to wear a binder device? What happens when you take it off? An excessively large implant exerts excessive pressure forever? Want to wear a binder device forever?

## Special Bras

Some women love them; other women hate them! Some need them; some don't. If you ask women about bras following their augmentation, I promise you'll hear answers all over the map! Some will say you absolutely must wear a bra, even a certain type. Others will say no; it's not necessary. Surgical garment companies love bras and support garments because they boost the bottom line! But every different manufacturer will tell you that its design is better, for several reasons. How many bras do you need? It depends on whom you ask. The companies will tell you several. You'll probably enjoy at least two, so you can wash one while using the other. The real bottom line?

**If a bra or a certain type of bra were best, everyone would be using it.**

*It just isn't so.*

**If special bras were really necessary at all, patients wouldn't do well without them.**

*And believe me, a lot of patients do great without them every day!*

**If you or your surgeon feel that you need them or like them, use them.**

*Just don't fool yourself into thinking they're really necessary from a medical standpoint, provided you apply certain surgical techniques.*

Some surgeons feel that a bra "holds the implant in place." My question is, "Why do you need to hold the implant in place?" If the pocket is created accurately in the right location, the pocket holds the implant in place! Other surgeons feel that the pressure of a bra decreases chances of bleeding and makes patients more comfortable. I can't envision depending on a bra to prevent bleeding. Bleeding is prevented at surgery! And comfort? Just ask several women, and you'll get several answers. Some are more comfortable with a bra, and some without. It's a personal preference.

What do we tell our patients? "You'll go home with a single piece of tape over your incision. In the first few weeks after surgery, you can wear or not wear a bra. It's your choice. Wearing or not wearing a bra won't affect your final result at all! If you're more comfortable wearing a bra, or if you want to create a certain look, go for it, the sooner the better. It's not necessary to worry about a bra harming your incision, even if it's an underwire bra and your incision is under your breast! On the other hand, if you're more comfortable not wearing a bra, don't wear one. You don't need it, especially in the first few weeks after surgery."

You need a bra, however, when you are engaging in *any activity that causes your breasts to bounce,* such as running, jogging, aerobics (even low-impact aerobics), horseback riding, etc. Why? Gravity alone, even with a bra, pulls breasts downward! Add the force of bouncing, and the migration will definitely start sooner! No way around it! If they're bouncing, they're sagging sooner — and more! What type of bra will prevent this? Any tight bra that prevents bouncing. Sometimes two jog bras, one size too small! Whatever it takes, stop the bouncing! This rule applies from now on if you want to minimize tissue stretch and potential sagging!

## RECOVERY TIMES AND LIMITATIONS

What is normal for recovery times? Which limitations are mandatory, and which are optional? Do all patients respond the same? What is a normal time to return to normal activities? To athletic activities? What does all this tell you about your upcoming surgery?

**The shorter and easier a surgeon describes your recovery time, the less trauma that surgeon is causing to your tissues.**

### Patient Variations

All patients don't respond the same after surgery. Some have a higher tolerance for discomfort than others. Some don't have any tolerance at all — for any discomfort. Some follow instructions better than others. Some remember what they've learned better than others. Most are impatient for things to get back to normal, regardless of how many times they've been told that tissue healing takes time.

If you have a very low tolerance for discomfort, you will have a more difficult recovery. You're likely to request more pain medications and use them more frequently and longer. Pain medications make you sleepy while they make you comfortable, and you won't get moving as well. Most of all, it's easier to take pain medications than to work through discomfort. All of these factors tend to lengthen your recovery.

**Pain medications are a very mixed blessing — the less the better, and the sooner you're off them, the better.**

But despite patient variations, you can bank on the following:

**The MORE YOU KNOW what to expect, the EASIER YOUR RECOVERY.**

**The *less we traumatize you*, the *faster and easier your recovery*.**

**The BETTER YOU FOLLOW INSTRUCTIONS, the EASIER AND LESS COMPLICATED your recovery.**

**The *higher your discomfort tolerance*, the *more rapid your recovery*.**

**The more RAPIDLY YOU RESUME NORMAL ACTIVITIES, the SHORTER YOUR RECOVERY.**

### Normal Activities

For the sake of discussion, let's define normal activities as:

1) Lifting your arms above your head,
2) Lifting normal weight objects,
3) Driving your car, and
4) Carrying out all normal (non-athletic) daily activities.

Before your surgery, specifically ask when you can begin each of these activities. From the answers, you'll learn a lot about your upcoming surgery.

**If you can't return to these normal activities within two weeks, something's not ideal.**

*Tissue injury, low pain tolerance, too many pain medications, a complication — something!*

**If you can return to all normal activities in less than one week, you've probably made good choices of surgeon and techniques.**

**If you can return to all normal activities in less than four days, you and your surgeon are both DYNAMITE!**

*It occurs routinely, in over 90 percent of our patients, even when placing the implant submuscular!*

**If you're told that expecting to return to normal activities in less than four days is unreasonable and just won't happen, you might want to continue your surgeon search!**

### One of Our Typical Patients Describes Her Recovery...

The following letter was written by one of our patients to thank someone for providing information about us. It is reprinted with the patient's permission.

*Jean:*

*Here is a brief synopsis of my BA experience with Dr. Tebbetts. He was Fantastic.*

*I flew in from the Midwest, and arrived on a Thursday. I had my consultation with him that Thursday afternoon. I stayed with a friend of mine in Dallas, so we went out that evening, had dinner, and went home. The next morning, I went in at 7:45 for surgery. Even the waiting experience was pleasant. I waited in a comfortable recliner while I was being prepped for my surgery. I remember waking up immediately after surgery, and Dr. Tebbetts asked me to see if I could raise my arms above my head. I did it with no problem. That afternoon I went to the place where I was staying, with my friend, and I rested most of the day. However, I could change my own clothes (over my head) and do many other things with no problem. I took my prescribed medication that evening only. The next day (24 hours post-op) I took Advil, and never took anything else beyond that. I showered, blow-dried my hair, went shopping, got dressed, all at 24 hours post-op. I remember that evening, I made myself a sandwich and had no problem reaching the bread, which was in a cabinet, well above my head. When I flew home (48 hours post-op), my children were not feeling well, and I was able to squat down and pick up my 20 lb son with no problem. I'm now 4 days post-op and I have been sleeping on my side for the last two evenings. I must say that if I had to repeat this experience, I wouldn't change a thing. Dr. Tebbetts and his staff were very helpful, and professional. I am extremely pleased with my choice. As for the look, the partial-submuscular, anatomical implants I received look great now, but I think that they will look even better when they drop in a few months. That's about it. Let me know if I can answer any other questions for you. Thanks again for helping me find Dr. Tebbetts!*

*Margaret*

*(names are fictitious to protect patient privacy)*

This letter describes a typical experience for the vast majority of our patients. Because there is a normal variation in patients' tolerance to discomfort and their ability to follow our postoperative instructions, we can't guarantee this experience for every patient. But our commitment to patient education and the surgical techniques that we use in every case offer this type of experience to every augmentation patient.

## Athletic Activities and Emotional Stress

Athletic activities and emotional stress increase your pulse rate. When your pulse rate rises, your blood pressure rises. A rise in blood pressure can cause internal bleeding in your breasts. Internal bleeding means another operation, tubes coming out of your body for a while, and a higher risk of capsular contracture. ***It just isn't worth it!***

Athletic activities include any activity that causes your pulse rate to increase significantly (more than 20 percent above your resting pulse rate) — running, fast walking, bicycling, aerobics of any kind, heavy or prolonged exercise of any sort.

Emotional stresses vary a lot, but the most likely involve personal relationships or severe job stresses. Believe it or not, these stresses can cause just as much pulse and blood pressure increase as athletic activities. Again, it's not worth it! Avoid emotional stress as much as possible.

**Avoid athletic activities of any sort and severe emotional stress for at least two weeks following surgery.**

**You should be able to start a gradual return to normal exercise activities beginning two weeks after surgery.**

*If it hurts, stop it and try again two days later! Your body is smarter than you! Listen to it!*

**If you aren't allowed to begin returning to athletic activities in less than four weeks, ask questions!**

*Why not? What's going to happen? Ask other surgeons!*

## RECOVERY QUESTIONS ... AND THE MESSAGE FROM THE ANSWERS

Before your surgery, ask questions about your recovery:

***What will my recovery be like?***

***Will I have bruising?***

***Will I have drain tubes coming out of my body?***

***When can I return to normal activities, drive my car, lift normal objects, raise my arms above my head, etc.?***

***When can I bathe?***

***Do I need special bandages, bras, or binders?***

***When can I return to athletic activities?***

**THE BETTER THE ANSWERS TO these questions, THE BETTER YOU'LL LIKE YOUR RECOVERY and, likely, your result!**

## GET SURGEONS TO COMMIT

If you get hedged answers to any of these questions from surgeons, persist. Ask the questions again. Ask for pinpoint answers. No surgeon can give absolute guarantees in any single case, but answers to these questions provide you with valuable information about what you can expect.

This subject isn't nuclear physics. Part of recovery is you, and part is your surgeon. What your surgeon does in the operating room can substantially affect your recovery. You can't see what the surgeon does in the operating room, but you can gain insight before surgery by asking about your recovery. Either way, once you choose your surgeon, the rest of recovery is up to you. ***Your job will be easier if you make the right choice of a surgeon.***

## THE NEXT STEP ...

You've now done a major portion of your homework — *learning information* about every aspect of augmentation so that you'll have *knowledge tools* when you begin to consult surgeons. In the next chapters, we'll locate qualified surgeons and help you with the steps in consultation and decision making.

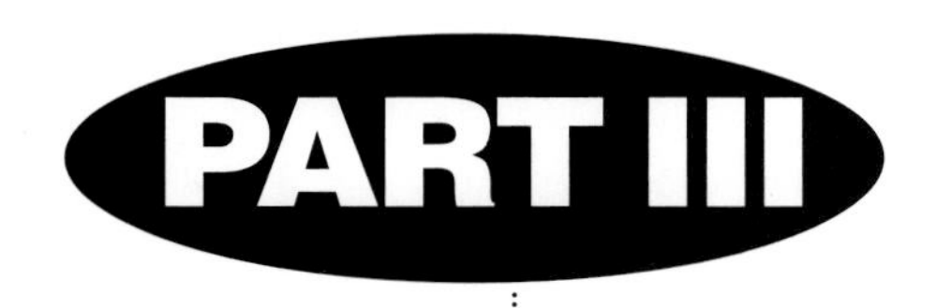

# USING YOUR INFORMATION: Consulting Surgeons And Making Decisions

[CHAPTER NINE]

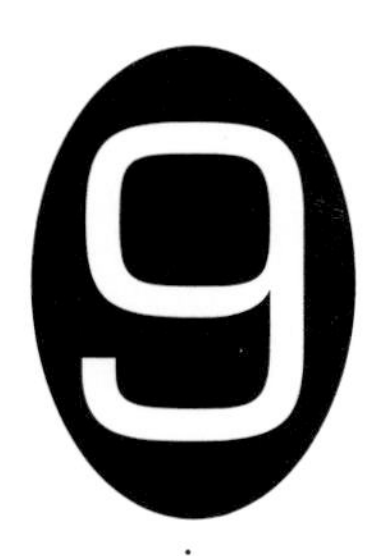

# FINDING QUALIFIED SURGEONS:

## Who Do I Call and Where Do I Go?

***"All surgeons are not equally qualified. Board certification is an essental criterion, but even board certified surgeons vary widely in qualifications and skills."***

The Yellow Pages are not the best resource! The only thing you'll really learn is which surgeons advertise there! You can definitely get names of surgeons from the Yellow Pages, but you'll learn very little about their credentials. A surgeon's basic credentials can tell you a lot, if you know what to look for!

Where did the surgeon train? How long? Is the surgeon board certified? By whom? What does board certification mean? What are the surgeon's other important credentials? Which credentials are important, and which are not? What are some important red flags? All of these questions involve surgeon credentials. Before you ever call a surgeon's office, you should check out the surgeon's basic credentials. Otherwise, you are more likely to waste valuable time and money or, worse yet, make poor decisions. Here are some things you need to know to check out a surgeon's credentials.

## A SITUATION YOU'LL FIND DIFFICULT TO BELIEVE...

**In most states in the United States, ANY PHYSICIAN who has completed four years of medical school and obtained an M.D. degree can LEGALLY ADVERTISE AS A PLASTIC SURGEON, or a neurosurgeon (brain surgeon), or any other type of surgeon — WITHOUT HAVING OBTAINED A SINGLE DAY OF SPECIALTY TRAINING!**

**Any physician can call himself or herself a plastic surgeon! LEGALLY!**

**Any licensed physician can advertise as a plastic surgeon without a day of specialty training in plastic surgery!**

**Any licensed physician can operate on you if you let them! LEGALLY!**

Can't happen, you say? It happens every day. Patients see an ad or hear a name, go to a surgeon, and submit to a procedure that changes their bodies forever! They do this without ever investigating the surgeon's credentials, without ever seeing more than one surgeon, without ever learning about the operation they're considering!

When a less-than-optimal outcome occurs (and "less than optimal" covers everything from not so good to complete disasters), unbelievably, many patients allow the same surgeon to operate on them repeatedly—often without ever seeking another opinion or researching the surgeon's credentials! After the downhill slide (things often get worse with each reoperation), ultimately something or someone must get the blame. Incredibly, it's usually the breast implant or the last surgeon who operated, trying to correct the problems! I've seen literally hundreds of such cases in my 20 years of practice. *Rarely have I seen a patient take responsibility for her lack of homework in selecting a surgeon!*

**Many patients spend more time shopping for a car than they spend selecting a plastic surgeon.**

**It's your body... you'll be looking at it for the *REST OF YOUR LIFE.***

***It's your job to select your surgeon.* Don't complain later if you neglect your responsibilities.**

**Selecting your surgeon is the SINGLE MOST IMPORTANT THING you can do to assure an optimal result!**

So how do you go about it? The first step is to understand how a plastic surgeon is educated and what various credentials really mean. What is board certification? What does it mean? Board certified by whom? Some credentials are meaningful; many are less meaningful. Once you understand basic credentials, you can assemble a list of surgeons who have meaningful credentials. Then you'll need to shorten the list by looking past board certification to other useful information. After you shorten your list, you can begin calling surgeons' offices and requesting information. Your final decision and surgeon selection should be a combination of 1) credentials, 2) quality of information you receive (written and spoken), and 3) your experiences during your consultations. This chapter will introduce you to surgeon credentials and other useful tools to help you begin your search for a surgeon.

## EDUCATING A PLASTIC SURGEON

After four years of college, most physicians (M.D.'s) complete four years of *medical school,* learning the basics of medicine. After medical school, most physicians who plan to specialize in a certain area then begin *residency training.* The length of residency training varies with the specialty. Plastic surgery and neurosurgery are among the longest residencies requiring *an additional six to eight years after medical school.* Many board certified plastic surgeons complete a 5-year general surgery residency, then complete an additional two to three years of plastic surgery training. Nevertheless, most plastic surgeons board certified by the American Board of Plastic Surgery have completed six to eight years of additional specialty surgical training after medical school!

**Most plastic surgeons who are certified by the American Board of Plastic Surgery have completed six to eight years of specialty surgical residency training after medical school.**

But remember! It is perfectly legal for a physician to set up a plastic surgery practice after four years of medical school without a single day of residency training in plastic surgery! Plastic surgery is an attractive specialty, and some physicians will shortcut the educational system any way possible! If a physician just skipped plastic surgery training (or some portion of it), the physician could begin doing plastic surgery six to eight years sooner—and could retire six to eight years sooner! It may be a great deal for the physician who may not even be aware of what he or she doesn't know, but it may not be a great deal for patients! Would you take your car for repair to a mechanic that you knew started yesterday with no mechanic school or experience?

General practitioners perform plastic surgery. Dermatologists perform plastic surgery. Gynecologists perform plastic surgery! Ear, nose and throat physicians (otolaryngologists) perform plastic surgery! Dentists perform plastic surgery! General surgeons perform plastic surgery! And the list goes on. Every specialty listed above has residency training, but none are as long or as comprehensive as plastic surgery residency! None focus on plastic surgery as much as a plastic surgery residency! Does that mean that none of these other specialists can do good plastic surgery? Not necessarily. But it's your job to decide how much training and experience you want your surgeon to have!

The following is my own perspective about surgical training. Many physicians who have completed medical school, with the help of a good book in the operating room (and some actually do this), can probably carry off a basic operation. If a physician has seen an operation performed several times or attended an instructional course of one or two days, so much the better. But neither compares with *six to eight years* of specialty training. Here's what I think:

**A little plastic surgical training may be adequate for a basic operation when the patient expects only a basic result.**

*Do you really want only a basic result?*

**You don't need in-depth surgical training until you need it!**

*A plastic surgeon with years of training has been there, seen that, done that, and, above all, doesn't panic when problems occur.*

**In surgery, the more you've seen, the more you know, and the better you deal with complex problems**

*You don't see much in a weekend course or minimal residency training.*

**They don't put student pilots in the seat of the space shuttle for a reason. Training, training, training, experience, experience, experience. I can't imagine having too much!**

*If you're on the shuttle and it crashes, you don't have to worry about it! If lack of training and experience cause a problem with your plastic surgery, you'll get to look at it every day for the rest of your life!*

**Ask every surgeon specifically: How many years of residency training did you complete? In what specialty? In what location?**

*Then check it out. Call the residency program and ask if the physician completed the program!*

## BOARD CERTIFICATION — WHAT DOES IT MEAN?

Board certification can mean a lot, or it can mean nothing. A "board" can be nothing more than an individual or organization that will issue a certificate to anyone who pays a fee! Means absolutely nothing! Many different "boards" exist, but you need to sort out which mean something and which don't!

**The key question to ask about board certification? Board certified *by whom*? By which board?**

The American Medical Association's Board of Medical Specialties (ABMS) determines which "boards" are recognized as the most qualified boards to certify medical specialists in a specific specialty including plastic surgery. You can access in-depth information about the ABMS at **www.abms.org** on the Internet.

Currently, the AMA Board of Medical Specialties recognizes only one board to certify plastic surgeons — **The American Board of Plastic Surgery (ABPS).**

At the present time, the American Board of Plastic Surgery has the most stringent requirements for board certification in plastic surgery of any organization that certifies plastic surgeons. Other "boards" exist, but, to my knowledge, none requires as much residency training, surgical experience and rigorous examinations as the American Board of Plastic Surgery. Details of the requirements for certification can be found on the ABPS web site at **www.abplsurg.org** on the Internet.

## How can I locate a plastic surgeon certified by the American Board of Plastic Surgery?

Plastic surgeons certified by the American Board of Plastic Surgery are listed in the Official ABMS Directory of Board Certified Medical Specialists published by Marquis Who's Who in cooperation with the American Board of Medical Specialties (ABMS). Instead of purchasing this $485 set of books, it's easier and cheaper to look up plastic surgeons in your area that are board certified by the American Board of Plastic Surgery on the following web sites or at the following numbers:

**The American Society of Plastic and Reconstructive Surgeons** at: **www.plasticsurgery.org/findsurg/finding.htm**, or call at **1-800-635-0635.**

**American Society of Aesthetic Plastic Surgery** at **www.surgery.org/enhanced** or call **1-888-272-7711.**

When you choose a surgeon who is a member of either of these organizations, the surgeon is certified by the American Board of Plastic Surgery. This means that the surgeon has graduated from an accredited medical school and completed at least five years of additional residency, usually three years of general surgery (or its equivalent) and two years of plastic surgery (many have completed 6-8 years of residency training). To be certified by the ABPS, a doctor must also practice plastic surgery for two years and pass comprehensive written and oral exams.

## AFTER BOARD CERTIFICATION, THEN WHAT?

**Board certification is not the only thing you should consider when selecting a surgeon.**

### Is board certification enough? What about experience?

Does board certification (even by the ABPS) guarantee you an expert in breast augmentation? Not necessarily. Board certified plastic surgeons do a wide variety of procedures. Some focus on reconstructive surgery, some on cosmetic surgery, and others combine both in their practices. We mentioned earlier that experience is important, but there's no specific amount of experience that guarantees a good surgeon or a good result. A lot has to do with the personality of the surgeon, and you'll need to judge that during your consultation. In Chapter 11, we'll give you more specific questions to ask your surgeon about experience.

What percentage of your practice is breast augmentation? How many augmentations do you average per year? Based on what you've already learned about surgical options in Chapter 6, you'll be able to quickly determine how much experience a surgeon has with different augmentation options.

### Subspecialization and the Surgeon's Curriculum Vitae

Some surgeons who perform only cosmetic surgery further specialize in specific types of cosmetic surgery. They will usually have more experience because that's what they do every day! They may have other credentials. Ask to see a copy of their curriculum vitae. It will list the surgeon's training in detail and all professional activities the surgeon has completed. Check out how many professional presentations the surgeon has given, courses taught to other surgeons, and professional papers published. Ask if they have a web site, and check it out for *content* (almost all have a lot of fluff).

## Hospital Privileges

Another important way to assess a surgeon's credentials is to ask where the surgeon has hospital privileges. If a surgeon has hospital privileges at an accredited hospital in the community, it means that the surgeon's credentials have been reviewed by other surgeons and physicians before allowing the surgeon to operate in that hospital. Credentialing committees usually do much more homework than you can do. Many plastic surgeons operate in their own facilities, but to assure peer review of the surgeon, the surgeon should have hospital privileges. Call the hospital to be sure.

## Professional Societies

There are many professional societies that use the name "plastic surgery." But, like the various "boards,"some are more meaningful than others. The two major societies in plastic surgery that require members to be board certified by the American Board of Plastic Surgery are 1) the American Society of Plastic and Reconstructive Surgeons (**www.plasticsurgery.org** or phone 1-800-635-0635) and the American Society of Aesthetic Plastic Surgery (**www.surgery.org** or phone 1-888-272-7711). Members of these societies also must adhere to a very stringent code of ethics and participate in continuing education. Other societies, including state and local societies, are less important when judging credentials.

## Who's Who in America

Marquis Who's Who, in cooperation with the American Board of Medical Specialties (ABMS), publishes a directory of board certified specialists with a summary of their credentials. This set of books is available at most libraries.

## Best Doctors in America

A Directory of the Best Doctors in America, published by Woodward-White, is also available at most libraries. Doctors are listed by specialty and by region. Combining Who's Who with Best Doctors gives you a good reference to locate experts in plastic surgery.

### Recommendations From Friends

These recommendations can mean a lot or very little! Depends on the friend, how much they know, and how much their surgeon educated them. If a friend is thrilled with her surgeon, ask why. Try to determine how much your friend really knows about augmentation. If you're impressed, add the surgeon to your list.

## CREDENTIALS AND SOURCES: A CHECKLIST

Credentials won't be the only thing you'll consider when selecting a surgeon. We'll cover a lot more in the coming chapters. But credentials are a start. Here's a useful checklist:

**Essentials:**

- ❑ Board certified by the American Board of Plastic Surgery
- ❑ Completed an approved residency training program in plastic surgery
- ❑ Member of ASPRS and ASAPS (see professional societies above)
- ❑ Has hospital privileges to do breast augmentation at an accredited hospital
- ❑ Curriculum vitae documents scientific presentations and publications

**Cream on Top of the Essentials:**

- ❑ Subspecializes in cosmetic surgery
- ❑ Subspecializes in breast augmentation
- ❑ Listed in Who's Who
- ❑ Listed in Best Doctors in America
- ❑ Recommended by a knowledgeable friend or physician

**Not as Reliable:**

- ❑ Advertisements
- ❑ Media coverage
- ❑ General physician referral services (most are paid by the surgeon to refer you)
- ❑ Recommendations from anyone without in-depth knowledge about augmentation

**Red Flags:**

- ❑ Completed residency training in a specialty other than plastic surgery
- ❑ Certified in an unrelated specialty
- ❑ Not board certified by ABPS
- ❑ No hospital privileges
- ❑ If you obtain any false or misleading information— claims that aren't true
- ❑ Unwilling to answer questions about credentials
- ❑ Unwilling to provide access to curriculum vitae

You can check basic credentials without even calling a surgeon's office using the sources and references in this chapter. List the surgeons, check with the ASPRS and ASAPS, and check Who's Who for a summary of the surgeon's education and board certification. Use the checklist above to compare credentials. Shorten your list of surgeons based on credentials *before* you call their offices for information, and you'll save a lot of time.

## HAVING LOOKED AT CREDENTIALS, WHAT'S THE NEXT STEP?

Now you have a list of surgeons with good, basic credentials. The next step on the stairs is contacting the surgeon's office for *information,* not necessarily an *appointment.* In the next chapter, we'll supply guidelines of what to look for when you call for information and what to look for in the information you receive.

[CHAPTER TEN]

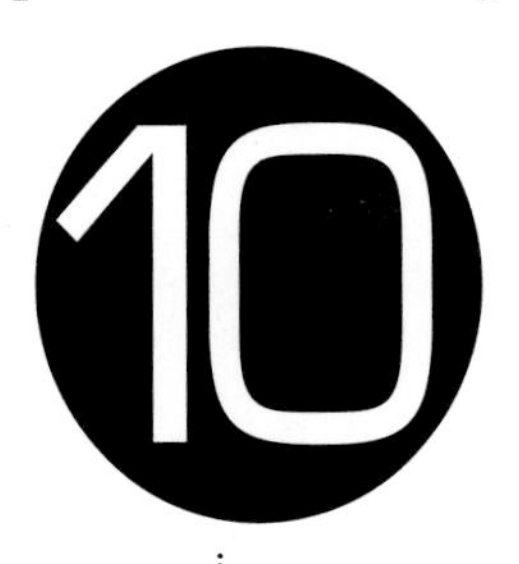


# INFORMATION FROM SURGEONS' OFFICES: Getting and Evaluating It

***"A surgeon's habits are reflected in every aspect of the surgeon's practice. The quality and detail of a surgeon's information materials should tell you a lot about the surgeon."***

You've obtained the names of several qualified surgeons, and you've checked their credentials. Now you're ready to call their offices and request information. Before you pick up the phone, do you know what to request? Do you know what questions to ask about breast augmentation? Do you want to simply request information, or would you like to spend some time on the phone talking with someone about breast augmentation? What do you hope to learn from your call? What would you like to get from the surgeon? To get the most from your time, you need answers to each of these questions — *before you call!* Other sources of information can also help — the Internet, the FDA, and implant manufacturers. Once you've gathered the information, what do you do with it? How do you evaluate information from surgeons? Before you visit a surgeon, gathering and evaluating information will make you better informed and better able to evaluate the surgeon during your consultation.

## CALLING A SURGEON'S OFFICE

When a prospective augmentation patient calls our office, these are the three most commonly asked questions:

***How much does it cost?***
***Which way does the surgeon like to do it?***
***Which type of implant does the surgeon use?***

In our opinion, these three questions are not the most important things you should focus on during your first call to a surgeon's office. Yes, you may want to know the answers to those questions eventually. But initially, you might ask yourself, "Before I ask the price, is this a surgeon that I would even *consider*?" You can help answer this important question during your first phone call to a surgeon's office!

Rather than asking questions on your first call to a surgeon's office, focus on *listening*.

## Listen for three things in your first call to the office: COURTESY, SERVICE, AND KNOWLEDGE

### Courtesy

How does the surgeon's office staff answer the telephone? If you select this surgeon, you'll be dealing with this staff before and after your surgery! Does the person who answers the phone have a name? What is it? Are you told? If not, I'd immediately hang up and try another surgeon!

Are you put on hold? For how long? Were you given a choice of a callback rather than holding? While wasting your time on hold (a discourtesy), is the surgeon trying to sell you additional operations with quasi- tasteful recorded commercials? Rather than listening to recorded commercials on hold, wouldn't it be nice to *get substance* and *information* without ever staying on hold? If your time is of no value to the surgeon now, how much more of your time will he or she waste in the course of caring for you?

Is the person on the other end of the line cheerful and enthusiastic, or is the attitude, "Yeah, what do you want?" Is the person appreciative that you chose to call this office? After all, you will be paying a substantial amount of money and could potentially refer more patients!

Is the person listening to you and your questions (a courtesy)? Or does the person immediately launch into something that sounds like a recorded answering machine, giving you answers to questions you didn't ask and don't need to know? What should you listen for?

***We're glad you called us.***

***We respect your time.***

***I am listening to you.***

***I'm going to do everything I can to help you and make you want to come and see us.***

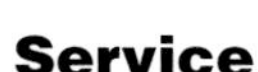

## Service

Plastic surgery, especially cosmetic plastic surgery, is a service-oriented business. At least, it should be. You aren't sick. You don't require emergency care. You are choosing to have an operation that is not medically necessary, taking certain risks, and spending a considerable amount of money in the process. Why shouldn't you expect good service?

**Service in plastic surgery means meeting your needs NOW, during your first call!**

To meet your needs, a surgeon's personnel must first show the courtesy of *listening* to your needs. What information are you seeking? What are you trying to achieve? If they don't listen, or they immediately try to sell you two more operations or services you didn't ask for, beware!

Service means making things easy for you. Is every single word or question difficult? If you ask whether the surgeon does augmentation, does it take a while to think of the answer? Does every question seem to be an imposition or a problem? Does the person offer to send you information? Is it sent it in a timely manner? Did someone call to be sure you received it? The only message you should hear is:

**I want to make this easy for you.**
***Let's get started.***

But what if you don't really know what you need.

**One of the highest forms of service is helping you understand what you might need in a knowledgeable, friendly, no-pressure manner.**

Which brings us to our next important point...

**To help you understand your NEEDS, a surgeon's staff must give you good INFORMATION using terms that are easy to understand, and that requires KNOWLEDGE!**

## Knowledge

One of the very best ways to judge a surgeon is to listen carefully to the surgeon's staff. The staff is a reflection of the surgeon.

**I've never seen a highly knowledgeable staff that worked for an average-level surgeon!**

It's difficult and time consuming for a surgeon to hire, train, and keep knowledgeable staff. If you find a knowledgeable, courteous, helpful staff, it probably didn't happen by accident. The kind of person who trained that staff is likely the kind of person you'd want doing your surgery!

**You won't believe how easy it is to distinguish FACT from FLUFF in plastic surgery. All you need to do is LISTEN.**

If it sounds too good to be true, it usually is! Is the surgeon trying to tell you there's only one best way to do augmentations? You already know that's not true! Is everything all roses with no thorns—all benefits with no tradeoffs? You already know that no surgical option is without tradeoffs. Does the surgeon tell you all augmentations are done a certain way? If so, you already know the surgeon is doing some of them wrong! Is the surgeon or staff willing to honestly and frankly discuss risks and tradeoffs?

**Are the surgeon and the surgeon's staff telling you things you need to know?**

*Does the answer sound reasonable? Pertinent?*

When you ask a question, is there a huge void on the other end of the line when it comes to substance, or do you want to pick up a pen and take some notes? Do the minutes pass quickly on the phone? Do you feel you are really learning something useful?

### Are the surgeon and the surgeon's staff willing to spend time with you?

*Knowledge doesn't come quickly.*

Are you getting the feeling that the person on the other end of the line would rather be doing anything rather than talking to you? Do you feel rushed? When you ask a question, do you hear a deep sigh, "Gawd, are you really going to ask me another question?" Or does the person make you feel like you can ask all the questions you want—they'll be happy to spend any amount of time required to answer them. If the office is extremely busy, do they offer to call you back at a mutually agreeable time to spend more time answering your questions? No office is perfect at every one of these items, but some are definitely more perfect than others!

### Do the surgeon and the surgeon's staff help you even if you don't really need an operation or if this surgeon is not the best doctor to do your operation?

*The ultimate in service and knowledge is not selling you an operation you don't need!*

Am I dreaming, suggesting that any surgeon's office might, in good faith and with nothing to gain, refer you to another surgeon or help you with a non-surgical service rather than suggesting an operation? It can happen. But don't hold your breath because it's rare. I've actually heard a well-known plastic surgeon say, "If they call my office, I assume they're looking for an operation, and I'm here to see that they get one!" That's not good service. That's greed.

## Does the surgeon offer you an opportunity to come into the office and spend a considerable amount of time with a patient educator at no charge?

*You'll always learn more in a face-to-face visit.*

Surgeons who use patient educators almost always have better informed patients. No surgeon can spend as much time with every patient as a staff of patient educators. The best plastic surgery practices want to help you understand as much as possible. You'll often find that you are more comfortable with a patient educator than with the surgeon. If you're more comfortable, you'll listen better and learn more! If given the opportunity, take it!

## Is the surgeon's staff willing to help guide you in the decision process?

Knowledgeable staff people are interested in helping you make the best decisions, so that you and the surgeon can make the best team decisions. The more they know about the different options, the better they can help you understand which options are realistic for you, helping guide you in the decision-making process. The very best staff people also always know when to stop and never exceed their own knowledge. There is always a point where the only correct answer is, "You'll need to discuss that with the doctor. That's something that the two of you will decide after your consultation and examination."

## Are you offered an opportunity to look at before-and-after pictures and speak with other patients?

We've already covered some of the pros and cons of before-and-after pictures. The most important thing to remember is that no other patient is just like you. Nevertheless, you want to be a bit skeptical if a surgeon can't or won't show you examples of results. Speaking with other patients can also be helpful. Not that you'll have the same experience, but hearing from another patient can sometimes make you more comfortable.

## COSTS: HOW DO THEY EXPLAIN THEM?

When you ask about costs, are the costs broken down or all lumped together? Are there different costs for different procedures and different types of implants? Although a package price may seem attractive, you don't really know what you're paying for. Costs should be broken down by surgeon fees, implant costs, laboratory fees, mammogram fees, electrocardiogram fees, anesthesia fees, surgery facility costs, and any hidden costs such as preoperative and postoperative medications. Just ask about costs, and see how much detail you hear! Ask about each item separately! Is each item included in the price you were quoted?

## WHAT TO ASK AND WHAT TO ASK FOR: A LIST OF QUESTIONS

When you first call a surgeon's office, the following questions will help you get what you need: 1) **verbal answers** that help you evaluate courtesy, service, and knowledge, and 2) **written informational materials**.

When you ask the following questions, listen carefully to the answers! Take notes, and keep the answers organized by surgeon. The answers are key to making good decisions when selecting a surgeon:

1) I'm interested in getting information about breast augmentation. Does Dr. X do breast augmentation?
2) How does Dr. X do breast augmentation?
3) Could you send me some information about breast augmentation and about Dr. X and your practice?
4) What are the risks involved in having breast augmentation?
5) Do you offer free consultations?
6) Do you have before-and-after photographs that I could see?
7) Would it be possible to speak with other patients of Dr. X who have had augmentations?
8) How long has Dr. X been in practice?
9) How many augmentations does Dr. X do every year?
10) Does Dr. X limit his practice to cosmetic surgery?

11) Where does Dr. X have hospital privileges?
12) Is Dr. X board certified? By which board?
13) How much will my augmentation cost?

After asking these questions, evaluate the answers. Did you get a little or a lot of information? Is the information quality or fluff?

## EVALUATING WRITTEN INFORMATION YOU RECEIVE FROM SURGEONS

When you receive written information from a surgeon, read it carefully. That's part of your job. At least 30 percent of patients never read information sent to them. If you don't read it, you can't use the knowledge (or lack thereof) to make better decisions!

In later chapters, we will emphasize repeatedly that:

**A surgeon's habits are reflected in everything a surgeon does. All you need to do is notice.**

*Informational materials reflect a surgeon's habits and commitment to educating patients.*

What should you look for in written information and brochures? The following are some guidelines:

**Is the information generic, or did the surgeon write the information personally?**

*If it's generic, you can tell. You'll probably see the same thing from other surgeons.*

**Does it appear and sound distinctively different compared to other surgeons' information?**

*If it doesn't sound different, it probably isn't much different! What might that say about your result?*

**What do the informational materials tell you about the surgeon's habits?**

*Is the surgeon compulsive and different? Better? What might that say about your surgery?*

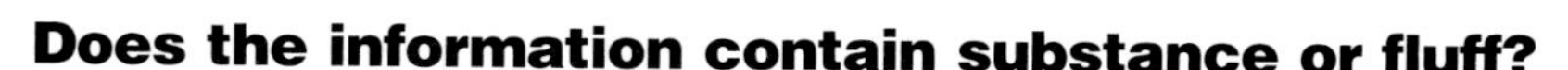

**Does the information contain substance or fluff?**

*If you took away the fancy look, what does it SAY? Fluff with little substance? What might that say about the surgeon?*

**Does the information address most or all of your questions and concerns? How well?**

*If only 50 percent of the answers are there, what might that say about the percent of knowledge?*

**Is the information written in easy-to-understand language? And, at the same time, is it informative?**

*If not, why not? Does the surgeon not know enough, or not care enough, or both?*

## THE INTERNET AS A SOURCE OF INFORMATION

Information from the Internet should be scrutinized using the same criteria as verbal and written information from surgeons. The questions listed earlier in this chapter apply to Internet information as well as verbal and written information.

Many individual plastic surgeons have web sites. When visiting these sites, continually ask these questions:

***How much is substance, and how much is fluff?***

***Have I seen and heard this before?***

***Is anything different?***

Check all Internet information against surgeon credentials obtained from sources listed in this chapter and in Chapter 9.

## RED FLAGS IN INFORMATIONAL MATERIALS AND SPOKEN ANSWERS

If you read or hear any of the following, beware! Every statement listed here is an actual statement that a patient has told us they have heard from a surgeon or a surgeon's staff!

### Regarding Training

Oh, don't worry about formal plastic surgery residency training. Dr. X did special training in cosmetic surgery under Dr. Y and Dr. Z, world famous cosmetic surgeons. Now he's the best in the world!

Dr. X is specially trained in cosmetic surgery, not plastic surgery.

I know that Dr. X is a dentist, but breasts are sometimes found in the mouth! Ha, Ha! That's why he does breast augmentations!

You don't need six years of training to do breast augmentations. It's a simple operation!

### Regarding Credentials

Dr. X doesn't operate in any hospitals, so he doesn't need hospital privileges.

Dr. X is certified by the X!*$$$$ board of plastic surgery—the most famous board in the world! (Only it's not recognized by the American Board of Medical Specialties.)

Dr. X has only been in practice two months, but he's invented a completely new procedure for breast augmentation that is the most advanced in the world!

You don't need to worry about credentials. Dr. X has operated on five Playboy models and six famous actresses! Sorry, we can't give you their names! But you see his work in Playboy and Penthouse all the time!

Don't worry about credentials. Dr. X is the most famous breast surgeon in New York City, the center of the plastic surgery world!

## Picking an Implant Size

Bring us a picture of the breasts you like, and Dr. X can make them for you!

Go buy a bra that's the size you'd like to be, and bring it with you to the office. We'll let you put implants in the bra and choose the size you'd like to be! See Chapters 4, 5, and 6.

Fill your bra with panty hose. When it's full, take the panty hose out and soak them in water. Squeeze out the water and measure it. That's the size we'll select for your implants!

Try on some breast enhancers in a bra the size you'd like to be. Tell us the size and we'll match your breast implant to it!

Fill plastic baggies with water (or peas, or anything else) and stuff them into a bra the size you'd like to be. Bring them to the office with you and well measure how much water is in the baggy and match your implant to that size!

## Sending You Information

You won't need any written information. We'll tell you everything you need to know when you come in. It'll only take 15 minutes.

Information? Sure we've got information we can send you! (Funny, it never arrives!)

You can get all the information you need on Dr. X's web site (sure, at www. whatinfo, justfluff.com).

We're just going to send you some brochures from the most prestigious plastic surgery society in the world.

You don't need any special information. Breast augmentations are pretty much all the same. Come on in, and we can get you taken care of!

### Selling You What You Didn't Ask About

Breast augmentation? Sure, we do that! But you'll probably want to think about liposuction and a facelift, too! Why have big breasts and not have a tiny butt and great looking face?

You don't want to just do your breasts. You'll need some liposuction to perfectly balance your figure!

Your breasts will look so good that no man can look you in the face unless we get you on our special skin care program and do a facelift!

### Discounts

Sure, we have discounts. How much can you pay?

If you choose two other operations at the same time as your breast augmentation, we can give you a huge discount!

This list could go on forever — but you get the messages!

## THE NEXT STEP...

Having gathered and evaluated information from the list of surgeons with good credentials, now you're ready to decide which surgeons you want to see in consultation, and prepare for the consultations well in advance.

[CHAPTER ELEVEN]

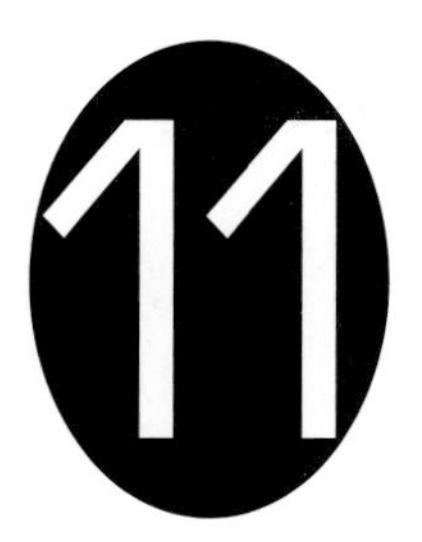


# CONSULTING WITH A PLASTIC SURGEON: Preparing and Doing It

***"A surgeon's habits are reflected in the surgeon's staff, information materials, office organization, thoroughness, and in the logic of what the surgeon tells you. Look, listen, and ask yourself if these are the characteristics you want in your surgeon."***

You've obtained names of surgeons (hopefully more than one), and you've checked their credentials (Chapter 9). You narrowed the list based on credentials, then gathered and evaluated information from each of their offices (Chapter 10). You narrowed the list again. Now it's time for the main event—your consultation with plastic surgeons. Notice I said plastic surgeon**S—plural**. You're cheating yourself if you don't consult more than one. No matter how great you may think one is, you don't really know if you don't compare!

## MAKING APPOINTMENTS

### Complimentary Consultations With a Patient Educator

Most busy, experienced surgeons offer complimentary consultations with a nurse or patient educator prior to seeing the surgeon. A patient educator consultation is a great opportunity for you for the following reasons:

- You have an opportunity to learn more before you see the surgeon.
- You'll be able to make better use of your time with the surgeon.
- You'll probably communicate better with most patient educators than with most surgeons.
- You have an opportunity to evaluate the surgeon, and, in general, the better the patient educator, the better the surgeon.
- You have an opportunity to save money on a surgeon consultation if anything is not right for you (the procedure, the information you hear or don't hear, how you're treated, and whether you're subjected to hard-sell techniques).

Most patient educators are willing to spend as much time with you as necessary, usually at least 30-45 minutes. The benefit is that you have that much additional time to gain information *before* you see the surgeon—regardless of how much time the surgeon spends with you!

**If you have an opportunity to consult a patient educator before consulting the surgeon — do it!**

*The best surgeons will almost always offer this service because they want you to know as much as possible.*

## Don't See the Surgeon Until You're Prepared

After visiting with patient educators in different surgeons' offices, you'll have a totally different perspective. There's a good chance you'll shorten your surgeon list, saving money and time in the process, based solely on your visit with the patient educators.

Don't make an appointment to see a surgeon until you're prepared. We'll give you a specific checklist later.

**The more PREPARED you are BEFORE meeting with a surgeon, the better you'll understand the surgeon, and the better you can evaluate the surgeon.**

## Best Times for Appointments

Your best chance for a thorough consultation is at a time when the surgeon is least likely to be rushed. Many surgeons operate in the morning and see patients in the afternoons. The majority of surgeons are chronically behind schedule and will keep you waiting. Ask if appointments are available in the morning or anytime on a day when the surgeon is not operating. You won't sit in the waiting room as long.

## Be on Time

It's reasonable to expect a surgeon to respect your time. It's also reasonable to respect the surgeon's time. The surgeon has set aside time to see you. If you're late, your consultation will either be more rushed, which usually happens, or you totally disrupt the schedule for the surgeon and all of the other patients being seen that day.

### Call If You Can't Make It

When you make an appointment with any professional and don't cancel if you can't make it, you are wasting that professional's time. A plastic surgeon has only two things to sell—expertise and time. Whatever the cost of your consultation, if you don't call to cancel in advance, you're costing the professional that much money. Always call if you can't make it or need to change an appointment time.

## SEEING WHAT THEY DON'T TELL YOU—THINGS TO NOTICE

### The Surroundings

A surgeon's office doesn't need to look like the Taj Mahal. If it does, you're paying for it. On the other hand, what you see is what you get. A plastic surgeon's office also shouldn't look like the offices of a general practitioner in a busy HMO.

**You're not going to a museum or estate. You're going to see a surgeon.**

*Statues, art, and expensive furniture don't tell you a thing about the quality of surgery you'll get, but guess who gets to pay for the décor? You!*

**A quiet, comfortable atmosphere that reflects good taste is all that's required. Anything more, and you're paying extra for the décor.**

*You want to spend your money on the surgeon, not the decorator.*

**If the office looks like it may not belong to a plastic surgeon, there's a message.**

*An overly "medical" appearing office is not typical of cosmetic surgery offices. Do you want someone operating on you that doesn't do those procedures very often?*

## The Organization

Watch the flow of the office and the flow of patients. Does it appear well-organized, or does it look like feeding time at a zoo? The organization and function of a surgeon's office should tell you a lot. If it's a zoo, just ask yourself how organized the surgeon is.

**The organization, function and flow of every surgeon's office is a reflection of the surgeon's habits.**

*Ask yourself if you want someone with these habits operating on you.*

## Information Versus Pressure Sales

Look around the office. Are you barraged at every turn with something trying to sell you another operation or service? Informational materials can be valuable, provided they aren't the same materials you see in other offices (generic materials personalized with a surgeon's name). As you look at materials and displays in an office, ask yourself:

***Are they trying to INFORM me or trying to SELL me?***

*If you're sold by good information, that's fine. That's what you're looking for!*

## Does the Surgeon Respect Your Time?

If you're on time and the surgeon keeps you waiting excessively, the surgeon is not respecting your time. Sure, problems occur in surgery, and patients before you want to talk about three more procedures than the one for which they made an appointment. But many surgeons are chronically rude and waste their patients' time.

**If everything else about your experience with the surgeon is great, and the surgeon keeps you waiting, you may be satisfied by an apology.**

**If anything else isn't great and you wait a long time, then you can probably conclude it's poor organization and rudeness.**

*Do you want someone operating on you who is poorly organized and rude?*

Our policy is that if we keep you waiting for a surgeon consultation longer than 10 minutes, you will not be charged for your consultation regardless of the reason. You won't get excuses. You'll get a free consultation! If more surgeons adopted that policy, more patients would be treated more courteously.

## BEFORE-AND-AFTER PICTURES, COMPUTER IMAGING

In Chapter 4, we discussed window shopping for breasts and the relative advantages and risks of using before-and-after pictures and computer imaging to make decisions. If you didn't read that section before, do it now! When you look at pictures or computer images, use the following checklist:

- ❐ Did the person in the picture look exactly like me before the operation? If not, I'm not going to look like her after my operation, even if everything is done exactly the same.
- ❐ Did the surgeon look at a magazine picture you brought and say, "Sure, we can make that breast! No problem?" If so, consult other surgeons.
- ❐ Did the surgeon say, "I'll use the pictures to help me understand what you'd like, and then I'll try to help you understand our best options and tradeoffs, given your tissues?" If so, GREAT!
- ❐ Were you given some excuse why there were no pictures for you to see? If so, consult other surgeons.

- ❐ Does every result look good? If so, you aren't seeing a range of results. Consult other surgeons.
- ❐ Did the book does not contain a wide variety of breasts, with some results better than others? If not, consult other surgeons.
- ❐ Did the surgeon or staff fully explain any question you asked about the pictures? If not, consult other surgeons.
- ❐ What about the quality of the pictures? Are they standardized? Good quality? Is the background consistent in all the pictures? *A surgeon's habits are also reflected in the quality of the picture as well as the quality of the result.*
- ❐ If you looked at computer images, remember that even a technician can produce changes on a computer that no surgeon can produce with living tissue.
- ❐ If the surgeon uses the imager to help you understand some points, fine. If a technician or the surgeon uses the imager to try to sell you something that doesn't make sense or sell you other non-breast operations, beware.
- ❐ If the surgeon morphs (changes the appearance of) your breasts on the computer and prints you a simulated before-and-after picture, don't look at it too much and try not to fix the image in your mind. Your result definitely won't match the image exactly.
- ❐ Don't count on getting the result you've seen from imaging. Once you've seen a simulated result, you tend to expect that result, even if the computer screen is covered with disclaimers informing us that this is only a simulation.

## PREPARING FOR MY VISIT — A CHECKLIST FOR MY CONSULTATION

### Are You Ready for a Consultation?

If you can check all of the items on the following checklist, you're ready to consult with a plastic surgeon!

- ❒ I've read Chapters 1 through 10.
- ❒ I made a list of surgeons and verified credentials.
- ❒ I called surgeons' offices and requested informational materials.
- ❒ I evaluated surgeons' staffs on the phone.
- ❒ I've gathered information from at least three surgeons with solid credentials, good informational materials, and knowledgeable staffs.
- ❒ I took advantage of visits with patient educators.
- ❒ I've made a specific list of questions I want to ask the surgeon.

## Questions to Ask Every Surgeon During the Consultation

If you don't already know the answers, review Chapters 1-10. Don't give clues. Ask the questions and take notes about the answers. You can review your notes and refer back to this book later.

- ❒ In what specialty was your residency training? How many years? Are you board certified? By whom?
- ❒ How long have you been in practice?
- ❒ Do you have hospital privileges? Where?
- ❒ How many breast augmentations have you done, and how many do you perform each year?
- ❒ What are the three most important things you'd advise me to think about with regard to breast augmentation?
- ❒ What is your preferred incision location? Why? How many of each location have you done? Can you show me pictures?
- ❒ Which do you prefer, over or under muscle? Why? Do you do both? How many of each have you done?
- ❒ What is your preferred implant? Why? Do you offer all different types of implants?
- ❒ Do you prefer round or anatomic implants? Why? Do you offer both? How many of each have you done?

- ❒ If you prefer round implants, how do you deal with the fill issue?
- ❒ Are round implants adequately filled with saline or silicone to prevent shell folding?
- ❒ Do you think shell folding can affect the life of the shell?
- ❒ If we overfill a round implant, are you willing to guarantee the implant if the manufacturer does not? What happens if my implant fails?
- ❒ What are the three worst things that can happen following my augmentation? What are the chances they will happen? Exactly what do we do in each case if they happen? What are the costs involved? Time off work, worst possible scenario?
- ❒ Would you ever recommend implant removal without replacement? If so, why? What affects how my breast will look if we had to remove implants?
- ❒ Does the size of the implant we choose affect my tissues as I get older? How?
- ❒ Do you charge me to replace my implant if it ruptures? Is there anything that can occur that you would charge me for in the future, including followup visits or surgery?
- ❒ Will anyone else perform any part of my surgery? Are they more qualified than you?
- ❒ When can I lift my arms above my head, drive my car, and lift my children or other objects?
- ❒ Will I have drains?
- ❒ Will I have bruising?
- ❒ Will I wear special bandages, bras, or binders? For how long?
- ❒ Why should I choose you to do my surgery?

## Things to Notice During the Surgeon's Examination

- ❒ Is the surgeon organized?
- ❒ Does the surgeon explain what he or she is doing during the examination?
- ❒ Does the surgeon measure your breasts? Measurements demonstrate minor differences that even the most experienced surgeon cannot see by simply looking at the breasts, and remember, a surgeon cannot improve what a surgeon cannot see. Some of the basic measurements are illustrated in Figure 11-1, A-E.
- ❒ Does the surgeon use a precise record in your chart where measurements and details are recorded while you are being examined? An example of our clinical evaluation sheet used during the examination is illustrated in Figure 11-2.
- ❒ Does the surgeon demonstrate and discuss the specific characteristics of your tissues during the exam, and how those tissue characteristics might affect your options and results?
- ❒ Does the surgeon explain during the exam how the width of the breast implant you choose might affect the result, depending on the width and amount of breast tissue that you have before surgery?
- ❒ Does the surgeon point out limitations of your tissues that might affect your choice of implant size or width?
- ❒ Does the surgeon demonstrate to you using your own tissues what might be achievable in terms of your result?
- ❒ Does the surgeon meticulously record the details of your examination during the examination? If not, how can the surgeon remember all the details of your exam later, after examining several other patients?
- ❒ Does the surgeon explain everything in terms that you clearly understand, and ask you if you had any other questions?
- ❒ Does the surgeon thank you for your coming for consultation?

**Figure 11-1.**

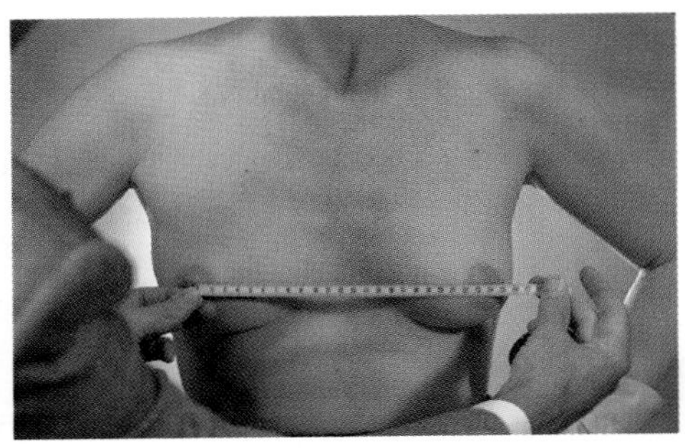

**A.**

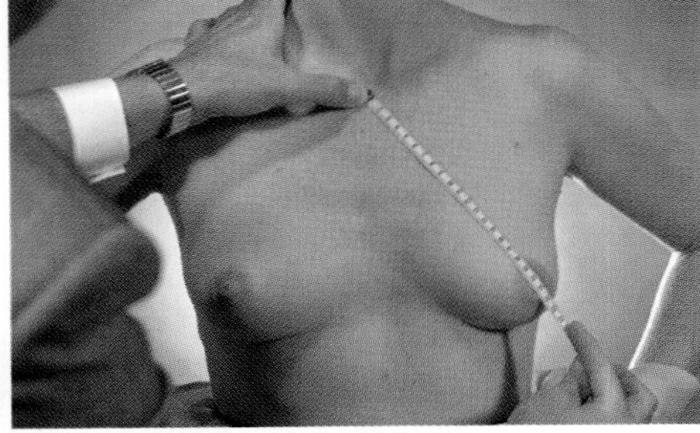

**B.**

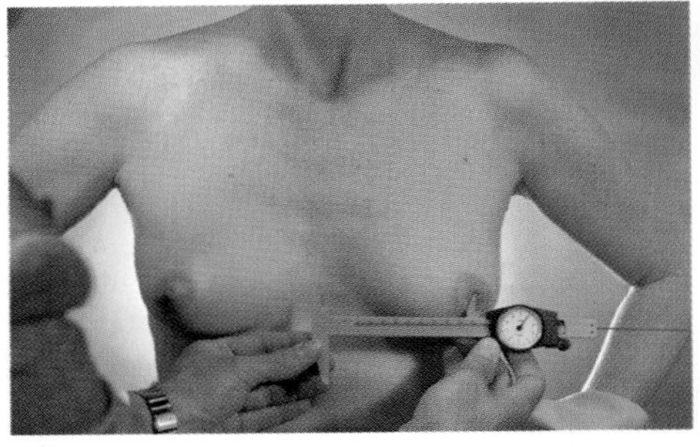

**C.**

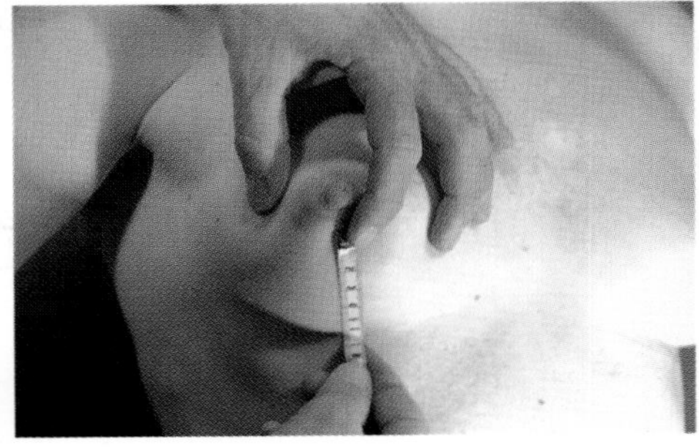

**D.**

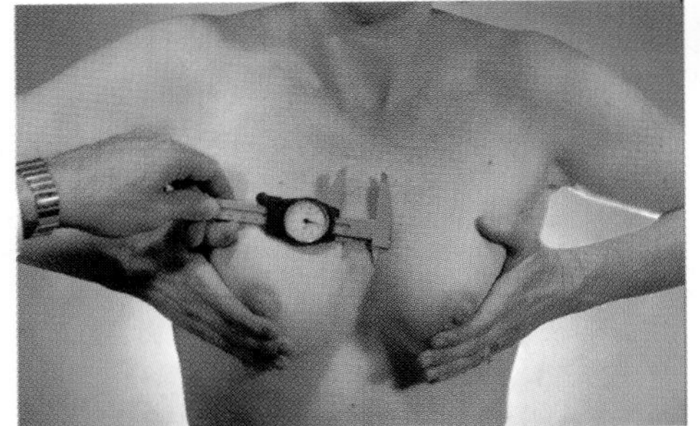

**E.**

**Precise breast measurements add accuracy and predictability to your augmentation — more than the most experienced "artistic eye".**

**Figure 11-2.**

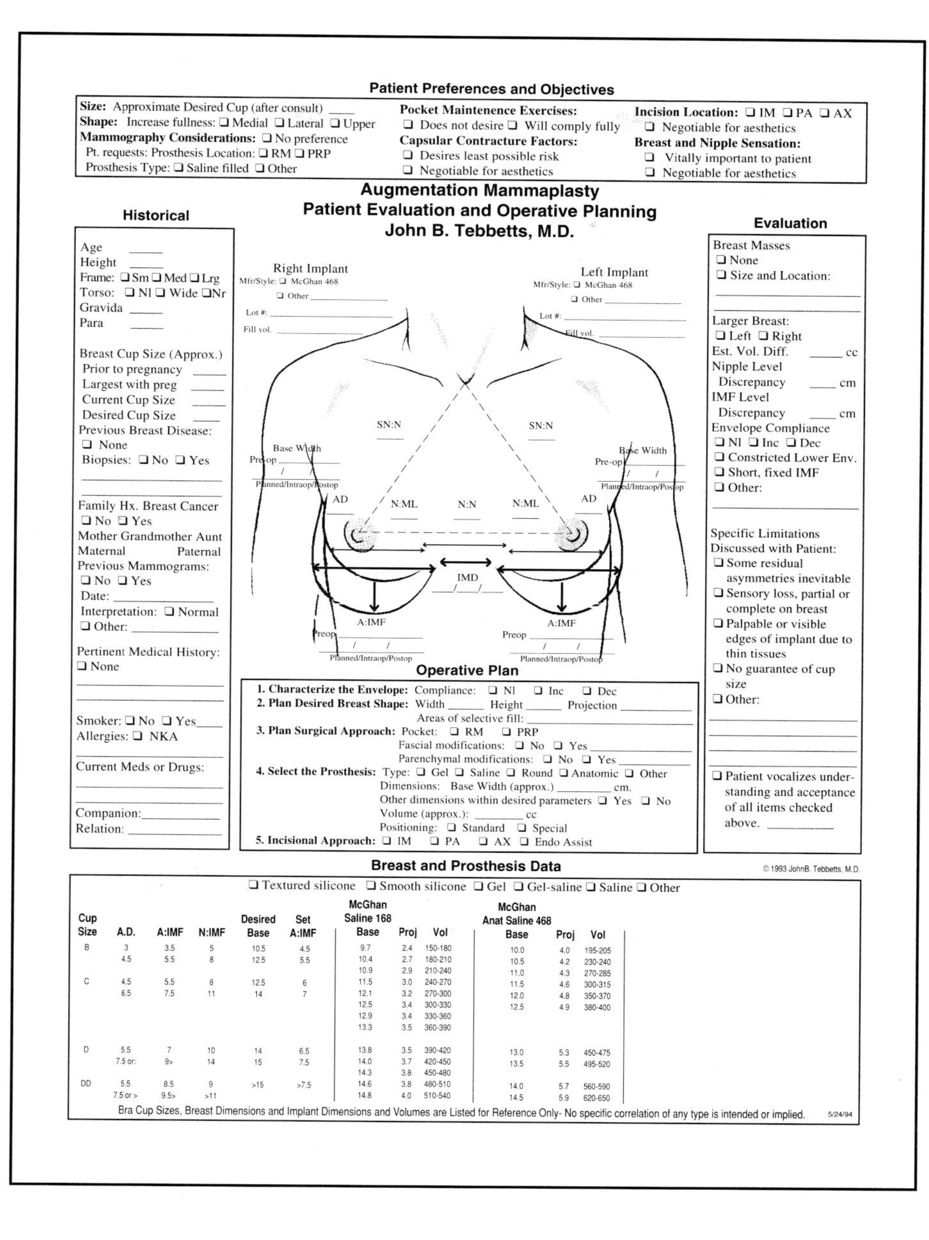

### Patient Preferences and Objectives

**Size:** Approximate Desired Cup (after consult) ____
**Shape:** Increase fullness: ❑ Medial ❑ Lateral ❑ Upper
**Mammography Considerations:** ❑ No preference
Pt. requests: Prosthesis Location: ❑ RM ❑ PRP
Prosthesis Type: ❑ Saline filled ❑ Other

**Pocket Maintenence Exercises:**
❑ Does not desire ❑ Will comply fully
**Capsular Contracture Factors:**
❑ Desires least possible risk
❑ Negotiable for aesthetics

**Incision Location:** ❑ IM ❑ PA ❑ AX
❑ Negotiable for aesthetics
**Breast and Nipple Sensation:**
❑ Vitally important to patient
❑ Negotiable for aesthetics

### Augmentation Mammaplasty
### Patient Evaluation and Operative Planning
### John B. Tebbetts, M.D.

#### Historical

Age _____
Height _____
Frame: ❑ Sm ❑ Med ❑ Lrg
Torso: ❑ Nl ❑ Wide ❑Nr
Gravida _____
Para _____

Breast Cup Size (Approx.)
Prior to pregnancy ____
Largest with preg ____
Current Cup Size ____
Desired Cup Size ____
Previous Breast Disease:
❑ None
Biopsies: ❑ No ❑ Yes

Family Hx. Breast Cancer
❑ No ❑ Yes
Mother Grandmother Aunt
Maternal Paternal
Previous Mammograms:
❑ No ❑ Yes
Date: ____________
Interpretation: ❑ Normal
❑ Other: ____________

Pertinent Medical History:
❑ None

Smoker: ❑ No ❑ Yes____
Allergies: ❑ NKA

Current Meds or Drugs:

Companion:____________
Relation: ____________



#### Evaluation

Breast Masses
❑ None
❑ Size and Location:

Larger Breast:
❑ Left ❑ Right
Est. Vol. Diff. _____ cc
Nipple Level
Discrepancy ____ cm
IMF Level
Discrepancy ____ cm
Envelope Compliance
❑ Nl ❑ Inc ❑ Dec
❑ Constricted Lower Env.
❑ Short, fixed IMF
❑ Other:

Specific Limitations Discussed with Patient:
❑ Some residual asymmetries inevitable
❑ Sensory loss, partial or complete on breast
❑ Palpable or visible edges of implant due to thin tissues
❑ No guarantee of cup size
❑ Other:

❑ Patient vocalizes understanding and acceptance of all items checked above. ________

#### Operative Plan

**1. Characterize the Envelope:** Compliance: ❑ Nl ❑ Inc ❑ Dec
**2. Plan Desired Breast Shape:** Width ______ Height ______ Projection ________
Areas of selective fill: ________
**3. Plan Surgical Approach:** Pocket: ❑ RM ❑ PRP
Fascial modifications: ❑ No ❑ Yes ________
Parenchymal modifications: ❑ No ❑ Yes ________
**4. Select the Prosthesis:** Type: ❑ Gel ❑ Saline ❑ Round ❑ Anatomic ❑ Other
Dimensions: Base Width (approx.) ________ cm.
Other dimensions within desired parameters ❑ Yes ❑ No
Volume (approx.): ________ cc
Positioning: ❑ Standard ❑ Special
**5. Incisional Approach:** ❑ IM ❑ PA ❑ AX ❑ Endo Assist

#### Breast and Prosthesis Data



❑ Textured silicone ❑ Smooth silicone ❑ Gel ❑ Gel-saline ❑ Saline ❑ Other

| Cup Size | A.D. | A:IMF | N:IMF | Desired Base | Set A:IMF | McGhan Saline 168 Base | Proj | Vol | McGhan Anat Saline 468 Base | Proj | Vol |
|---|---|---|---|---|---|---|---|---|---|---|---|
| B | 3 | 3.5 | 5 | 10.5 | 4.5 | 9.7 | 2.4 | 150-180 | 10.0 | 4.0 | 195-205 |
| | 4.5 | 5.5 | 8 | 12.5 | 5.5 | 10.4 | 2.7 | 180-210 | 10.5 | 4.2 | 230-240 |
| | | | | | | 10.9 | 2.9 | 210-240 | 11.0 | 4.3 | 270-285 |
| C | 4.5 | 5.5 | 8 | 12.5 | 6 | 11.5 | 3.0 | 240-270 | 11.5 | 4.6 | 300-315 |
| | 6.5 | 7.5 | 11 | 14 | 7 | 12.1 | 3.2 | 270-300 | 12.0 | 4.8 | 350-370 |
| | | | | | | 12.5 | 3.4 | 300-330 | 12.5 | 4.9 | 380-400 |
| | | | | | | 12.9 | 3.4 | 330-360 | | | |
| | | | | | | 13.3 | 3.5 | 360-390 | | | |
| D | 5.5 | 7 | 10 | 14 | 6.5 | 13.8 | 3.5 | 390-420 | 13.0 | 5.3 | 450-475 |
| | 7.5 or: | 9> | 14 | 15 | 7.5 | 14.0 | 3.7 | 420-450 | 13.5 | 5.5 | 495-520 |
| | | | | | | 14.3 | 3.8 | 450-480 | | | |
| DD | 5.5 | 8.5 | 9 | >15 | >7.5 | 14.6 | 3.8 | 480-510 | 14.0 | 5.7 | 560-590 |
| | 7.5 or > | 9.5> | >11 | | | 14.8 | 4.0 | 510-540 | 14.5 | 5.9 | 620-650 |

Bra Cup Sizes, Breast Dimensions and Implant Dimensions and Volumes are Listed for Reference Only- No specific correlation of any type is intended or implied. 5/24/94

***Did your surgeon record precise measurements and other information on special record sheets during your examination?***

## What About Costs?

During your consultation visit, you need to inquire about costs. At this stage, you are gathering information. In Chapter 13, we'll discuss costs, costs analysis, and financing alternatives in more detail. From your surgeon or the staff, you'll need costs for each of the following items:

- ❒ Surgeon fees
- ❒ Laboratory fees (for lab work prior to surgery)
- ❒ Electrocardiogram fees (if needed)
- ❒ Mammogram fees (if surgeon requires mammogram)
- ❒ Surgery facility fees
- ❒ Costs of implants
- ❒ Anesthesia fees
- ❒ Medications fees or costs (for before and after surgery)
- ❒ Any other fees

**If a surgeon offers a "package price," always insist that the price be broken down into the categories listed above.**

*If you don't, you won't be able to analyze what you're paying for and compare to other surgeons. See Chapter 13.*

**Always ask for a written quote for costs signed by the surgeon or a staff member.**

*And ask how long the prices on the quote apply.*

## A Post-Consultation Checklist for Evaluation

In the next section, "Your homework after the consultation," is a checklist. Before your consultation, review the checklist thoroughly so that you'll notice all of the items listed.

## YOUR HOMEWORK AFTER THE CONSULTATION

### Doing your homework after the consultation is just as important as doing it before the consultation.

*Record your impressions while they are fresh in your mind.*

As soon as possible after your consultation, complete the following checklist, making brief notes beside each item. Don't procrastinate. Do it as soon as possible!

- ❒ Did you see the surgeon within 10 minutes of your appointment time?
- ❒ Was the staff courteous, efficient, and knowledgeable?
- ❒ Were the surroundings pleasant, comfortable, and not excessive?
- ❒ Did anyone try to sell you operations or services that you weren't interested in?
- ❒ How thorough was the surgeon?
- ❒ Did the surgeon use a specific checklist during your exam or just rely on memory?
- ❒ How well did the surgeon explain the issues?
- ❒ Did the surgeon measure your breasts? Did the surgeon explain the importance of the measurements?
- ❒ What did the surgeon tell you specifically about your tissues?
- ❒ Did the surgeon present you several options and discuss the tradeoffs of each?
- ❒ Did the surgeon discuss possible outcomes and tradeoffs with respect to your specific tissues?
- ❒ How did you select an implant? Were your tissues a major consideration?
- ❒ Was the surgeon glad to see you?
- ❒ Was the surgeon's personal appearance neat, and did it reflect attention to detail?

- ❒ Did the surgeon seem to really care?
- ❒ Was the surgeon precise, with a lot of attention to detail?
- ❒ How long was the surgeon willing to spend with you? Did you feel it was enough time?
- ❒ Did the surgeon seem irritable, uncomfortable, or impatient when you asked questions?
- ❒ Did the surgeon say, "Thank you for coming to see me"?

### Think About the Person You Just Met With and What You Heard!

It's your job to evaluate surgeons. Focus on substance instead of *hype* and *fluff*.

**You'll recognize a great surgeon without the surgeon having to tell you.**

**Gorgeous and charming don't contribute to what you'll get in the operating room.**

*Ask yourself how much substance is behind the appearance and charm.*

**Caring, thoroughness, and substance definitely contribute to what you'll get in the operating room.**

*How much of each did the surgeon have?*

**Remind yourself: This person will be changing my body forever, and I'll look at it every day.**

*Are you comfortable?*

**Were you offered options? A surgeon can't offer what the surgeon doesn't know how to do.**

*There is definitely not one best way to do an augmentation if you know all the different ways.*

**Were you told there was only one best way?**

*Ask yourself why.*

**Did you honestly and frankly discuss complications and what would be done?**

*If the worst occurred, would you want this person to take care of you?*

**Did you discuss your tissues and how implant selection would affect them over time?**

*If you didn't, you are very likely to make* ***BAD TEAM DECISIONS!***

Repeat this process for each surgeon that you consult. Make your notes, and file them with the information you obtained from each surgeon. When you're done, you will have all of the information that is reasonably necessary to make good decisions about surgeon selection. If you shortcut any of the steps, you may shortcut your quest for the best breast.

## THE NEXT STEP...

Now that you've completed your surgeon consultations, it's time to finalize your choices.

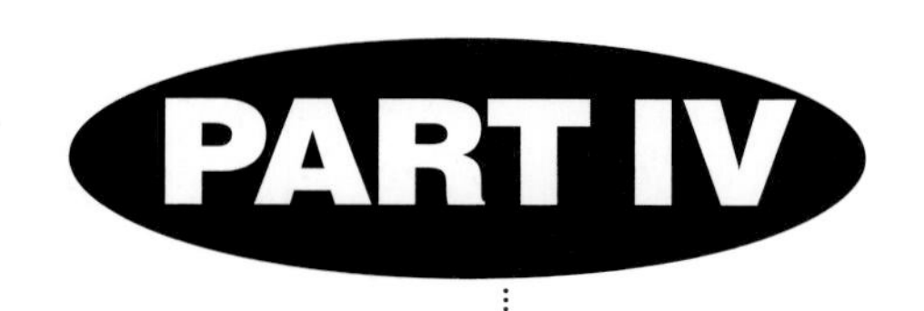


# PUTTING IT ALL TOGETHER:
## Finalizing Your Decisions and Preparing For Surgery

[CHAPTER TWELVE]

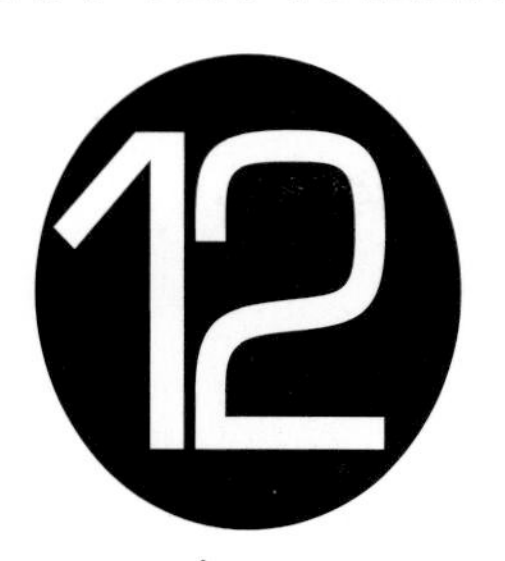


# PUTTING IT ALL TOGETHER: Making Your Selections

***"After doing your homework, make your choices in the following order: Your surgeon, type and size of implant, pocket location, and incision."***

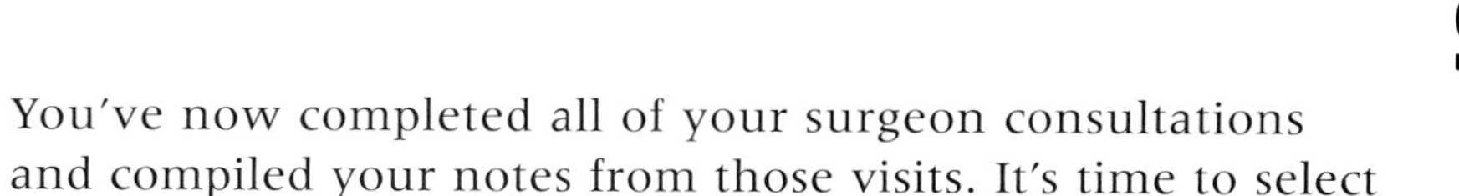

You've now completed all of your surgeon consultations and compiled your notes from those visits. It's time to select your surgeon!

## WHAT TO DECIDE FIRST? DOES IT MATTER?

Yes, it matters. If you make the right choice of surgeon, the rest is easier. The best surgeon should always present you with options and should discuss the tradeoffs of each option or set of options. Together, you'll make team decisions. You'll need to decide the following things, in order:

***Who is my surgeon?***

❒ Dr. X
❒ Dr. Y
❒ Dr. Z

***What type and size implant?***

❒ Smooth
❒ Textured
❒ Round
❒ Anatomic
❒ Filler material
❒ Size

***Which pocket location?***

❒ Retromammary (behind breast tissue only)
❒ Partial retropectoral (behind the pectoralis muscle)
❒ Total muscle coverage (behind pectoralis and serratus muscles)

***Which incision location?***

❒ Inframammary
❒ Periareolar
❒ Axillary
❒ Umbilical

Figure 12-1 summarizes the basic decisions sequence in a flow chart diagram.

**Figure 12-1.** **PATIENT DECISIONS IN BREAST AUGMENTATION**

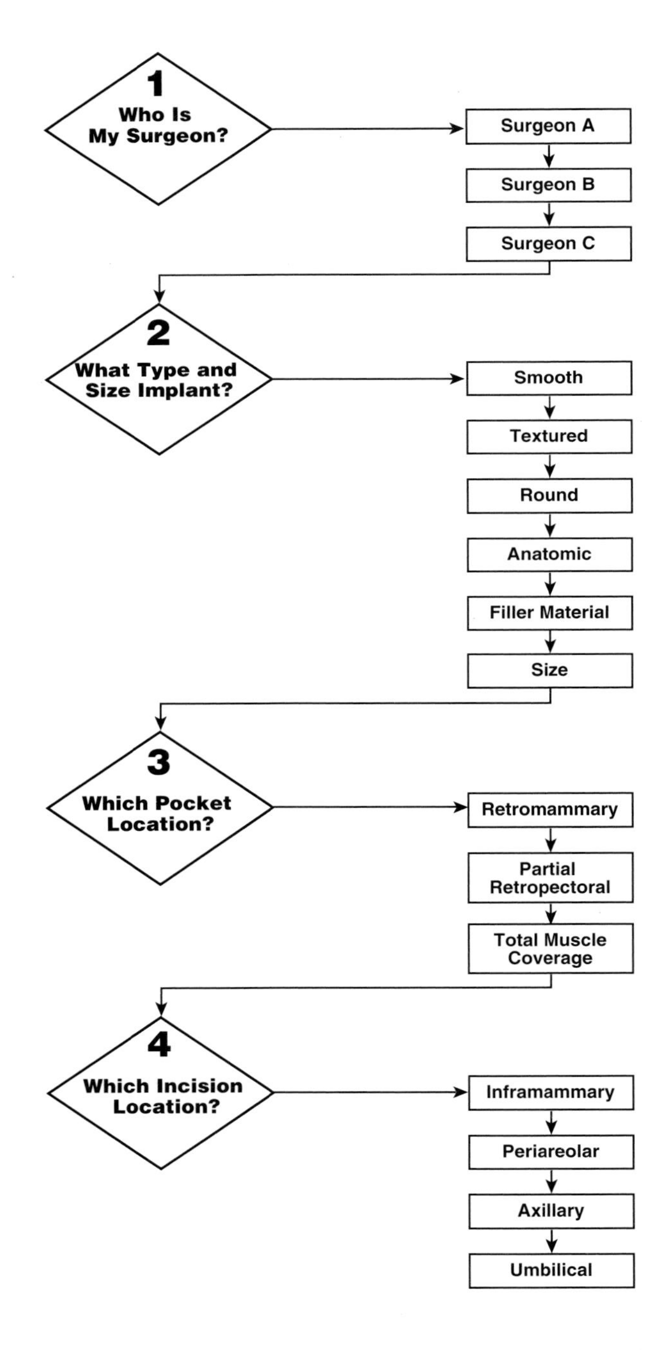

## PICKING YOUR SURGEON

**If you've done your homework, picking your surgeon is usually easy.**

Chances are good that you already know who you want to be your surgeon. One surgeon will often clearly stand out above the others, but if you are fortunate enough to have more than one surgeon who meets most of the guidelines we've given you, read on.

### How Do You Know Who's Right? The Comfort Level

First, review your checklists from Chapter 11. If you evaluated each surgeon objectively, using the criteria in the checklists, one surgeon will usually meet several criteria that other surgeons don't meet. If a surgeon clearly meets more criteria, go with that surgeon. But if you've found two or more surgeons who meet all of the objective criteria, it's time to go with your gut feeling.

**Select your surgeon based on objective criteria from your homework.**

**Assuming equal qualifications (and that doesn't often exist), go with your gut feeling.**

*Who makes you most comfortable?*
*(Never place comfort above qualifications!)*

Which surgeon listened to you best? Which do you feel best understands what you want? Which surgeon presented you the most options with the best explanation of tradeoffs? Which surgeon seemed to care the most? Which was most thorough? We've mentioned all of these criteria before, but these are the ones that should weigh heavily on your gut feelings.

If you're still not sure, make a second visit to each surgeon you're still considering. Focus on which surgeon pays the most attention to detail. Which surgeon is more patient, answering your questions, and reviewing points you've already discussed?

Look for distinguishing points to help with the final decision. ***Always focus on substance.***

In the following sections, place a checkmark beside your choices.

## PICKING THE IMPLANT

### What Type and Size Implant?

❒ ***Smooth***

Do you prefer a smooth surface implant? Why? Don't make this choice believing that you'll be less able to feel the implant because it isn't so. Tissue coverage is the main issue that affects whether you can feel an implant. The fact that a smooth wall implant can move around more than a textured is a positive and a negative. The main worry is whether smooth implants really are as good at preventing capsular contracture.

❒ ***Textured***

Most surgeons believe that textured surface implants offer a decreased risk of capsular contracture. Scientific studies confirm it! From the standpoint of logic, you should probably have a solid reason NOT to select a textured implant.

❒ ***Round***

Easier to use than an anatomic, hence, preferred by many surgeons. The main question is how to deal with the fill issues with current round implants. If you fill it to manufacturer's recommendations, the shell folds and risks visible rippling and shell failure. If you overfill, you void the manufacturer's warranty.

❒ ***Anatomic***

Looks more like a breast. More demanding of the surgeon. Offers better long-term control of upper breast fill and breast shape. Best in first-time augmentations until a surgeon has plenty of experience, then okay for reoperations. Fill volumes are defined differently by the manufacturer. You don't need to overfill (and you shouldn't) to prevent rippling and shell folding, so you don't risk shell folding, and you still get the warranty!

❒ ***Size***

If your envelope has been stretched by pregnancy, you'll need enough to fill the envelope adequately for the best result. If you've not been pregnant, a good rule of thumb is to think about enlarging the breast the amount it would enlarge during pregnancy — about a cup size. If you want an especially large breast, you must accept the inevitable consequences of your decisions. The larger the implant above 350cc, and the thinner your tissues, the greater your risks of complications, additional surgery, visible implant edges, and rippling. You need to consider what you want, and balance that with what will happen to your tissues as you age, especially with a larger implant. Best choice? Ask your surgeon to enlarge your breast proportionate to your figure, not too large — and don't ever discuss ccs. You'll definitely be happier 10 years or more later! Don't be too concerned when you hear many women say they want to be larger. They aren't thinking about the long-term consequences.

## PICKING THE POCKET LOCATION

❒ ***Retromammary*** (behind breast tissue only)

Logical if you have more than two cm. of pinch thickness of the tissues higher on your chest above your breast tissue. If your surgeon doesn't measure tissue pinch thickness, how do you know? A visual guess isn't as good as a measurement, and this has a lot to do with whether you'll see the edges of your implant. If you have adequate thickness of tissue coverage, in front of muscle offers the surgeon better control of breast shape, more control of upper fullness, and fewer tradeoffs (except, possibly, more interference with mammograms).

❒ ***Partial retropectoral*** (behind the pectoralis muscle)

If you don't have more than two cm. of pinch thickness, put the implant partially behind the pectoral muscle, regardless of the tradeoffs. You may have some distortion of the breast when the muscle contracts (that's not often), and the distance between the breasts may widen slightly over time, but both of these tradeoffs are better than putting an implant under tissues that are too thin!

❐ ***Total muscle coverage***
(behind pectoralis and serratus muscles)
This is not usually a good choice for augmentation because it has too many tradeoffs that affect the lower, outer shape of the breast and the shape and position of the fold beneath the breast. It is sometimes useful in reconstruction cases.

## PICKING THE INCISION LOCATION

❐ ***Inframammary*** (in the fold under the breast)
The most commonly used incision in breast augmentation offers surgeons the greatest degree of control in the widest range of breast types and implant types and sizes. The standard by which all other incisions must be measured. The only reasons to NOT have an inframammary incision are 1) you absolutely do not want a scar on the breast or 2) you have a documented history of hypertrophic (heavy) scarring from a surgical procedure (not an accident).

❐ ***Periareolar*** (around the areola)
A good selection if you have a history of hypertrophic scarring, or if you just prefer this location. The implant has more exposure to bacteria in breast tissue by this approach, but no scientific studies prove a higher risk of infection or capsular contracture. Nipple sensation is an issue. Nursing should not be an issue if the procedure is performed properly.

❐ ***Axillary*** (in the armpit)
The ideal location if your main goal is to get the scar off the breast. Much better control during surgery compared to the umbilical approach. The entire pocket can be created under direct vision by the surgeon using endoscopic instruments. This scar is not visible in over 90 percent of patients, even with the arms raised.

❐ ***Umbilical*** (around the belly button)
Attractive to some surgeons from a marketing standpoint, you'll find that the vast majority of highly experienced surgeons feel this approach offers much less control compared to other

approaches and unnecessarily traumatizes abdominal tissues. The entire pocket is created by tearing tissue with an expander balloon and by forceful, manual movement of the inflated device. You'll have injury with discomfort and bruising in the upper abdomen unnecessarily, and, in a few cases, you can have permanent deformity of the upper abdomen. You can't judge by pictures because many of the irregularities under the breast or in the abdomen aren't visible in standard pictures. You get all of the benefits of the umbilical approach without the tradeoffs and risks by selecting an axillary incision!

## WHAT ABOUT COSTS?

We'll cover costs in the next chapter, and discuss options for dealing with costs.

## THE NEXT STEP...

Congratulations! You've done your homework and made your choices! Now it's time to prepare for your surgery.

[CHAPTER THIRTEEN]

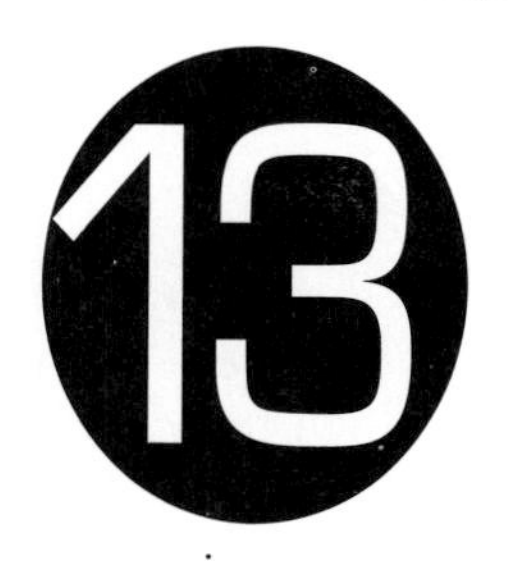


# PREPARING FOR SURGERY: What Should You Do?

***"You are ultimately responsible for thorough planning that assures optimally safe surroundings and the most pleasant experience."***

Now that you've selected your surgeon, it's time to prepare for surgery. Preparations begin with money—what are the costs, which are justified, and where does the money come from? Next, you'll need to check into the surgery facility to be sure that you're not having surgery in someone's back room (don't laugh; it happens every day in bargain basement situations). Finally, it's important to clearly understand the scheduling policies and procedures of your surgeon and make all necessary arrangements in an organized manner. A lot of arrangements are required. Preparation and organization prevent glitches that can interfere with your surgery.

## COSTS

Part of preparation is paying for your surgery. During your visits with surgeons, you collected a specific breakdown of costs from each surgeon. You've probably noticed that we didn't go into detail about *analyzing costs* while *choosing a surgeon*. The reasons?

**If you want the best result, cost should not be the only determining factor in choosing your surgeon.**

*Choose based on qualifications, and then address the costs.*

**Consider costs LAST. You can always *save* to afford the *best*.**

**You can't pay enough later to undo problems from "bargain" surgery, but you *will* pay to *correct* them!**

Are we saying that costs don't matter? No! Costs certainly DO matter. But you're not going shopping for a dress! You're asking someone to permanently make changes in your body! If costs seem unreasonable or totally out of line with other quotes, investigate! Way too high or way too low is worth looking into! Ask questions! Why the high cost? Or, how can you get such a bargain? Look carefully at the breakdown list of costs we provided. Don't just accept a "package deal" if it seems out of line.

### Bargain Surgery

Is there such a thing as "bargain surgery?" Undoubtedly, you can find low-cost plastic surgery! But a bargain? A bargain is *value* at a *lower than expected price!* The key word in this definition is "value." If, in fact, you get top-quality surgery at a lower-than-expected price, then you're getting a real value! But it's not often that you get a "steal" when buying surgery. When bargain surgery seems attractive, ask yourself:

**Am I getting top-quality surgery for this bargain price?**

*How do you know? What might you be giving up?*

**How is the bargain surgeon able to offer such a good price?**

*Cheaper implants? "Back room" surgery, instead of an accredited surgical facility? Not many cases scheduled? Less qualified?*

**How many professionals (or anyone, for that matter) do you know who do more work for LESS money — at the same quality level?**

*I don't know a single one! Less money — less work — or less quality!*

Most of the better surgeons we know charge similar surgical fees. We don't know any top-quality surgeons who offer bargain basement prices. In fact, we don't even know any above average surgeons who offer extremely low prices. If you encounter prices that are substantially lower than other surgeons you consult, beware. You may find some surgeons who do equivalent quality surgery at a lower price than other surgeons, but how do you really know until they've already operated on you? Once they've operated on you, you'll definitely have to live with the "bargain."

Our favorite answer when asked about surgeons and prices is:

**If there is anyone who knows what a surgeon is really worth, it's the surgeon.**

*To some degree, a surgical fee is a reflection of what the surgeon thinks the surgeon is worth.*

### How Much Difference Is There, Really?

"After all, this is just a breast augmentation, and breast augmentations are simple." Believe it or not, I've heard more than a few patients and surgeons make this statement. My response?

**Anything seems simple if you don't know enough to understand why it's not simple.**

*If augmentations were really simple, all results would be outstanding, and you'd see very few reoperations.*

**Your best chance for a good result is at the first surgery.**

*After that, everything gets more difficult and risky, with more tradeoffs and more costs.*

Few patients appreciate the importance of getting a good result at the first operation! We can't overemphasize this important point! If you require a reoperation, even the best surgeon is working with previously operated tissues. Things are always more difficult, and every aspect of a reoperation is less predictable. All augmentations and all surgeons are not the same. No surgeon can offer an augmentation without risks and tradeoffs, but some surgeons have better results with fewer problems compared to other surgeons!

**There is a huge difference in the range of quality of augmentation results. Never doubt that fact!**

*Don't let cost prevent you from getting the best result at the first operation, regardless of the time required or the arrangements you need to make.*

## Costs by Category — The Details

Fees for all cosmetic surgery are paid prior to surgery. We're not aware of a single quality cosmetic surgeon who does not follow this policy. To fully understand costs of your surgery, look at the breakdown of costs associated with first-time (primary) breast augmentation surgery:

**Surgeon fees** — These fees vary with the qualifications and experience of the surgeon. Cost range: $2000 - $5000; Average $3000.

**Laboratory fees** (for lab work prior to surgery) — Some basic lab tests are usually required, even if you're perfectly healthy. A routine blood count (to assure that you're not anemic or have an undiagnosed infection or other problem), and routine blood chemistry (to check factors that could affect how you react to sedative drugs or anesthesia) are common. Some surgeons require HIV testing. Some surgeons don't feel that any lab tests are necessary in a healthy individual. We disagree. To make this surgery as completely safe as possible, leave no stones unturned. Check everything. It's not worth risking a problem! Costs of lab tests? Range: $25-$200; Average $75.

**Electrocardiogram fees** (if needed) — If you are over 40 years old or have any history of any type of heart problem, your surgeon may require an electrocardiogram. Cost range: $100- $200 (including interpretation by a cardiologist); Average $150.

**Mammogram fees** (if your surgeon requires mammogram)— Many surgeons require routine mammograms before a breast augmentation, regardless of your age or family history of breast cancer. Some surgeons do not feel that routine mammograms are necessary. It's true that breast cancer is exceedingly rare in women below the age of 30-35 years, but it happens. We require mammograms on every patient because operating in the area of an undiagnosed breast cancer can have significant effects on whether that cancer can be cured. We want to take no unnecessary risks with a totally elective operation, even if a mammogram increases the costs. Have your mammogram at a breast center where they are familiar with breast augmentation patients. Cost Range: $50-$150; Average $75.

**Surgery facility fees**— This fee is the fee that a hospital or outpatient surgery facility charges for the costs of the facility and supplies required to do your surgery. If a surgeon operates in an office facility, this fee may be lumped with other fees. If this fee is excessively low, beware! The only way to substantially lower this fee is to use fewer or cheaper supplies, have fewer or less qualified personnel, or to have less equipment or cheaper equipment in the facility. Fully accreditied facilities with adequate, qualified staff and equipment must charge fees that allow them to remain in business. Cost range: $900- $1,500; Average $1,200.

**Costs of implants**—Implant costs vary widely. In Chapter 4 we discussed many of the factors affecting implant costs. Cheaper implants are usually cheaper. Enough said! If an implant fails sooner because it was cheaper with respect to quality, you didn't get a bargain. What you got was another operation with substantial costs and risks. Check carefully into implant costs and manufacturer before you implant this device! Cost range: $400- $1,400 per pair; Average $1,100.

**Anesthesia fees**—Fees for anesthesia vary according to the type of anesthesia (general versus local) and increase with the level of person giving the anesthesia [surgeon's staff, nurse (R.N.) employed by the surgeon, certified registered nurse anesthetist (C.R.N.A.), and anesthesiologist (M.D.)]—in that order. Most state-of-the-art facilities require that C.R.N.A.s or anesthesiologists to administer anesthesia—particularly general anesthesia. Cost range: $250- $750; Average $350.

**Medications fees or costs** (for before and after surgery)—Costs of medications that are required before and after surgery vary a lot from surgeon to surgeon. The more medications a surgeon requires you to take, the more you'll spend! The most common medications required for breast augmentation surgery are antibiotics and pain medications. Other medications are optional, and the necessity varies with the surgeon. The less trauma a surgeon causes, the less medication you will need. Cost range: $15- $200; Average, less than $40.

**Any other fees**—Always ask if there are any other fees! If other fees are charged, they are unusual, and you should carefully investigate the value of those charges. Special circumstances exist, but always check out any unusual fees.

### The Totals

Adding individual costs listed above, you'll find that an augmentation at today's prices will cost between $3,740 and $9,400, with an average of $5,940. What a range! In our opinion, if you pay more than $7,000 for a top-quality augmentation, you are paying too much. If you pay less than $4,500 today, beware!

## FINANCING FOR COSMETIC SURGERY

Financing options are available for patients desiring breast augmentation who cannot or don't wish to pay with cash or check. Common options include credit cards, bank financing, and finance companies specializing in cosmetic surgery. Let's examine these options.

**Credit cards**—A good option for those who 1) want to take advantage of payments over time or 2) want to take advantage of special perks associated with certain credit cards (airline free travel miles, for example). The downsides? Most credit cards charge high rates of interest compared to bank financing and other financing options. Spending limits may not be adequate to charge all surgical costs.

**Bank financing** — Banks usually offer better interest rates compared to credit cards, depending on your credit rating and banking relationships. Check with your bank or ask your surgeon about banks that finance cosmetic surgery.

**Finance companies** — Until recently, most finance companies that offered financing for cosmetic surgery charged exceedingly high interest rates and offered financing only when a patient selected a surgeon that had an agreement with the finance company. Needless to say, if a finance company is taking a portion of a surgeon's fee to refer you to the surgeon, you are hardly choosing a surgeon based on all of the information we've given you. Always choose your surgeon based on *qualifications* we've listed for you — *then arrange financing!* Today, there are better financing options for patients than before, but you must be very careful. Be sure that you understand the interest rates, payment options, and late or default penalties before arranging any financing. With better financing companies, the interest rate you'll be charged is directly related to your credit rating. The better your credit rating, the lower the rate of interest. Remember, the money you are borrowing is unsecured. If you don't pay, what can the finance company repossess? As a result, you'll pay higher interest rates compared to a secured loan.

## The Realities of Financing

**You can't afford what you can't afford.**

*Financing increases the costs for your surgery. Be sure your budget can support the increase!*

For many women, the best financing option is to save until you can pay cash or check for your breast augmentation. Meanwhile, you can learn more and better research your options, and the options only get better. If you choose financing, be absolutely sure that your income and budget will support the payments, and be sure that getting the operation a bit sooner is worth the increased cost of financing! If you find good financing and feel that's the best option for you—fine—but be sure to look at the total cost with and without financing, so you can place a dollar value on having the operation sooner!

## SURGERY FACILITIES

For the greatest safety, you want to have your breast augmentation in an *accredited surgical facility*. What does that mean? How do you know? What difference does it make? What type of accreditation is adequate?

### Facility Accreditation

"Accredited" means that a surgical facility has passed rigorous examination to assure that the equipment and procedures of the facility meet standards for optimal safety. To become accredited, a surgery facility must conform to a huge number of rigorous standards and requirements. Once the facility meets written standards, examiners perform an on-site inspection visit to assure full compliance with all standards, regulations, and requirements.

### Who Accredits Surgery Facilities? How Do You Know?

The two most well-known and well-respected accrediting bodies are the Joint Commission on Accreditation of Hospitals (JCAH) and the American Association for Accreditation of Ambulatory Surgery Facilities (AAAASF). The regulations are as long as the names—a pain to those who must pass examination but an asset to patients. The JCAH usually accredits hospital facilities and hospital-based outpatient surgery facilities. The AAAASF specializes in accrediting outpatient or ambulatory surgery facilities, regardless of where they are based. How do you know if a facility is accredited? Ask to see the accreditation certificate of the facility where you'll have surgery. Often it's posted in the facility. Your surgeon should know.

## What Accreditation Is Adequate?

If you want to assure that a surgical facility is properly equipped and staffed, and follows procedures for optimal safety, we'd look for a facility accredited by the JCAH or AAAASF. Other accreditation bodies exist, but these two are most widely respected at this time. If a facility is not accredited, or if it is accredited by a less well-known organization, be very careful. How important is accreditation?

**Would you climb aboard the space shuttle if you were not sure the equipment and check-out procedures were optimal?**

*An accredited surgical facility assures you that specific, high standards have been met.*

One of the requirements of accreditation is to assure that personnel are trained, and procedures and equipment are in place to deal with any emergency from a power outage to cardiac arrest. Ask your surgeon for additional information about surgical facilities and emergency contingency plans. If you have doubts, ask other medical personnel you know or other surgeons about a facility.

**If a facility is *not accredited,* ask to see the facility. Then visit an *accredited* facility.**

*With no special expertise, you should notice a significant difference.*

If you're not comfortable with a surgical facility, don't have surgery there. This is an important area that's often overlooked by patients — especially patients seeking bargain surgery. It's your job to ask and assure that you're having surgery under the best circumstances. If a problem occurs and you haven't done your homework to assure that you're in the best of surroundings, it's too late.

## WHAT TO LOOK FOR IN A SURGERY FACILITY— THE THINGS WE THINK ARE IMPORTANT

When we designed our outpatient surgery facility, we tried to put ourselves in your place. What would we want if we were coming to this facility to have surgery? And how could we make it totally state-of-the-art medically, but make you feel less apprehensive compared to a hospital type setting?

The surroundings and personnel in a surgery center can have a significant impact on your experience as a patient. If the surroundings and personnel are warm and personal (Figure 13-1), more like at home, you'll be more comfortable. The rooms where you will change and prepare for surgery need not be extravagant, but should be comfortable (Figure 13-2), with reading material, television, and personnel immediately available. Computer information systems should be state-of-the-art (Figure 13-3), and the nursing station (Figure 13-4) should be immediately adjacent to your preparation and recovery rooms.

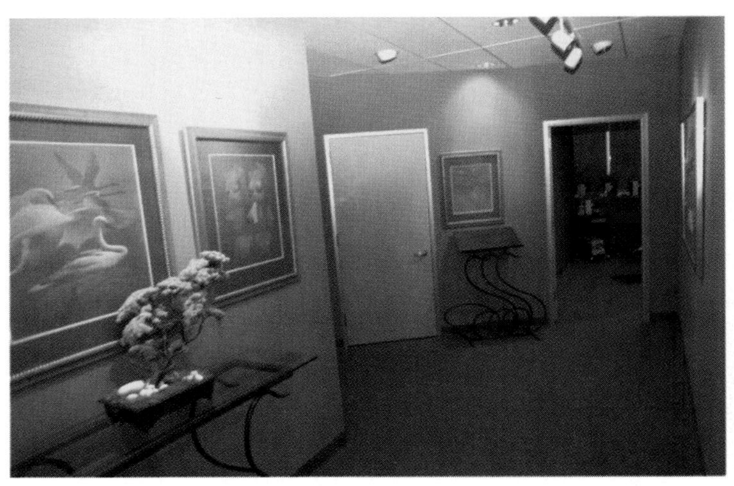

**Figure 13-1.**

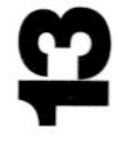



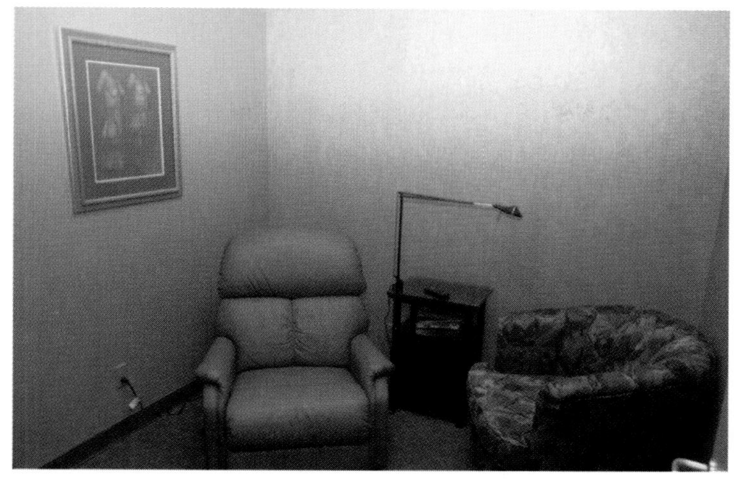

**Figure 13-2.**

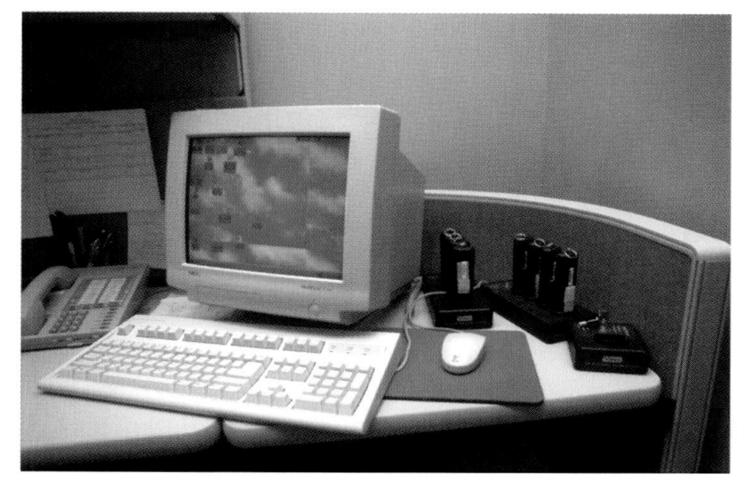

**Figure 13-3.**

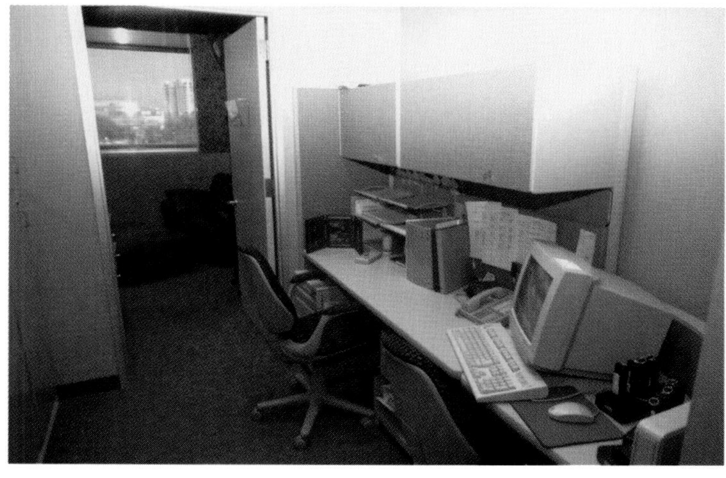

**Figure 13-4.**

The operating rooms should appear state-of-the-art, spotlessly clean and equipped with the most up-to-date equipment (Figure 13-5, A-D). Ideally, computer systems will also be present in the operating rooms that allow the surgeon access to your preoperative photographs and patient data (Figure 13-6). The recovery area should be immediately adjacent to the operating rooms (Figure 13-7) and should be state-of-the-art equipped.

**Figure 13-5.**

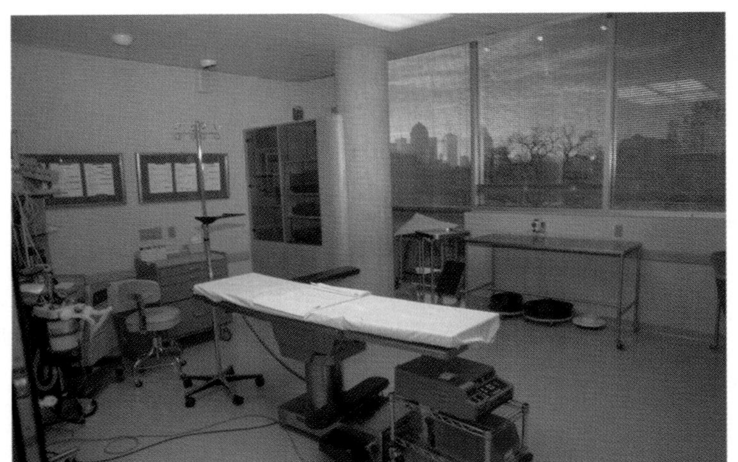

**A.**

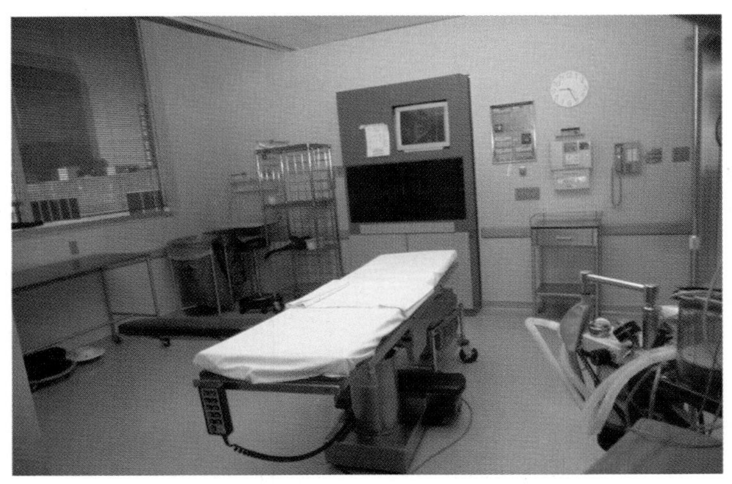

**B.**

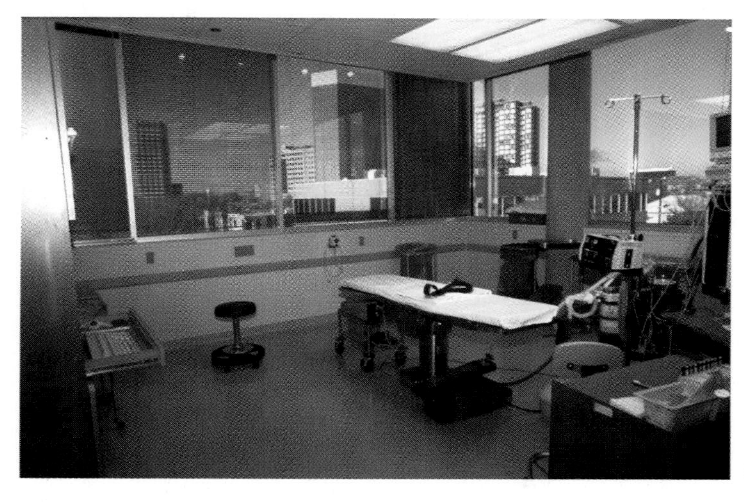

C.

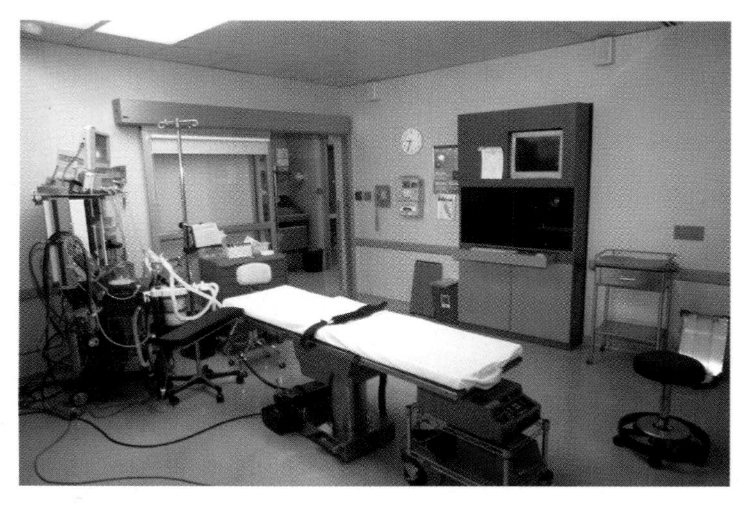

D.

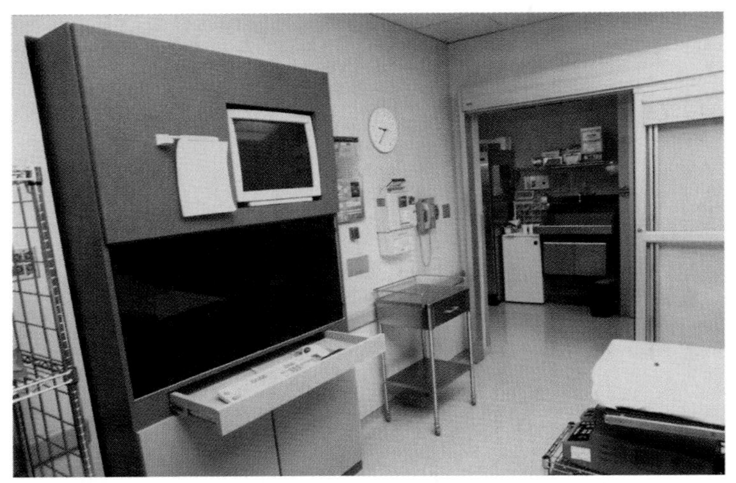

**Figure 13-6.**

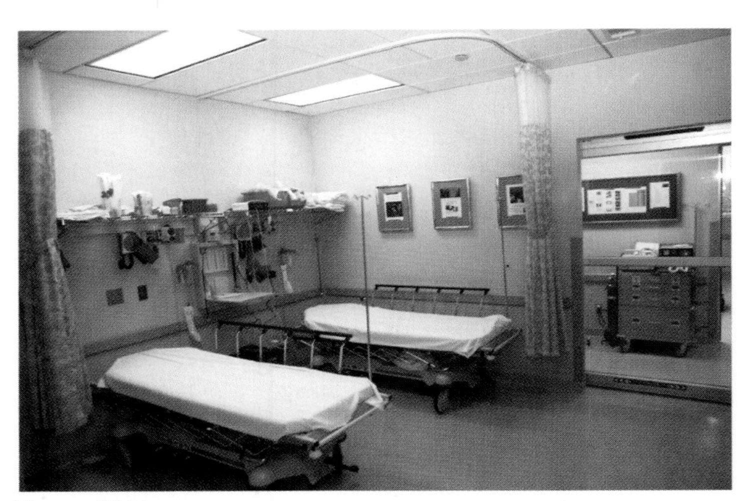

**Figure 13-7.**

Some facilities may also provide overnight accommodations with immediately adjacent, one-on-one nursing care for patients who need overnight care after more extensive procedures (Figure 13-8 A,B). Some centers also provide other special services, such as makeup and skin care after surgery (Figure 13-9), but these ancillary services are certainly not essential.

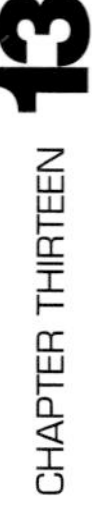


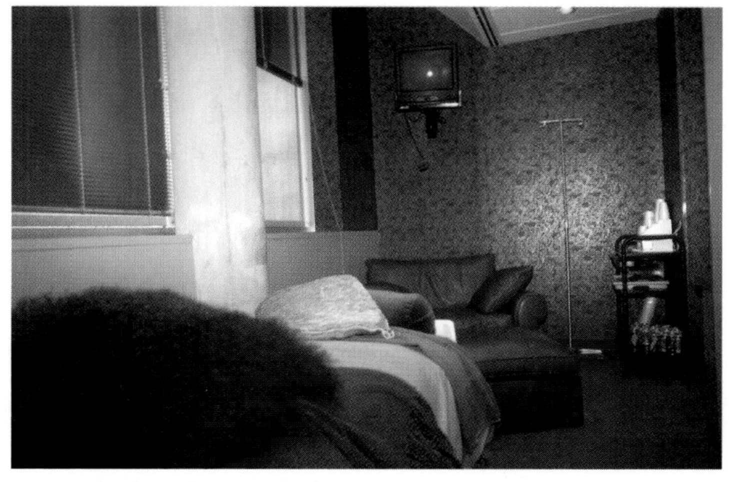

**Figure 13-8.**

**A.**

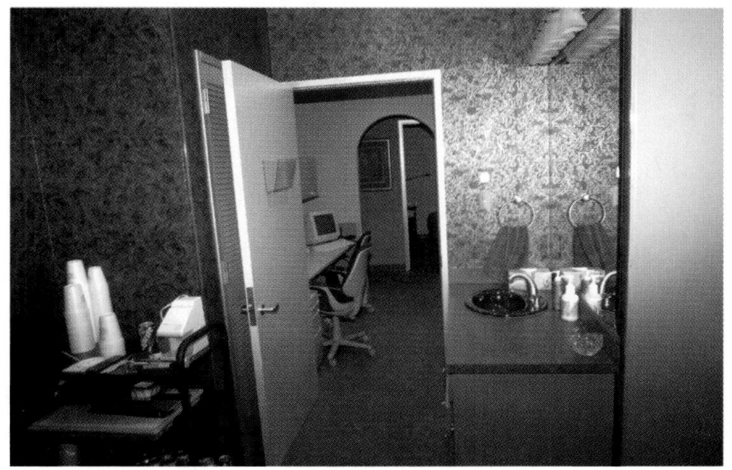

**B.**

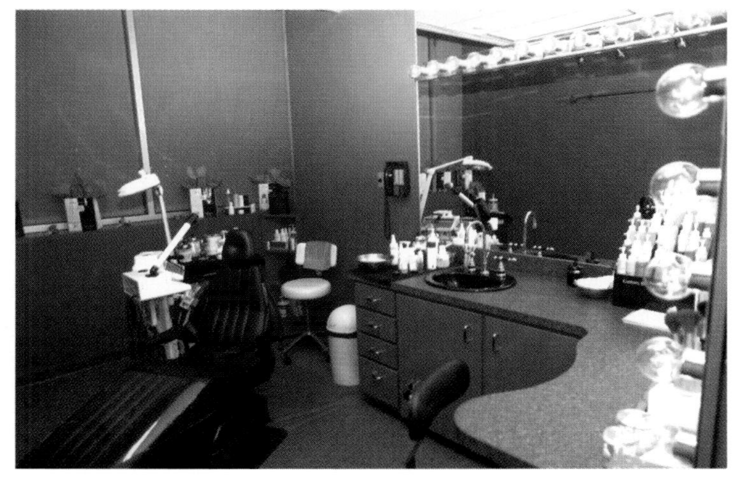

**Figure 13-9..**

## SCHEDULING POLICIES AND PROCEDURES

When you are ready to schedule your surgery, the surgeon's staff will help with all the necessary arrangements. Specific scheduling policies and procedures are necessary to assure that arrangements are correct to the smallest detail. These procedures can vary among different surgeons, but each of the following activities should occur before arrangements are final.

### A Surgical Arrangements Checklist...

- ❑ Select a date for surgery.
- ❑ Review surgeon's financial policies and policies for refunds.
- ❑ Pay scheduling deposit if surgeon requires.
- ❑ Sign informed consent documents and operative consent forms.
- ❑ Review and sign implant manufacturer's documents:
    - ❑ Implant package insert
    - ❑ Terms of implant guarantee
    - ❑ Manufacturer's consent forms (if applicable)
    - ❑ Verify that surgeon will register your implants with the national implant registry.
- ❑ Schedule lab tests and mammography.
- ❑ Review medications to avoid and medications to take before surgery.
- ❑ Review instructions for the night before surgery.
- ❑ Review instructions for the day of surgery.

### Selecting a Date for Surgery

Check your schedule carefully before discussing dates with your surgeon's staff. Select a time at least one month in advance that allows you to have surgery without interfering with any other activities. Depending on the time required for recovery (you should already know this from information you've gathered from your surgeon), you'll need from three to 10 or more days

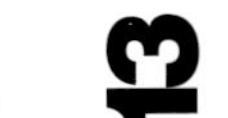



off work. Try to select at least *two time periods* when you could have surgery and recover, *the first period at least one month in advance*. You need some flexibility to fit your surgeon's schedule.

Discuss available times with your surgeon's staff. The staff should be helpful and offer you alternative times, but you should also try to be helpful and flexible, if possible.

**If you have a very specific time that you want to have surgery, the further in advance that you schedule, the more likely a busy surgeon can meet your needs.**

**If you are pressured to schedule, or if you hear, "Why don't we just do this tomorrow?"**
**RUN AWAY!**

*The best surgeons usually can't operate on you the next day!*

### Financial Policies and Conditions of Refunds

If you did not already receive written information from your surgeon detailing financial policies and procedures, ask for a written summary when you schedule. Every credible surgeon should provide you specific, written information that details all financial policies. Conditions for refunds vary from surgeon to surgeon, but you should know the details before you schedule! What if your child becomes ill the day before surgery? What if you just decide you'd rather have your hair done than have surgery on the day it's scheduled? Which fees are payable in advance of surgery, and when are they due? The answers to each of these questions should be spelled out in written financial policies. Read the information carefully. You'll be required to follow these policies!

### Scheduling Deposits

Most busy, experienced, highly-qualified surgeons require a scheduling deposit when you select a surgery date and schedule your surgery. An average scheduling deposit is 10-20 percent of the surgeon's fee, payable at the time of scheduling to reserve a surgery date. If a conflict occurs that prevents your having surgery on the date scheduled, most surgeons will reschedule your surgery once, but the scheduling deposit is usually non-refundable if you cancel more than once. Scheduling deposits are necessary because you are reserving the surgeon's time and the time of many personnel. If you cancel, the surgical facility must pay these personnel, and the surgeon wastes time that could have been spent productively.

### Signing Informed Consent Documents

Informed consent documents and operative consent forms are essential to document your understanding and acceptance of the potential benefits, tradeoffs, and risks associated with your surgery. You will be required to sign these forms prior to surgery. Ideally, you should discuss the information contained in these forms with your surgeon and the surgeon's staff well in advance of surgery. Most surgeons provide you copies of all operative consent forms well in advance of surgery. Information on these documents should not be new! You should have heard all of it before, during your patient educator visits and surgeon consultation.

**Read all informed consent documents and operative permits carefully well in advance of your surgery.**

*Write down any questions, and be sure they are answered to your satisfaction before signing any documents!*

When you read all of the risks and possible problems in the informed consent documents, don't be surprised if you feel a bit frightened. You should! These documents are designed to present you the very worst-case scenarios and risks, regardless of how rarely they may occur. If you don't understand or feel that you can't accept any of the information in the informed consent documents, discuss your concerns with your surgeon, or don't have the surgery! The time for understanding is before your surgery!

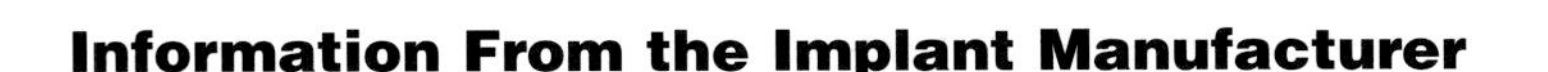

## Information From the Implant Manufacturer

At the very least, your surgeon should provide you 1) a copy of the package insert that comes with your implants, 2) terms of the implant guarantee, 3) any required manufacturer's consent forms, and 4) verification that your implants will be recorded in an implant registry program. The package insert contains a lot of information from the manufacturer that you should read and understand before having an implant device placed in your body. Terms of implant guarantees vary widely and are critically important. Read the guarantee carefully before you accept a surgeon's recommendation of implant! If the manufacturer requires additional consent forms, wonderful! That means the manufacturer cares about your being informed! Finally, ask your surgeon if your implant information will be recorded at surgery and forms completed and submitted to assure that your implants are registered in the national implant registry program. If you have any questions about any of the information contained in these documents, ask your surgeon or contact the manufacturer before you sign or have surgery!

## Scheduling Lab Tests and Mammography

Most surgeons require blood tests within two weeks of your scheduled surgery. Mammograms and electrocardiograms are usually acceptable if they have been performed within one year of your surgery date. Your surgeon's staff will assist with arranging for all necessary tests prior to surgery. Remember that these tests are important to assure your safety! Be absolutely certain to keep your appointments to have these tests done on schedule!

## Medications to Avoid and Medications to Take

Every surgeon should provide a list of medications to avoid prior to surgery. The exact medications can vary from surgeon to surgeon, but some important basics:

**Be sure that your surgeon is aware of all medications that you are taking.**

**Avoid all medications that contain aspirin for at least two weeks prior to surgery.**

*Read the labels carefully for all over-the-counter medications. Many contain aspirin.*

**Be very careful about herbs and herbal medicines.**

*If you are using any herbal preparations, discuss them with your surgeon!*

Aspirin and aspirin-containing products can interfere with your blood-clotting mechanisms and cause bleeding during and after surgery! Even one aspirin can cause problems within two weeks of surgery! Some herbs and herbal medicines can cause similar problems. Other medications can interfere with your anesthesia or produce undesirable effects if combined with anesthetic drugs. Your surgeon can't prevent these problems if you don't make the surgeon aware of medicines or herbs that you are taking before surgery.

### Instructions for the Night Before

Normally, you'll be somewhat apprehensive the night before surgery! Some patients are virtual basket cases! Generally, the better informed you are, the more comfortable you'll feel the night before surgery, but some apprehension is natural. Your surgeon will provide specific instructions for the night before surgery, but the most important basics are:

**Never eat or drink anything after midnight the night before surgery.**

*If you do, material in your stomach can cause you to regurgitate, aspirate, and possibly die during surgery!*

Sound drastic? It is drastic! Something as simple as having an empty stomach when you receive any sedative or anesthetic medicine is critically important to your safety! Don't cheat. Even if you think you're going into withdrawal without your coffee or Diet Coke in the morning!

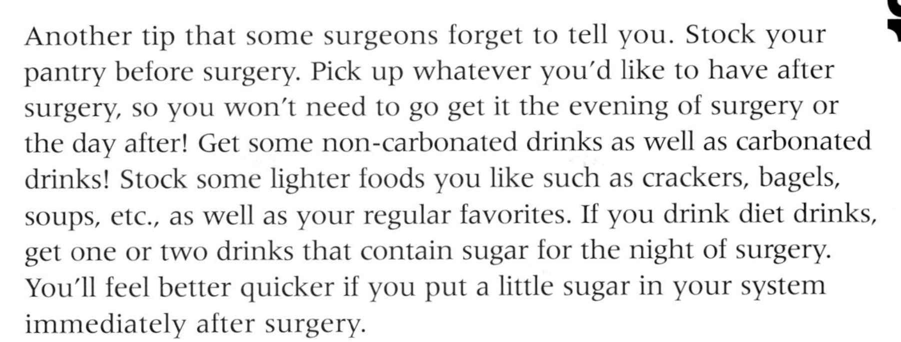

Another tip that some surgeons forget to tell you. Stock your pantry before surgery. Pick up whatever you'd like to have after surgery, so you won't need to go get it the evening of surgery or the day after! Get some non-carbonated drinks as well as carbonated drinks! Stock some lighter foods you like such as crackers, bagels, soups, etc., as well as your regular favorites. If you drink diet drinks, get one or two drinks that contain sugar for the night of surgery. You'll feel better quicker if you put a little sugar in your system immediately after surgery.

Ask your surgeon to give you any prescriptions you'll need after surgery so that you can pick them up before surgery. Just one less thing you'll need to worry about!

## Instructions for the Day of Surgery

You should receive specific instructions for the day of surgery, and these instructions can also vary among different surgeons. A couple of essentials:

**Wear very comfortable clothing like a jogging suit that buttons or zips up the front.**

*You won't enjoy tugging something on over your head.*

**Make arrangements for someone to drive you home from the surgery facility and be with you overnight.**

*You'll receive medications that make driving yourself unsafe!*

**Leave off your eye makeup, otherwise you'll wake up with it in your eyes!**

*Protective eye lubricants during surgery make a total mess of makeup!*

**Leave your jewelry and valuables at home!**

Some surgical facilities prefer that you don't wear any type of makeup, nail polish, or belly button rings, but most facilities can work around these things that make you feel and look better! Just ask, or read the instructions you're given!

## THE NEXT STEP...

Believe it or not, it's time to do it! You've gone through all the steps to get to the top of the stairs in the best possible manner, and now you're there! Try to relax as much as possible with the assurance that you've done your part toward getting the best breast! In the following chapters, we'll tell you what to expect during your recovery and suggestions for living with your new breasts!

[CHAPTER FOURTEEN]

# RECOVERY: What to Expect

***"The better your surgeon performs, and the better you follow instructions, the more rapidly you will recover. Full normal activity in 3 days or less is routine in over 90% of our patients."***

Recovering from an augmentation is different than preparing for it! During preparation, there were many things that you could actively do to change the course of events. During recovery, your body does most of the work automatically—provided you don't expect everything to happen quickly and provided you don't mess with the autopilot! If you understand what's normal, what to expect, and some of the reasons behind the "do's" and "don'ts," the recovery process will be smoother.

**The better your surgeon performs, and the better you follow instructions, the more rapidly you will recover.**

*Full, normal activity in 3 days or less is routine in over 90% of our patients.*

## RECOVERY IS VARIABLE

Is recovery similar from patient to patient? Sometimes, but not necessarily! What is recovery like? The answer varies from patient to patient and from surgeon to surgeon. If you understand some of the reasons for variations in recovery, the whole process should be easier.

### Patient Variations

Your body and your breast tissues are different than other women. The tighter your breast skin envelope and the more surgical manipulation required, the more tightness and tenderness you can expect following surgery. Everyone has some tightness and tenderness, but the amount varies according to what's required of your tissues. Generally, if you've had children prior to your augmentation, your tissues have been previously stretched, and you'll feel less tightness for a shorter time. If your skin is very tight and has never been stretched by pregnancy, you'll feel tighter longer.

Some patients are more tolerant of discomfort than others. Some patients are better able to get moving after surgery despite discomfort. Some patients follow instructions better than others.

**Your individual pain tolerance, motivation, and ability to follow instructions will affect your recovery.**

*Adopt a positive attitude, follow instructions, and get well sooner!*

## Surgeon Variations

A surgeon can't change what you bring the surgeon to work with. But *how* the surgeon works with what you bring can affect your recovery. **The less surgical trauma the surgeon causes to your tissues, the easier and shorter your recovery**. Hopefully, you learned from Chapter 8 how to ask the right questions about recovery before surgery to help select a surgeon who minimizes surgical trauma.

If your tissues are thin and submuscular placement of the implant was necessary for adequate tissue coverage of your implant, you'll have more tenderness compared to patients whose implants are placed over the muscle. But this is a short-term inconvenience for long-term protection against seeing edges of your implant and possibly a greater risk of capsular contracture! If your surgeon used blunt dissection techniques, you can expect more tenderness and the possible inconvenience of drain tubes for a few days.

**The easier your surgeon expects your recovery to be, the shorter the list of postoperative instructions.**

*The more the surgeon can do in the operating room, the less you'll be burdened with after surgery.*

Surgeons' postoperative instructions vary a lot. The most important thing to remember is to follow your surgeon's instructions! A surgeon knows what is done in the operating room, and because of that, what needs to be done or not done after surgery!

**Don't try to outthink your surgeon! Follow your surgeon's instructions!**

*And don't follow your friend's postoperative instructions if she had a different surgeon.*

If you talk to several women who've had breast augmentation, you'll find a tremendous amount of variation in their recovery experiences. If your surgeon is giving you instructions that sound a lot simpler than what you've heard, be grateful! Your surgeon is probably doing a lot of things in the operating room that allow you to have an easier and shorter recovery! If you hear from another patient that you shouldn't lift your arms, lift your child, or drive your car and your surgeon is telling you it's okay to do all these things immediately, go for it! Your surgeon just made your life easier! On the other hand, if your surgeon tells you NOT to do these things, there's a reason! Always follow instructions!

### Your Surgeon's Staff

Your surgeon's staff is an extension of your surgeon! The goal is to help you get better sooner, so it's important to follow the staff's advice and instructions as well! When a person calls to check on you, listen carefully to that person's questions and instructions. The information you convey will help the staff make the best recommendations to speed your recovery. Some surgeons have better staff than others. The more knowledgeable the surgeon's staff, the better they can help answer your questions and give you optimal advice. If you're in doubt about anything after speaking with staff, ask to speak directly with your surgeon or ask for an appointment to see your surgeon.

## THE MOST IMPORTANT DOs

The following is a checklist of the most important DOs that apply to almost all postoperative augmentation patients:

- ❑ Follow your surgeon's instructions to the letter! Don't try to outthink your surgeon!
- ❑ Stay hydrated! Drink plenty of fluids for the first few days after surgery.
- ❑ Eat! And eat well! You need nutrition to heal!
- ❑ Never take any pain medication on an empty stomach—it'll get even emptier!
- ❑ Resume normal activity as soon as possible, following your surgeon's instructions.
- ❑ Read your postoperative instruction sheets. They'll help you expect what's normal!
- ❑ Expect to be frustrated that your tissues don't change according to your schedule.
- ❑ Expect to be too big, too high, and too tight for a few weeks.
- ❑ Expect differences and constant changes in size and shape of your breasts for three to six weeks.
- ❑ Get out of the house and do something. Staring does not reduce swelling and tightness.
- ❑ If anything seems wrong, check your written instructions and information, then call your surgeon!

## THE MOST IMPORTANT DON'Ts

Your surgeon may give you a longer list of things to avoid, but the following is a basic checklist of don'ts that we use following augmentation:

- ❑ Avoid any type of aerobic activities or anything that creates a significant increase in your pulse for two weeks. Walking is okay; fast walking is not. Sex is okay, but olympic sex is not!

- ❑ Don't lift heavy objects (over 30-40 lbs.) or strain hard for two weeks.
- ❑ Don't take too many pain pills. Pain pills can constipate you.
- ❑ Avoid whatever else your surgeon tells you to avoid.

## PAIN MEDICATIONS—RELIEF VERSUS RECOVERY

**Pain medications are a two-edged sword. The less you need, the better!**

*They're necessary for relief, but they can interfere with recovery!*

Pain medications definitely relieve discomfort, but they all have side effects that can interfere with recovery. The stronger the pain medication, the more relief of discomfort, but the more side effects! One of the most important things you can do to get better is to get moving! The trick is to use enough pain medications to dull the discomfort at first. As soon as you get moving, things get better, and you'll need less pain medication!

**The three worst routine side effects of pain medications are: Drowsiness, nausea, and constipation.**

*If you're sleepy, nauseated, and constipated, nothing's going to get moving!*

**If you don't get moving, your recovery will definitely be longer and more difficult.**

*Get moving doesn't mean trying to be Olympo-woman. Just resume normal activities!*

Any pain medication can cause nausea if you take it on an empty stomach. I can't tell you how many patients have told us that they are "allergic" to codeine or Demerol! When asked what type of allergic reaction they've had, the answer is almost always the same, "It makes me nauseated!" Nausea to pain medications is not an allergic reaction. It's a side effect. The stronger the pain medication, the more likely it will cause nausea, especially if taken on an empty stomach.

**Always put something in your stomach before taking pain medications.**

*Crackers, toast, bagel — just something!*

Pain medications can be extremely habit forming quickly. If you insist on stronger, narcotic pain medications, you're often creating a problem instead of solving one. Using today's surgical techniques, you should not need any pain medications that are stronger than codeine or a codeine-equivalent drug. Over 90 percent of our patients take codeine, synthetic codeine or codeine-equivalent strength medications for 48-72 hours, then switch to Extra Strength Tylenol. At least 50 percent don't take any prescription pain medication after 48 hours! You may require more than this, but you shouldn't require stronger narcotic drugs. There are countless examples of patients who have become addicted to stronger pain medications such as Demerol, Tylox, Percodan, or Valium after taking them for as little as seven days! Don't be one of them!

## WHAT TO EXPECT THAT'S NORMAL

**If you know what to expect that's normal, you'll be less frightened or concerned.**

*If you're more knowledgeable and less concerned, recovery is much easier!*

When you get concerned about something, first consult the following checklist! Everything on this list is normal following augmentation, so expect it! And continue to expect it for at least six weeks after surgery! If it's gone before then, you'll be pleasantly surprised!

- ❏ They don't match! My breasts are a different size and shape! And they're different every day!
- ❏ They're too high!
- ❏ They're too big!

- ❑ They're too tight!
- ❑ They're too swollen!
- ❑ They're too firm!
- ❑ I hear sloshing inside my breasts!
- ❑ They don't move!
- ❑ They're numb or they're too sensitive or I have weird sensations!
- ❑ I can't lie on them because they feel like basketballs!
- ❑ My waist has disappeared!
- ❑ The magic time when they'll feel like they belong to me is three months!

Remember, ***breasts never match!*** God couldn't make them match, and neither can your surgeon. Early after your surgery, one will always swell more than the other, adding to the difference. All of that is normal! Your breasts are supposed to feel *too big, too tight, too firm, too swollen, and weird!* Remember, yesterday you didn't have this much inside your breast. It takes your skin envelope time to adapt and stretch, and until it does, you'll feel all these sensations! After surgery, with or without drain tubes, you'll produce a little fluid inside the pocket, around your implants. This fluid, combined with a small amount of air that stays in the pocket from surgery, can produce a sloshing sound that you may or may not hear for a week or two after surgery. Don't worry. Your body will absorb all of this in due time! As long as your skin is tight from being filled, your breasts won't move normally. When the skin stretches, they will move!

The larger your implants or the tighter your skin envelope, the more stretch the implant will put on sensory nerves. When nerves are stretched, they usually do one of three things: Go numb, get more sensitive, send weird sensations to your brain, or all three. Sensory changes are very variable and very unpredictable—regardless of the surgical technique. Sensory changes can take a long time to resolve, as much as two years in rare cases. Most patients' sensory changes are resolved by one year, but some take even longer. Other patients experience virtually no problems with sensation. It's just very unpredictable!

There is something magic about three months! At about three months, most of our patients feel their implants are a normal part of their body. They stop referring to "them" and start talking about "my breasts!" The reason that this time period is magic is because your tissues will require about 3 months to return to a more normal state that you don't constantly notice as "different."

## WHAT'S NOT NORMAL ... CONTACT YOUR SURGEON

If you develop any of the following, you should contact your surgeon:

- ❑ Fever higher than 102 degrees or fever with chills
- ❑ One breast that is much, much larger than the other
- ❑ One breast that appears much more bruised than the other
- ❑ Noticeable redness and tenderness in any area of the breast
- ❑ Any drainage from your incision area after three days
- ❑ Any unusual discomfort
- ❑ Any breathing problems
- ❑ Any other symptoms that your surgeon advises you to call about

## A TYPICAL RECOVERY WITH OUR PATIENTS

The following is a description of a routine recovery in our augmentation patients.

## The Night of Surgery

You leave the surgery facility a bit drowsy, but comfortable. When you arrive home, make yourself comfortable on the couch or in bed. Drink some liquids and eat a few crackers, or some toast or a bagel. Just get something in your stomach. If you are uncomfortable, take a pain pill after getting something in your stomach, and expect to relax and get drowsy afterwards. You'll probably doze on and off in the afternoon and evening. You will have already raised your arms to shoulder height or above your head before you left the surgery center, but after you're home, do it again at least three times before bedtime! At first, just lift your arms until they are level with your shoulders. If you feel tightness but no pain, go ahead and lift them above your head. Lower them, and repeat two more times. Repeat this entire sequence three times before bedtime, and you'll be amazed at how much easier the rest of your recovery will be!

When you feel really hungry, provided you didn't have nausea with lighter foods and drinks, eat whatever you'd like. Don't pig out, but feel free to eat anything that sounds good! When you're ready to go to sleep for the night (provided you've put food in your stomach), take two pain pills and enjoy your rest. If you awake during the night, rearrange yourself to get comfortable, and try to go back to sleep without additional pain pills. Sometimes, hugging a pillow to your chest can make you feel more comfortable. If you want to slip into a soft bra or jog bra, feel free to try it. You can't harm anything! Most of our patients are more comfortable without a bra, but you can treat your breasts as normal breasts. Wear or not wear a bra according to your comfort!

## The Morning After Surgery

When you awaken in the morning, you'll feel stiff! That's normal! Roll to your side and sit up to get out of bed. Relax in a comfortable chair or on the couch, and have a light breakfast of whatever you like. As soon as you get something in your stomach, take one pain pill, and enjoy the rest of your breakfast. When you feel the pain pill taking effect (you'll feel less stiff with less discomfort), get into a very warm shower and let the water run over your shoulders, chest and breasts for five to 10 minutes. Then, gradually lift your arms above your head and wash your hair! Yes, you can do it! You won't believe how much better you'll feel after getting your arms moving! Expect to feel some tightness at first. That's normal. You won't hurt anything by moving your arms and lifting them above your head!

If you're feeling good, it's fine to go out to shop, to a movie, or anything else you'd like to do. Don't plan a whole day of anything. You'll get tired easily for the first two or three days, so plan to do something, then come home and relax. There's no reason you can't drive as soon as you feel like it. Most of our patients drive within the first three days, but not if you're taking any prescription pain pills! The sooner you can switch to Extra Strength Tylenol or Advil, the better. Whenever you feel discomfort, try two or three of these over-the-counter medications instead of prescription pain pills. Save your prescription pain pills for bedtime, so you'll sleep better.

While we're on the subject of pain pills, you should be aware that some surgeons do not recommend Advil or other forms of ibuprofen because they feel that these medications can interfere with normal blood-clotting mechanisms. Over the past 10 years, we have used Advil and other forms of ibuprofen in over 1500 patients, have had no increased rates of bleeding, and find these medications invaluable in shortening recovery and avoiding the side effects and addiction potential of stronger medications.

As soon as you feel like picking up normal weight objects or your small children, do it! Most of our patients with small children are able to pick them up by the day following surgery! Again, you won't hurt anything by picking up normal weight objects. Just avoid heavy objects and straining.

Be sure to drink plenty of liquids, and take it easy on prescription pain medications to avoid constipation. Remember, we want everything moving!

## The First Two Days Following Surgery

Don't be surprised if you feel bloated! You received fluids during surgery, and you'll accumulate some swelling around your breasts and chest. As this swelling gravitates downward, you'll begin to feel that your waist is getting bigger. Don't panic! All this will resolve, and you'll go to the bathroom more often, over the next two to four days.

**The first two days following surgery are filled with the most nuisances and discomfort.**

*After two days, start thinking three weeks.*

Immediately, try to get back into most of your normal activities. The sooner the better! Just plan your days to allow for some rest if you get tired in the afternoons.

## The First Three Weeks

**Listen to your body when it comes to all activity.**

*If something is too stressful, stop and try it again tomorrow!*

Your body will tell you what you need to know if you'll just listen! That doesn't mean to stop everything at the least sign of discomfort. Go ahead and move. But if something hurts, back off! Try again tomorrow or the next day! Whenever you're comfortable, sex is fine! You probably won't be overly amorous if someone puts too much pressure on your breasts the first few days, but there are ways around too much pressure! "Looks good, feels bad" takes on a whole new meaning until your breasts feel better! Your significant other may require some coaching and understanding (or a leash) at first! Be creative when you feel like it, but save Olympic-level sex for a few weeks down the road.

During the first three weeks, your breasts will feel very tight! For most patients, the worst tightness is in the first three days, but this begins to decrease a lot after the first week! If your skin was very tight before surgery, expect the tightness to take longer to resolve! You'll get used to it more after three or four days, and it won't constantly occupy your mind after the first week. By three weeks, you'll notice some tightness, but you won't think about it much.

If you heard some sloshing in your breasts, that will usually be gone in three weeks or less. Numbness, excessive sensitivity, and strange feelings (like pin pricks or electric shocks) are all normal. Most of these sensory changes won't disappear in the first three weeks. They take much longer to return to normal. Don't make any judgements about sensation for at least six months to one year, because sensation will continue to improve.

Wearing a bra is totally up to you. If you're more comfortable in a bra (any type), wear it. If you want to create a certain look, wear it. If you're more comfortable *out of a bra*, don't wear one. Despite anything you might hear, *a bra should not affect the results of your surgery* the way we perform the surgery. We've used this regimen in over 2,000 patients, and have found that you know better about what makes you comfortable than anyone else. It's up to us to find ways to give you the choice of bra or no bra according to your comfort.

**By the end of three weeks, most of the worst nuisances are over, but your breasts still won't feel like they really belong to you!**

*After three weeks, start thinking three months.*

## The First Three Months

Most of the time during the first three months, you'll refer to your breasts as "them." They simply won't feel like they belong to you. There are "things" inside your breasts. After the first three weeks, the skin begins to relax faster, but you don't notice day by day. As the skin relaxes, the excessive upper fullness begins to decrease, provided you haven't selected an excessively large implant for your tissue characteristics. The implants aren't really "dropping," but they appear to be. What's really happening? As the lower skin stretches, it's not pushing back against the implant as hard between the nipple and the fold under your breast. As pressure on the lower implant decreases, the filler inside the implant is not pushed upwards as much by pressure of the tight lower skin, and the filler redistributes into the lower part of the implant and the breast. As upper fullness decreases some, you may feel that you breasts are getting smaller. They're not, but you may think so because most of the time you're looking down at them. Check out a side view in the mirror. You'll see that you're gradually getting more fullness in the lower breast! This progression happens in every augmentation patient and more in some than others! Expect it, and don't worry that your breasts are getting smaller.

Suddenly, shopping is a lot more fun! Although your breasts will continue to change during the first three months, it's a totally new experience to go shopping, wear anything you want, and look fabulous! Different patients feel comfortable shopping at different times, but when you feel like it, do it!

A patient gave us a great description of how augmented breasts feel during the first three months. She said that "they are like trying to dial a phone with false fingernails. They just feel weird until you get used to them." That's what over 90 percent of patients tell us! They're not painful. You just notice them! Toward the end of the three-month period, you'll begin to notice them less, and one day, all of a sudden, you don't notice them at all. They're just part of you!

## The Years That Follow

**Once you no longer notice your breast implants, you'll almost totally forget them.**

*Provided you don't develop capsular contracture and provided you have made wise choices about implant size.*

Once your tissues heal and adapt to your implants, your breasts will no longer seem foreign to you. You incorporate the new you into your body image automatically! Your breasts are just your breasts. The implants are no longer an issue, and they usually don't even cross your mind.

If you escape the low risk of capsular contracture, and you'll usually know by the first 6 months to 1 year, your breasts won't change much, and they will seem totally normal. If you made good choices about implant size, your breasts will mature at about the same rate as a normal breast the same size. You may develop slightly more sagging over time, just as any normal, larger breast does with aging, but your breast looks a lot better while it is aging! The larger the implant you selected, and the thinner your tissues, the more sagging and thinning of your tissues you can expect with time.

## AND THE LAST STEP

After recovery, you'll enjoy living with your new breasts. In the next chapter, we'll discuss living with your breast implants and the care and maintenance of the best breast!

[CHAPTER FIFTEEN]

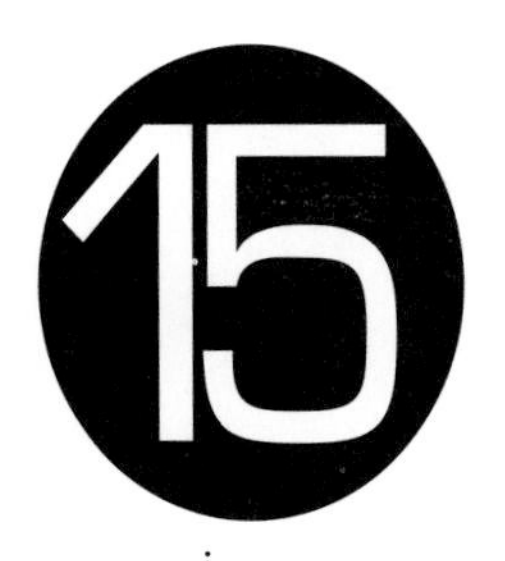


# FOLLOW-UP: Living With Your New Breasts

***"You don't need to 'baby' your implants. They should withstand any type of normal, vigorous activity."***

**Living with your new, augmented breasts is very similar to living with a normal breast, except that augmented breasts may require more maintenance.**

*More maintenance is the tradeoff for feeling better about you and feeling more normal!*

## ROUTINE MAINTENANCE

### Follow-up Visits With Your Surgeon

**Your surgeon can't give you optimal care if you don't show up for follow-up visits.**

Routine follow-up visit schedules vary among surgeons. We like to check our patients within the first two days following surgery, then at three weeks, three months, one year, and every two years thereafter. We also instruct every patient to come in at any time they have *any question or problem whatever*! One of the biggest problems with augmentation patients is failure to show up for follow-up visits. You think, "I'm doing great and don't have any problems, so I don't need to waste time and make a trip to see my surgeon!" ***Wrong!*** Even if the visit is routine, your surgeon will be able to take better care of you and identify potential problems sooner if you do your part and show up. A surgeon should never charge you for follow-up visits following augmentation because they are part of the original deal. Take advantage of your surgeon's efforts to take the best possible care of you, no matter how well you think you're doing.

### Supporting Your Breasts

Your breasts are supported primarily by your breast skin. As you get older, this skin usually becomes thinner and does not provide as much support. The larger your implants, or the larger an unaugmented breast, the more weight in the breast, and the more gravity will pull and stretch the skin over time, allowing your breast to sag.

**Breasts that are supported SOME of the time sag less than breasts that are supported NONE of the time.**

*Sagging—how much and when—depends on your tissue characteristics, the size of your implants, your age, and how much you support your breasts.*

Supporting your breasts, especially during activities that stress the skin and accelerate sagging, can decrease the amount of sagging and when it occurs. You can't totally escape the inevitable effects of gravity pulling on breast weight over time, but you can help. What happens if you never wear a bra? Check out pictures in National Geographic of women who live in cultures where the breast is never supported. Aging is inevitable, but supporting the breast, at least some of the time, can delay the inevitable and reduce sagging.

**If your breasts are bouncing, they are sagging faster than if they are not bouncing.**

*Support your breasts during any activity that causes bouncing.*

Whenever you are doing any activity that causes your breasts to bounce, wear a bra, or even two jog bras if necessary, to immobilize the breasts as much as possible. Bouncing puts more stress on the skin in your lower breast and causes it to stretch more rapidly and to a greater degree. That stretch is what allows your breasts to sag. Bouncing is bad! Aside from activities that cause bouncing, wear a bra at least some of the time. At other times, enjoy your breasts. You don't need to wear a bra all the time!

## Self-Examination

Breast self-examination is an essential activity for every woman. One out of every 10 or 11 women in the United States will develop breast cancer during their lifetime, and breast self-examination is one of the keys to early detection and cure.

Ask your gynecologist, family physician, or plastic surgeon to demonstrate optimal techniques. Perform breast self-examination every month about two weeks after the beginning of your menstrual period.

Your breast implants will not interfere with self-examination because the implants are *behind, not within*, the breast tissue. All of your breast tissue is in front of your implants and is totally accessible for examination by you or your physician. In fact, provided you don't have excessive firmness from capsular contracture, many physicians feel that breast examination is easier with implants in place.

Your breasts will feel different after you have implants. If you are thin and can feel your ribs with your fingers, you will probably be able to feel at least some part of your implants behind your breast. Wait until about three months after surgery to allow all swelling to resolve, then ask your surgeon to demonstrate how to feel the edges of your implant in the lower or outer breast. Once you recognize implant, you can distinguish it from anything else that is abnormal in either breast.

### Physician Examination

**Every woman should have a thorough breast examination at least once every two years from age 20 to 35, and annually thereafter, by your family physician or gynecologist.**

Most women have breast exams at the time of routine gynecologic examinations. You will also have breast examinations at the times of your follow-up visits with your plastic surgeon. Most women who have breast augmentation have more frequent and more total breast examinations compared to the general population, provided they keep their follow-up appointments.

In addition to regular self-examination and physician examinations, you should immediately see your plastic surgeon, gynecologist, or family physician at any time that you notice anything substantially different in either breast, or if you feel any mass or lump in either breast.

### Mammography

Mammography recommendations differ among surgeons and other physicians. We require mammograms before any augmentation, regardless of the patient's age. Following augmentation, we recommend waiting one year to allow all postoperative changes to resolve, then repeat a mammogram whenever it is convenient to establish a new baseline mammogram with your implant in place. Thereafter, you need mammograms annually or every other year after age 40, depending on the recommendations of your surgeon or gynecologist. If you have other risk factors, such as family history, that may increase your risks of breast cancer, more frequent mammograms will probably be necessary.

**Mammograms for augmentation patients should be performed in a state-of-the-art breast center where all personnel are familiar with techniques of optimal imaging for breast augmentation patients.**

*If you ever hear any negative comments about augmentation during a visit to a mammogram facility, seek another facility because the personnel may not be familiar with optimal techniques.*

Whenever you have a mammogram, ask the facility to fax a copy of the report to your plastic surgeon for your medical record.

### Recreation and Athletics

**Breast implants should not limit any type of recreational or athletic activities.**

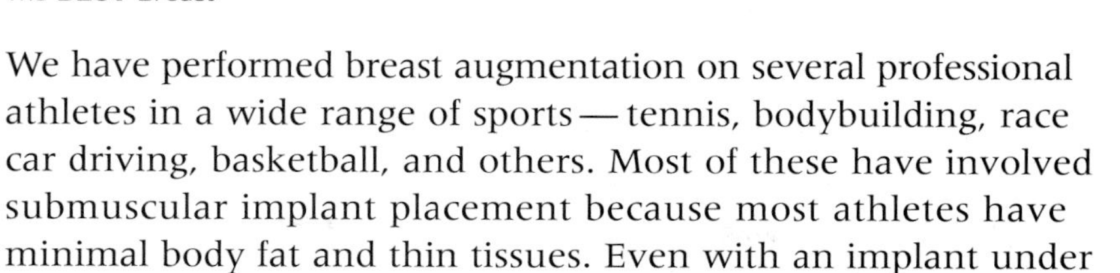

We have performed breast augmentation on several professional athletes in a wide range of sports — tennis, bodybuilding, race car driving, basketball, and others. Most of these have involved submuscular implant placement because most athletes have minimal body fat and thin tissues. Even with an implant under the pectoral muscle, these athletes don't miss a beat! Neither should you!

Theoretically, any high-impact blow can rupture an implant. A high-speed automobile accident or other severe trauma can rupture implants. But a lot of force is required, far more than you will encounter in any normal athletic activity.

## DURABILITY, RUPTURE, DEFLATION

Today's state-of-the-art implants are much stronger and more durable than you might think. I've demonstrated the strength of McGhan Anatomic Saline Implants by filling an implant and standing with my full weight on the implant without rupturing it. Nevertheless, implant shells can fail, usually due to folding from underfill (see Chapter 4), but also from rare manufacturing defects or valve failure. High-energy impact can also cause implant rupture, but even the most vigorous physical or sexual activity is unlikely to damage an implant without damaging you first. McGhan guarantees its implants for your lifetime, so any implant failure is more of a nuisance than a real problem.

**You don't need to "baby" your implants. They should withstand any type of normal, vigorous activity.**

*However, your implants were not designed to withstand closed capsulotomy, the practice of forcefully squeezing your breast to correct capsular contracture!*

We advise every augmentation patient that implant rupture is nothing more than a huge nuisance. I can replace any saline implant in less than 15 minutes and any silicone gel implant in less than 30 minutes in the operating room if implant replacement is all that's required, and you'll experience virtually no discomfort after surgery. The nuisance is filling out the necessary paperwork for the implant guarantee and doing the necessary preparations and laboratory tests prior to surgery. We never charge any patient on whom we performed an augmentation to replace the implant later if replacement becomes necessary. McGhan's guarantee covers all expenses for 10 years. Thereafter, you would have to pay only for a surgery facility and anesthesia but no surgeon fees.

Replacement of a ruptured silicone gel implant, though slightly more involved than replacement of a saline-filled implant, is easy and routine for a qualified surgeon, provided you didn't have a previous closed capsulotomy performed on your breast. Closed capsulotomy is a forceful squeezing of the breast that some surgeons used (and some still use) to correct an excessively hard breast caused by excessive contraction or tightening of the capsule (lining) that forms around breast implants. Closed capsulotomy is attractive to patients by avoiding surgery, but it can be very painful, cause bleeding and other complications, and does not predictably correct excessively firm breasts. In order to make a breast feel softer, closed capsulotomy produces tearing of the capsule (lining) surrounding the breast implant. Provided you didn't have a closed capsulotomy that disrupted the capsule around your implant, silicone gel that escapes from the implant is still surrounded by the capsule and is easy to remove. The only time that gel removal is complicated is following a closed capsulotomy when gel has been forced outside the capsule into the breast tissue. Never let anyone perform a closed capsulotomy on your breast!

With new, state-of-the-art *cohesive gel* anatomic implants from McGhan, gel migration is virtually a non-issue, even if the implant shell disrupts (see Chapter 4). The gel is so cohesive (sticky) that it is almost impossible to force it out of the shell, even if the shell is cut.

**If you ever have any type of problem with implant deflation or rupture, insist on a qualified surgeon.**

*Implant deflation or rupture is no big deal if your surgeon knows how to deal with it.*

Anything can be difficult if you don't know how to do it, and the last thing you need is someone who doesn't know how to easily manage problems!

### The Three S's — Sex, Scuba Diving, and Skydiving

For some reason, we get more questions about these three activities than all others combined. Implants can withstand almost any sexual activities. The pressure changes that occur with scuba diving, skydiving, or airline travel are of virtually no consequence to state-of-the-art breast implants. Go for it! You shouldn't need to worry about your implants.

## IF PROBLEMS OCCUR ...

We can't comprehensively address every problem that can potentially happen with a breast implant, but Chapter 7 covers most problems in detail. The following is a summary overview of some problems for your review.

### Excessive Firmness

Capsular contracture usually occurs in the first six months to one year following augmentation. If you notice one breast becoming noticeably firmer than the other, contact your surgeon. The best treatment is to completely remove the capsule and replace the implant, hoping that your body won't do it again. If it does, we recommend removing both implants rather than increasing risks with repeated surgeries.

### Displacement

If implants significantly displace from their desired position, the deformity is often difficult to treat. To reposition implants, the surgeon must close a portion of the pocket. That's relatively easy. Keeping it closed to prevent recurrent displacement is not easy.

The larger the implant, and the thinner your tissues, the less likely you'll get a long-term correction. Don't cause the problem with excessively large implants to begin with.

### Change in Size or Shape

A dramatic change in size usually means an implant leak or rupture. Treatment? Replace the implant.

A dramatic change in shape usually indicates that an area of the pocket has closed or the capsule is squeezing on the implant, affecting its shape and its position. The best treatment is to partially or completely remove the capsule and replace the implant.

### Tenderness

Tenderness in the breast is usually a response to hormonal changes that occur with aging or with changes in hormone or birth control medications. Tenderness can also occur in response to caffeine, chocolate, and other medications.

During the first three months following augmentation, tenderness can be due to the implant stretching nerves, usually at the sides of the breasts. After three months, nerve stretch tenderness is unusual. If you develop severe capsular contracture that causes excessive firmness of the breasts, the breasts can become tender.

**More than three months after augmentation, if you don't have capsular contracture or an excessively large implant stretching breast nerves, tenderness is usually not due to your implants.**

If you develop tenderness, pay close attention to whether it changes during your hormonal cycle. If it does, it's usually due to hormonal changes. If it is constant and persists, contact your surgeon or gynecologist.

**Breast cancer almost never causes tenderness. That's the good news!**

### "I've lost sensation"

Read more about sensation and sensory changes in Chapter 7. Most patients lose some sensation immediately after augmentation, and most get significant return of that sensation six to 12 months following surgery. Many patients lose no sensation whatever, and some patients actually develop hypersensitivity. Sensation just isn't very predictable!

Sensory changes are common, regardless of the incision location, type of implant, or whether the implant is above or below muscle. Sensory changes are very unpredictable and depend on several factors, many of which you and your surgeon can't control.

**Generally, the larger the implant, the larger the pocket the surgeon must create, the more stretch on nerves, and the more sensation you'll lose.**

*If you don't get the sensation back in two years, don't expect it to return.*

### "I want them larger"

**Many patients want larger implants after their tissues have stretched and adapted to their current implants.**

*Very few patients think about the consequences of placing larger implants.*

Every surgeon has heard this request from patients following augmentation. Perhaps it's due to the "if a little is good, a lot is better" rationale. Perhaps it's due to women feeling that their breasts are getting smaller as the excessive upper fill in the breast redistributes more into the lower breast. Placing larger implants doesn't solve either problem. This move just creates new questions and problems. How much is enough? How will we know? Are you willing to accept all the risks of your first surgery again, plus some new risks? Remember:

**You can't KEEP a lot of fill in the upper breast by placing larger implants.**

*Over time, and with aging, your lower breast skin will stretch, and you'll always lose some upper fullness.*

**With larger implants, sagging will occur sooner and more, and you face added risks of implant edge visibility, visible traction rippling of the breast, thinning of your breast envelope tissues, and other surgical complications.**

**Is it really worth it?**

*Past a proportionate amount of enlargement, bigger is definitely worse, if you think past dinner.*

### One Is Different Than the Other

One breast is always different than the other! No surgeon alive can make two breasts exactly match. Don't expect your breasts to match. If they are close, wonderful! That means you're like every other woman who has a normal amount of variation between the size and shape of her breasts.

Don't fall into the trap of thinking that if one is smaller than the other, the solution is simple. Just put more implant, or more filler in the current implant, in the smaller breast. It's not that simple. The smaller breast has less skin. If you try to put more filler into less skin, you'll often get permanent, excessive bulging in the upper breast. A difference in *shape* with more upper bulging on one side is much more noticeable than a difference in *size*.

**Remember, a difference in size is normal. Every woman has it.**

*Don't chase small differences in size and shape. You could end up looking worse!*

### Complications — When to Quit

Although we've mentioned this before, it's important to mention again. A huge majority of patients have absolutely no problems whatever with their implants. But a few patients have a lot of problems — usually the result of *bad team decisions* by the patient and the surgeon.

There are worse things than removing and not replacing breast implants. You may not like your breasts as well, but if you seem to have persistent or severe problems, there's a very logical solution. Get rid of your implants. Over 90 percent of the implant "horror cases" we've reviewed could have been averted if someone, either patient or surgeon, had said, "Enough! Let's get them out!" If you used good judgement in your initial selection of implant, your breasts should not look any worse than they would look after a pregnancy.

## THE LAST WORD

We'll stop where we started!

**The BEST BREAST is the natural female breast until nature misses a beat, takes a toll, or a woman decides that it's not.**

**It's normal to want to feel normal. It's also normal to want to be the best that you can be.**

*Breast augmentation can help with those normal goals.*

Whether breast augmentation is right for you is a personal decision. Whether you get the best breast depends on: How much you know, how well you do your homework, how well you make decisions, how qualified and skilled your surgeon is, and Mother Nature factors that neither you nor your surgeon can control. One thing is for sure. You're better prepared now than when you started, and you have a better chance of getting the **BEST BREAST**!

[CHAPTER SIXTEEN]

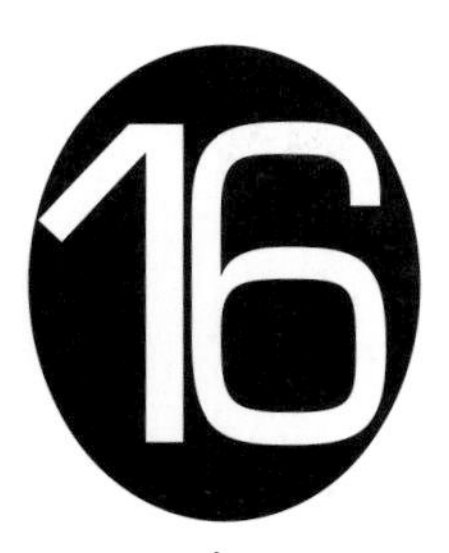


# BREAST AUGMENTATION: 11 Important Visual Lessons

***"Perfection or change to a different breast is never an option. Improvement in the existing breast is the only realistic alternative. When looking at pictures, look for breasts that look like your breasts BEFORE surgery."***

Pictures best illustrate some of the most important principles in augmentation. Pictures can also be misleading and confusing. *What you see* depends on *what you know*. The more you know, the more thoroughly and systematically you can evaluate pictures. Many of the terms and concepts used in this chapter have been explained in earlier chapters, so this chapter will be most meaningful and useful if you have read the previous chapters.

These visual lessons in augmentation focus on important concepts that every augmentation patient should know.

**Every woman's augmentation result is determined by two factors:**

**1) What the woman WANTS, and**
**2) What the woman's body (her TISSUES) will ALLOW HER TO HAVE (what the surgeon has to work with).**

As you look at any pictures of augmentation results, remember:

**This woman's breasts are unique in shape and appearance, different from any other woman.**

*This woman's* ***tissues*** *are different from any other woman.*

*This woman's* ***wishes*** *are different from any other woman.*

It's impossible to look at a catalog of breast pictures, and pick out what you'd like to have, unless your breasts are exactly the same as the woman's in the picture *before* surgery. It's also impossible to know exactly what the woman in the picture requested. What she wanted might be very different from what you want. And, most importantly, the characteristics of her breast tissues are not exactly like yours.

We have chosen each set of images to make a point. Each breast is not the most beautiful breast or the most "perfect" breast. Any experienced surgeon can select a large number of "best" results, but if education is the goal, you need to see a full range of breast types, results, and common problems. As you study the lessons, focus on the *message* of each image. Don't necessarily ask yourself whether you particularly *like* the breast. Remember, what you see in a "before" image is all the surgeon had to work with. *Perfection* or a *change to a different breast* is *never* an option. *Improvement* in the *existing breast* is the only realistic alternative.

## LESSON 1:
### Each woman's breasts have unique tissue characteristics. The skin envelope and breast tissue are different in every woman. A surgeon can only work with what the patient brings (her unique tissue characteristics). Ideal choices are different for each woman, depending on her wishes and her tissues.

This important principle is illustrated by the following "before and after" case studies. Compare each case to the other cases. Focus on the substantial differences between each patient's tissues *before* augmentation, and how those differences affected the result. Concentrate on the two major components of the breast: The skin envelope and the *breast tissue (parenchyma)* that fills the skin envelope. For each different combination of skin envelope and breast tissue, we will emphasize principles that affect the choices of implant and technique in each different type of breast.

### Skin Envelope: Tight, Unstretched
### Breast Tissue: Minimal

(Figure 16-1 A,B)

When the skin is tight and thin, with minimal breast tissue to cover a breast implant, the most important considerations are:

1) Avoid an excessively large implant. The skin will stretch only a moderate amount without permanently damaging or thinning the skin. Choose an implant that will not cause excessive skin stretch.

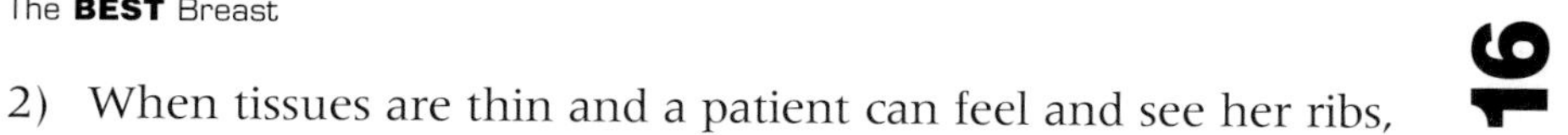



2) When tissues are thin and a patient can feel and see her ribs, she will also be able to feel the edges and possibly the shell of her implant, regardless of the type of implant chosen.

3) Positioning the upper portion of the implant under the pectoralis muscle (in a submuscular pocket location) reduces the risk of the upper edge of the implant being visible.

4) Thin tissues will not support the weight of an excessively large implant as a patient ages. With an excessively large implant, the breast will sag more, the skin will become thinner, implant edges can become visible, and visible rippling can occur from the weight of the implant pulling on the thin overlying tissues.

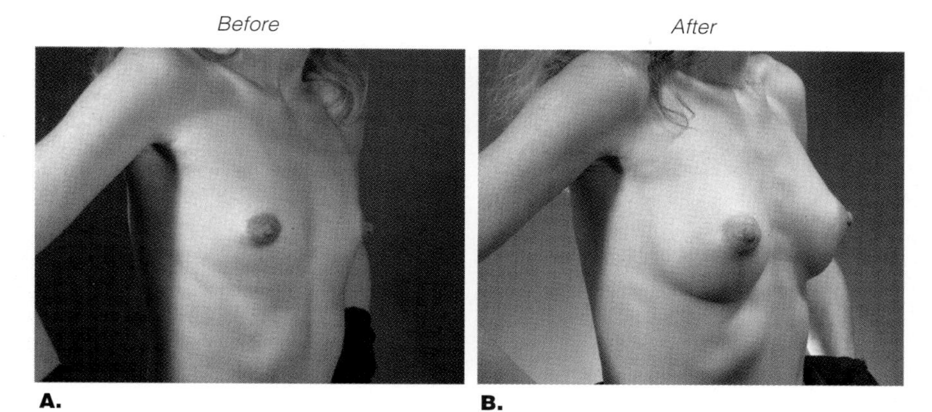


**A.** **B.**

**Figure 16-1.**

## Skin Envelope: Stretched, Looser
## Breast Tissue: Minimal

(Figure 16-2 A-C)

Breast enlargement with pregnancy usually stretches the skin, leaving the skin envelope looser. The breast tissue inside the envelope often shrinks following pregnancy. The result is less filler in a larger, looser skin envelope. The most important considerations with loose skin and minimal breast tissue are:

1) Adequately fill the loose envelope for the best result but avoid overfilling. An excessively small implant will fill the lower breast, but leaves the upper breast empty (the "rock-in-a-sock" look). When the loose envelope skin is thin (note the patient's visible ribs), the goal should be to provide just enough fill (implant size) to expand the envelope for a natural upper breast profile. Any implant larger than that required for adequate fill will cause excessive stretching and further thinning of the envelope as this patient ages, and risks all of the same long-term problems described for Figure 16-1, #4.

2) A thin skin envelope with minimal breast tissue covering the implant almost guarantees that the patient may feel some portion of the implant, just as she could feel her ribs beneath the thin tissues.

3) Notice the extremely thin skin in the cleavage area between the breasts. If the implants selected were wider than the existing breast tissue (Figure 16-2, C), the edge of the implant would be visible beneath the thin skin between the breasts. To avoid a visible implant edge between the breasts, an implant was selected that was slightly narrower than the patient's breast tissue. The patient had to choose between a) narrowing the gap between the breasts more and risking a visible implant edge, or b) accepting a slightly wider gap between the breasts and avoiding a visible implant edge. She chose option b.

*Before*

**A.**

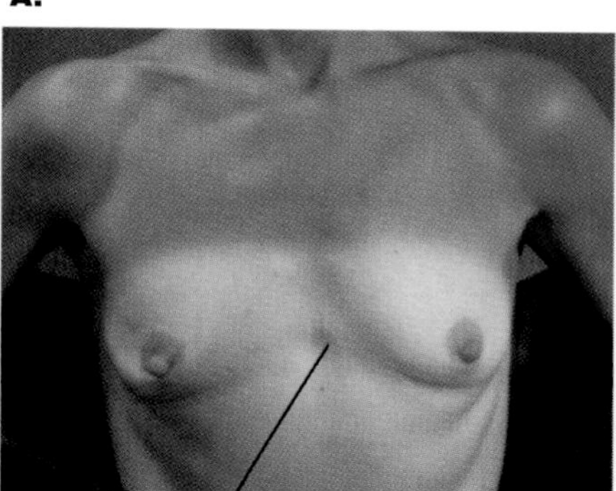


*After*

**B.**

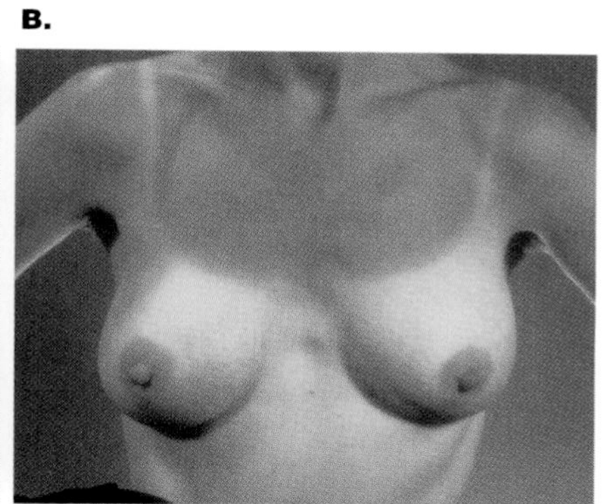

**C.**

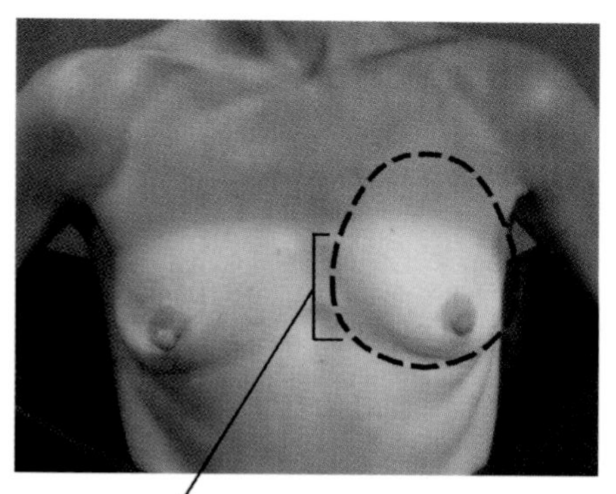


**Figure 16-2.**

**Skin Envelope: Stretched, Looser**
**Breast Tissue: Moderate**
(Figure 16-3 A,B)

1) When more breast tissue is present in a stretched envelope, the breast tissue provides more cover for the implant and the patient is less likely to feel portions of the implant.

2) The combination of skin already stretched by pregnancy with adequate breast tissue to cover an implant is ideal for augmentation.

3) The patient and surgeon can select from a wider range of implant sizes or widths without risking implant edge visibility when more breast tissue is present (a wider base width of the breast mound in front view).

*Before* *After*

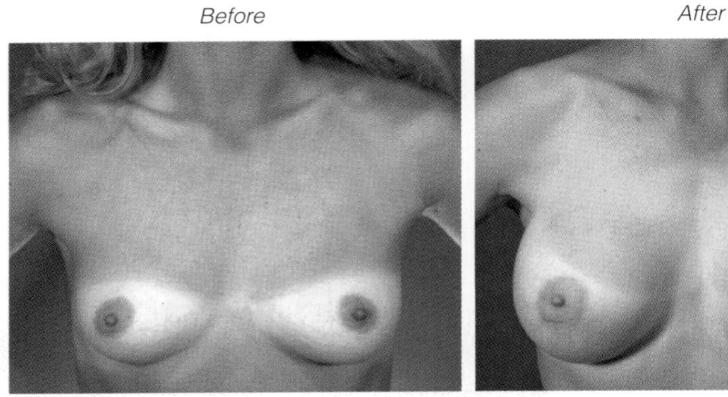

**A.** **B.**

**Figure 16-3.**

**Skin Envelope: Very Loose**
**Breast Tissue: Moderate**
(Figure 16-4 A,B)

1) The larger a breast, whether normally or during pregnancy or nursing, the more the skin envelope stretches. This patient's stretched skin envelope could be the result of gravity pulling on a moderately large breast as she aged, or could have resulted

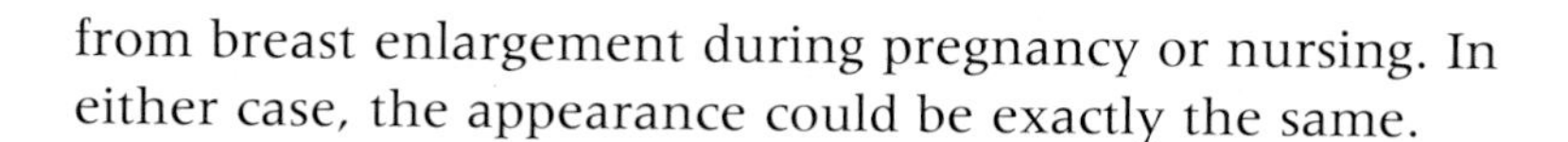

from breast enlargement during pregnancy or nursing. In either case, the appearance could be exactly the same.

2) Although it's important to adequately fill a stretched envelope for an optimal result, when we see sagging of the breast *before* surgery, the skin envelope tissues are sending a message. *The skin envelope did not support the weight of the patient's own tissue, or it wouldn't have stretched and allowed the breast to sag!*

3) Although this stretched envelope could accommodate a very large implant and maintain a natural appearance, what will the excessively large implant cause when placed in an envelope that has already proved that it cannot support the weight of the patient's own tissues? More sagging and more tissue thinning!

4) The key to a good long-term result in this type of breast is to select an implant that will provide *improvement* in lift and fill and *avoid selecting the largest implant* that the envelope could accommodate. The largest implant might look good, but only for a while. It would rapidly cause more stretch, more sagging, with loss of fill in the upper breast, thinning of the skin envelope, and increased risks of visible rippling in the upper breast. Excessive sagging could necessitate a breast lift procedure (mastopexy), with additional tradeoffs of more scars on the breast and possible increased loss of sensation. Making the right choices is important at the first operation!

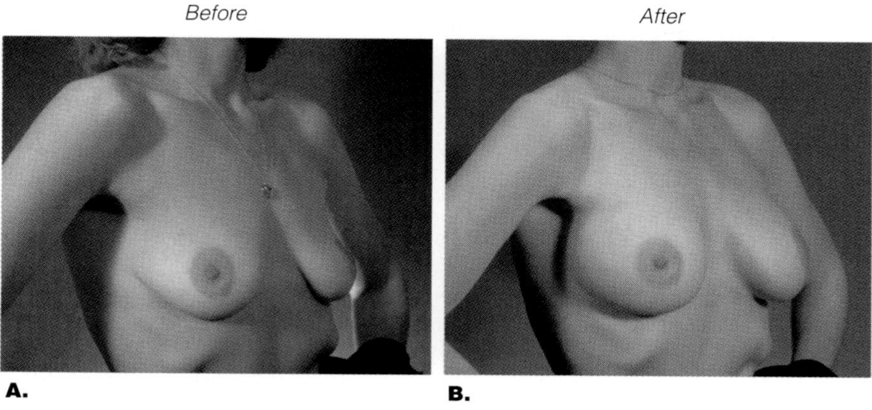


**A.** **B.**

**Figure 16-4.**

## LESSON 2:
## A woman's breasts are never the same on both sides, and no two women have breasts that are exactly the same. No surgeon can make both breasts exactly the same; differences will always exist after surgery. Each type of breast presents unique problems, and every correction involves limitations and tradeoffs.

In each of the following cases, we will point out the unique characteristics of the patient's *tissues*, the different *problems* that each patient's tissues present, and the *corrections* that were achieved by augmentation. In each case, we will also emphasize the *limitations* that each patient's tissues imposed, and the *tradeoffs* that were present during the decision-making process.

These different patients prior to augmentation emphasize the extreme variations in breast characteristics from one woman to another (Figure 16-5, A-J). To further appreciate the differences, pick one characteristic at a time from the following list, then scan up and down the left and right rows, comparing that one specific characteristic from patient to patient.

- **Breast size**
- **Breast shape**
- **Nipple location on one side compared to the other (one higher or lower)**
- **Nipple tilt (pointing up or down)**
- **Nipple orientation (pointing inward or outward)**
- **Breast size variation from side to side in each patient in front view**
- **Width of the breast in front view**
- **Gap between the breasts in front view**
- **Sag of the breast in side view**
- **Upper breast fullness in side view**

All breasts look different *after* augmentation because all breasts look different *before* augmentation. *A surgeon can only improve what the patient brings. A surgeon cannot exchange a patient's tissues for a different set of tissues.* In the before-and-after illustrations that follow, notice that each result is only an improvement over what the patient has before surgery. The appearance of the breast before surgery is a major factor affecting the appearance of the result. Breast augmentation surgery offers improvement, not perfection.

**Figure 16-5.**

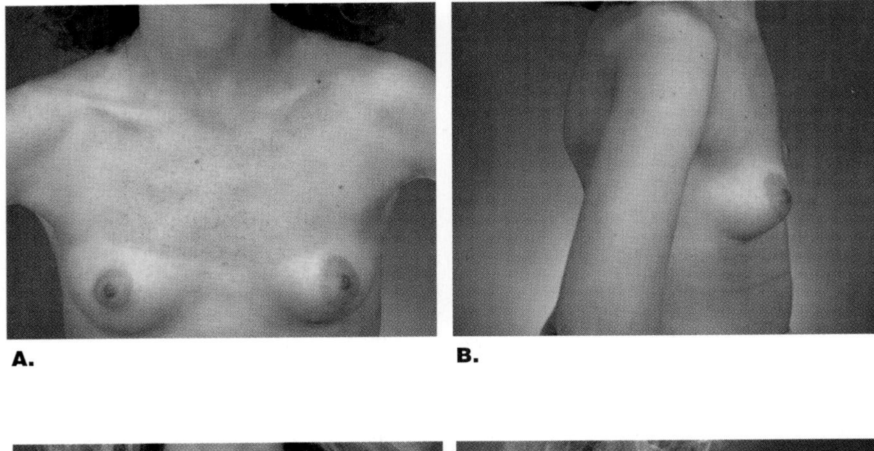

A. B.

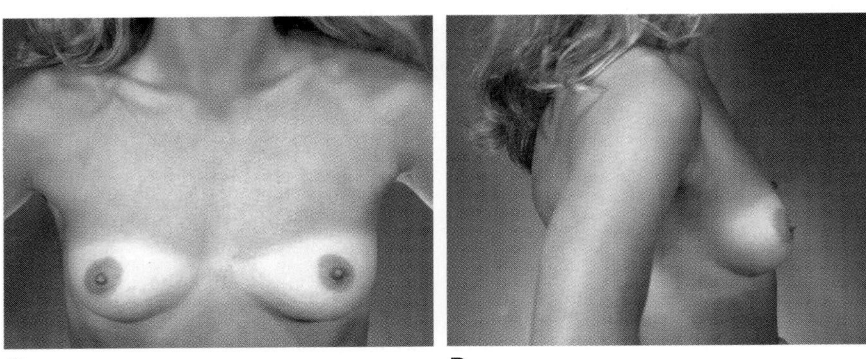

C. D.

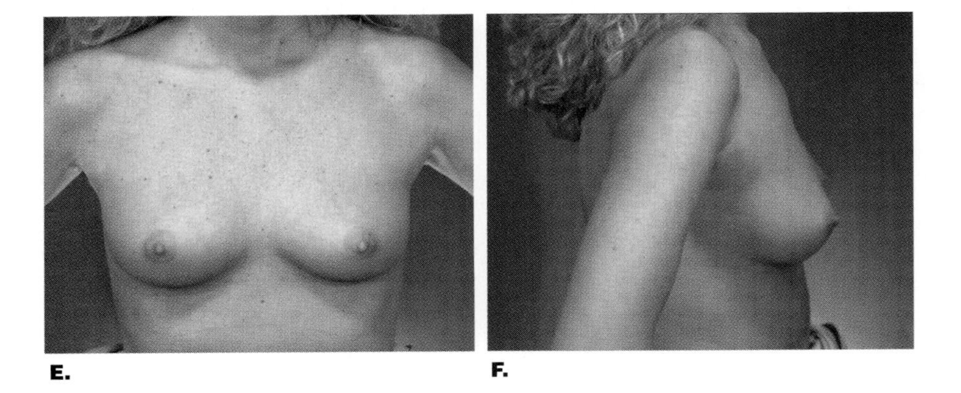

E. F.

***Breasts differ tremendously from woman to woman.***

**Figure 16.5 (continued)**

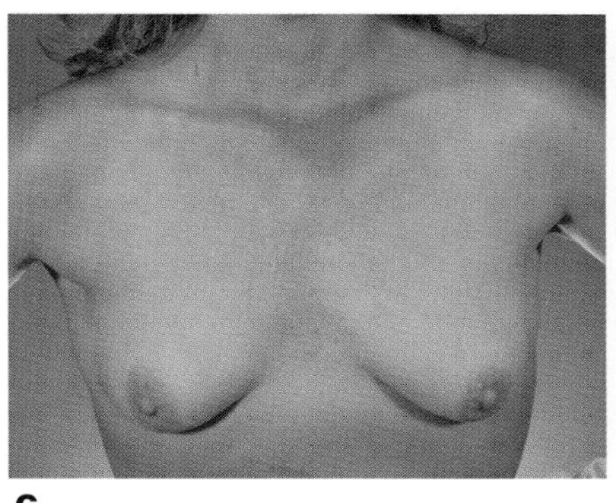

**G.**

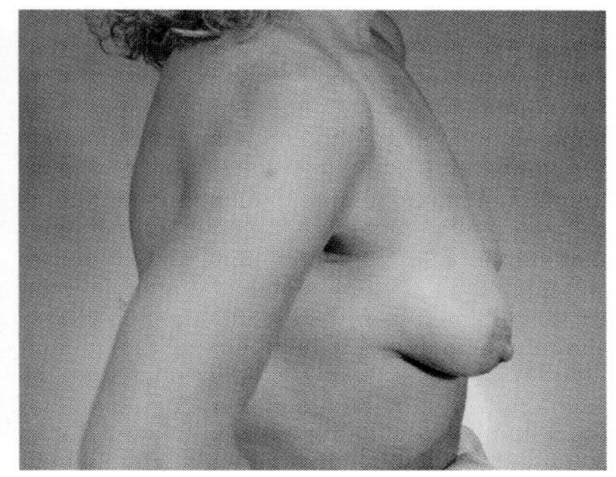

**H.**

**I.**

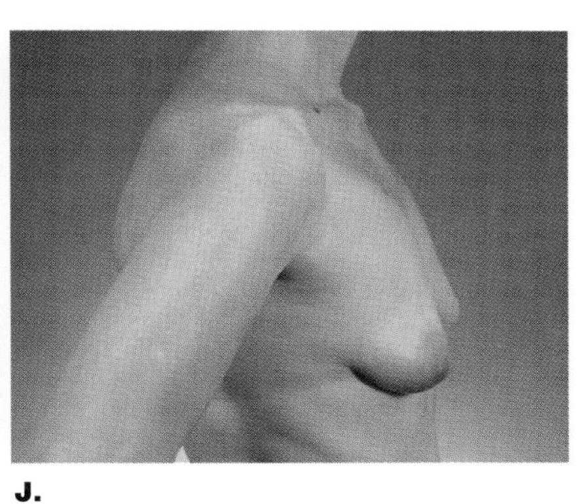

**J.**

Select one characteristic from the following list. Then scan up and down the left and right columns on these pages. Notice how each characteristic varies from breast to breast.

- Breast size
- Breast shape
- Nipple location on one side compared to the other (one higher than lower)
- Nipple tilt (pointing up or down)
- Nipple orientation (pointing inward or outward)
- Breast size variation from side to side in each patient in front view
- Width of the breast in front view
- Gap between the breasts in front view
- Sag of breast in side view
- Upper breast fullness in side view

## Figure 16-6

### *Tissues:*

No pregnancies, skin envelope not stretched, minimal breast tissue, thin tissues.

### *Problems:*

Breasts too small for torso, left smaller than right, left higher than right, left nipple higher than right, wide gap between the breasts, inadequate upper fullness.

### *Corrections, Limitations, Tradeoffs:*

Size and proportion improved, left nipple higher than right (patient declined lifting the right nipple to avoid more scars and possible loss of sensation), gap between breasts narrowed some. Patient elected to accept a slightly wider gap following surgery rather than risk a visible implant edge in the cleavage area if we had selected a wider implant to further narrow the gap.

**Figure 16-6.**

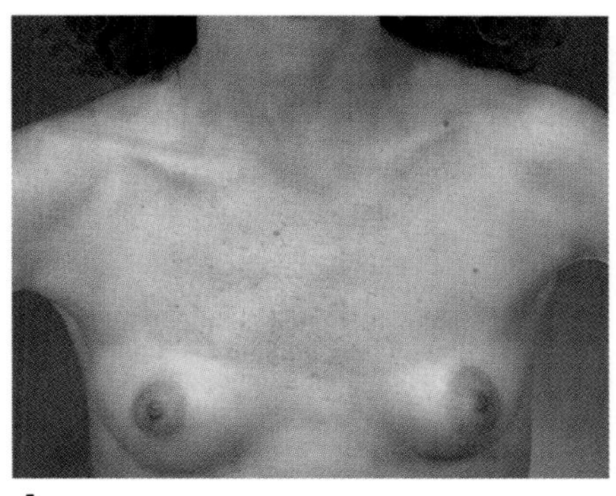

**A.**

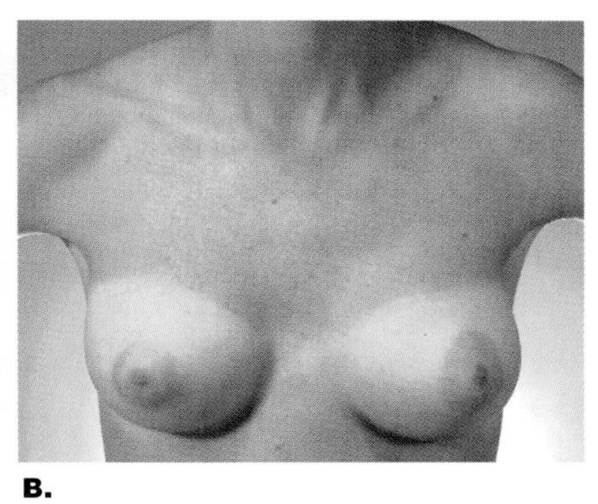

**B.**

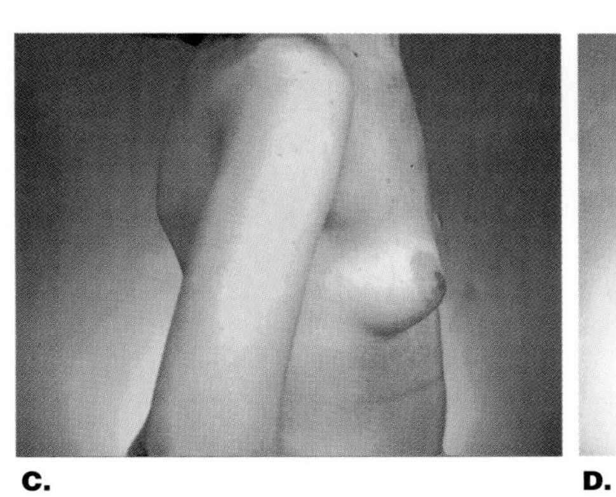

**C.**

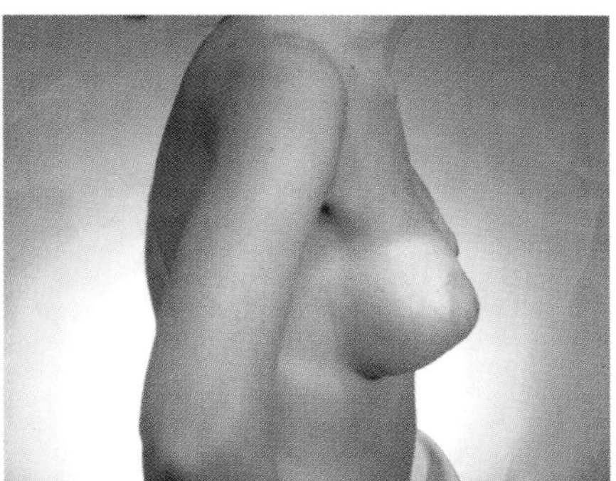

**D.**

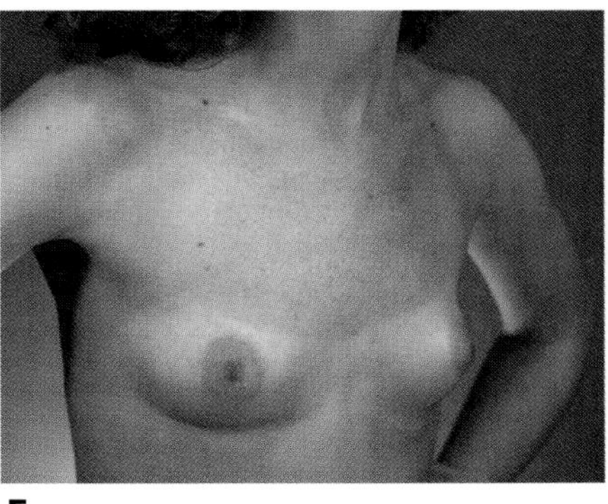

**E.**

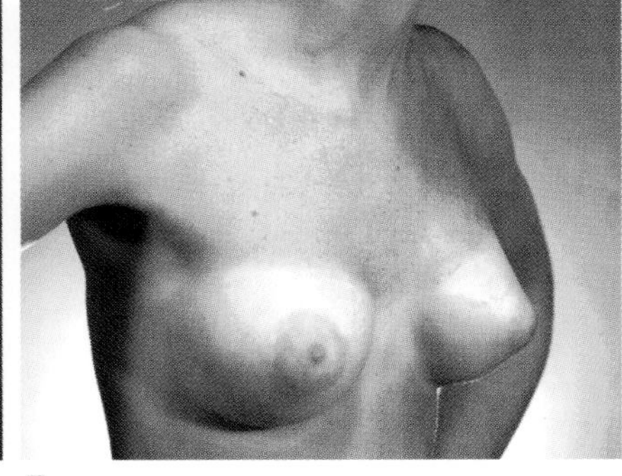

**F.**

## Figure 16-7

### *Tissues:*

Two pregnancies, skin envelope moderately stretched, moderate breast tissue, tissues thin (note visible ribs beneath breasts). Problems: Loss of upper fullness, loss of forward projection, excessively wide gap between the breasts or not enough cleavage.

### *Corrections, Limitations, Tradeoffs:*

Improved upper fullness, cleavage, and projection. Better overall proportion with torso by widening breasts at the sides. In front view, widening the breasts at the sides improves the balance of breast width with hip width and makes the waist appear smaller.

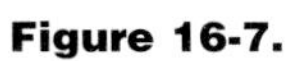

**Figure 16-7.**

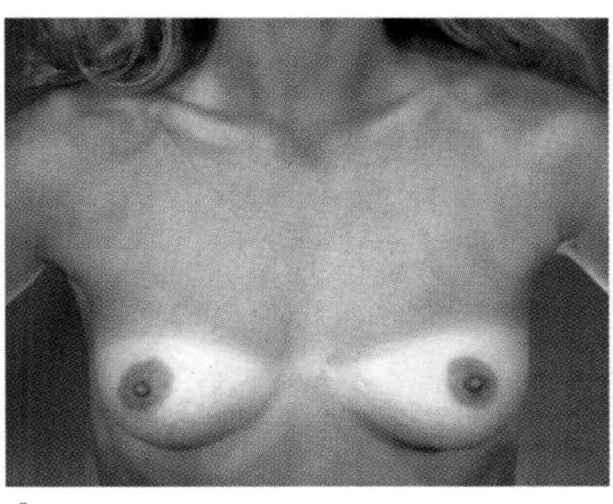

**A.**

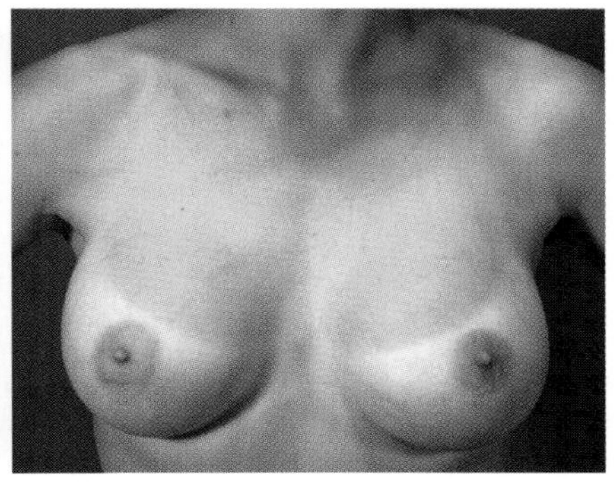

**B.**

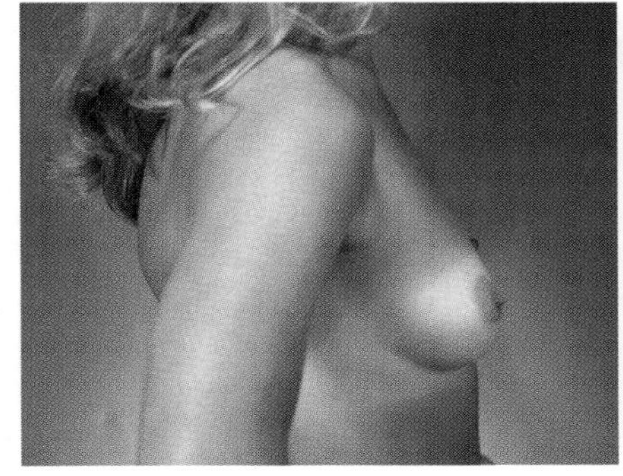

**C.**

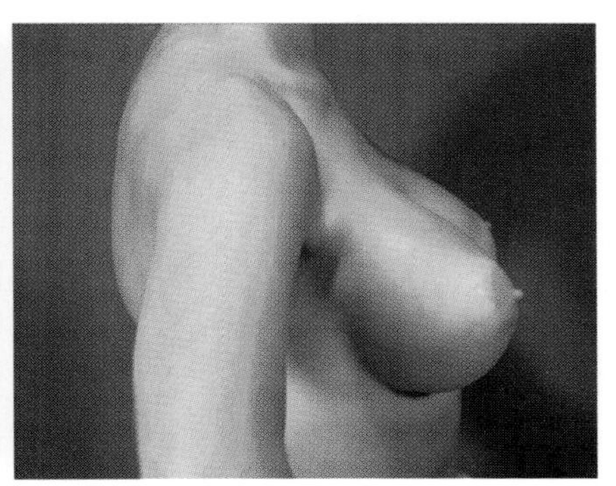

**D.**

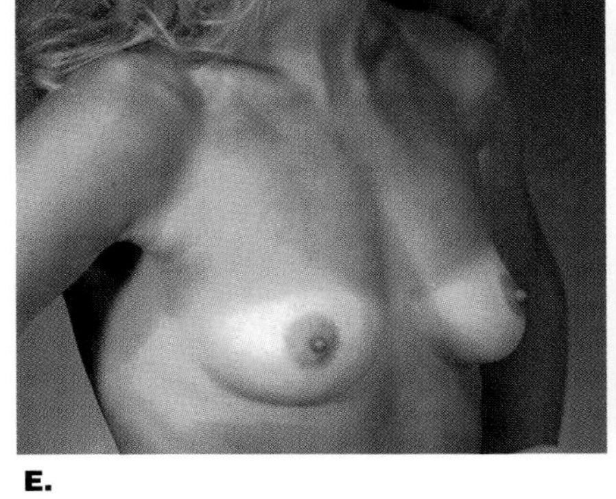

**E.**

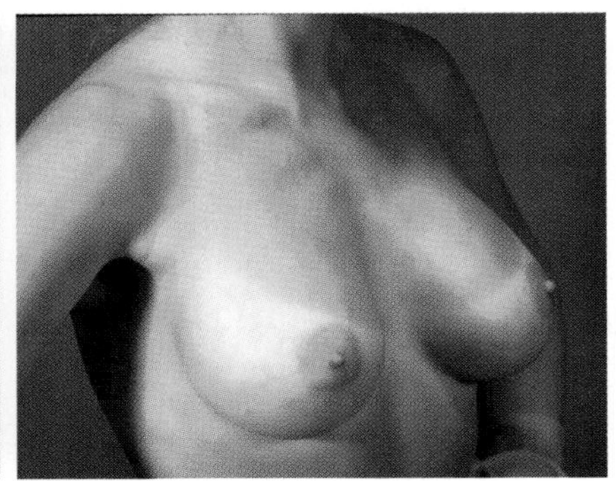

**F.**

## Figure 16-8

### *Tissues:*

Two pregnancies, stretched envelope, minimal breast tissue.

### *Problems:*

Very narrow breasts in front view with wide gap between breasts, thin skin in gap between breasts, thin skin envelope with ribs visible, breasts too triangular or "pointy" rather than round in front view, no upper breast fullness, down-pointing nipples.

### *Corrections, Limitations, Tradeoffs:*

Overall improved appearance, with a rounder, fuller, lifted appearance. Gap between breasts narrowed some, but limited because of thin skin between breasts and risk of visible implant edge if wider implant were used to narrow the gap more. Dramatic improvement in upper fullness and overall breast shape while preserving a natural breast appearance after augmentation.

**Figure 16-8.**

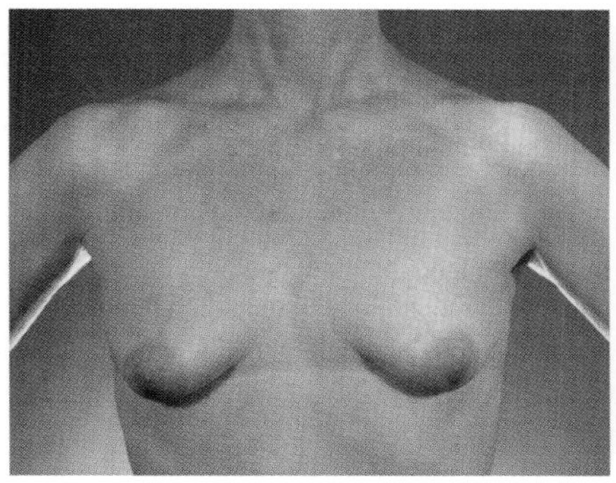

**A.**

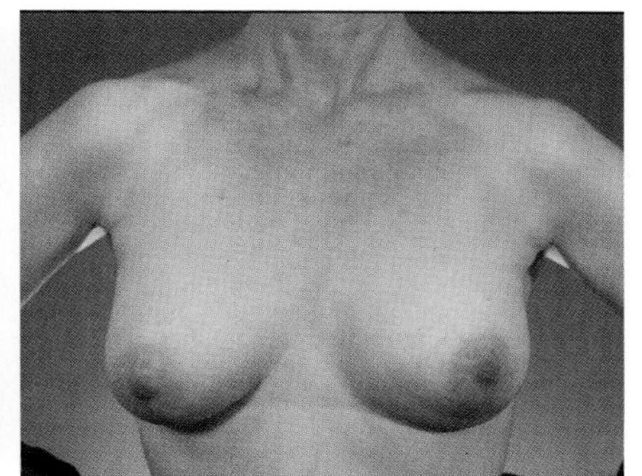

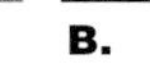

**B.**

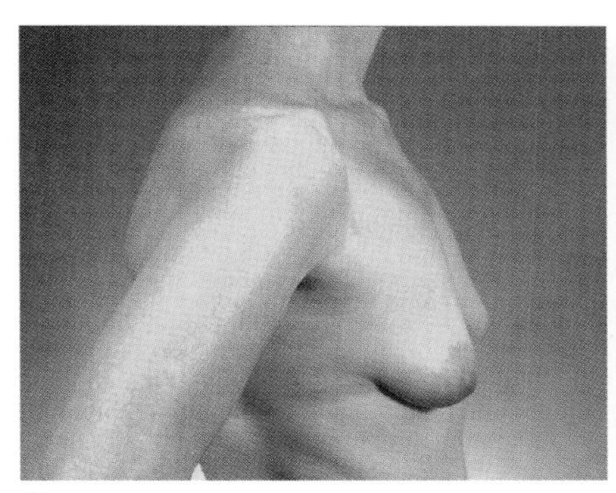

**C.**

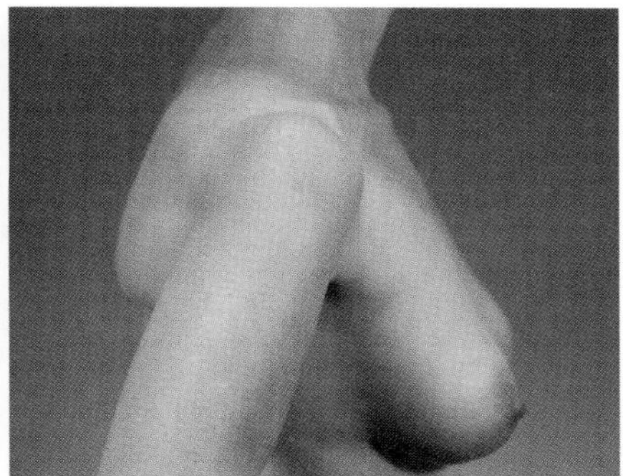

**D.**

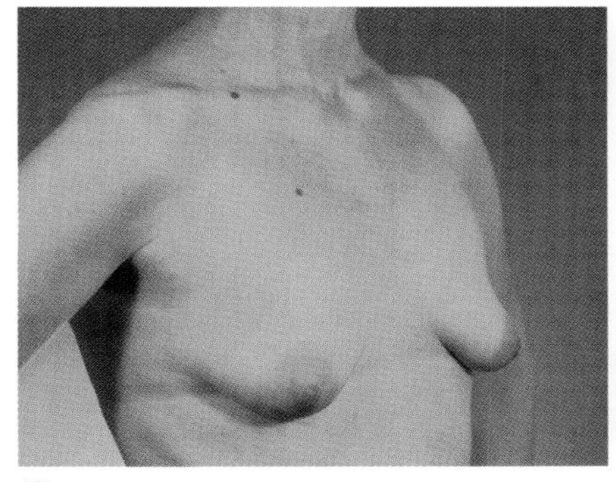

**E.**

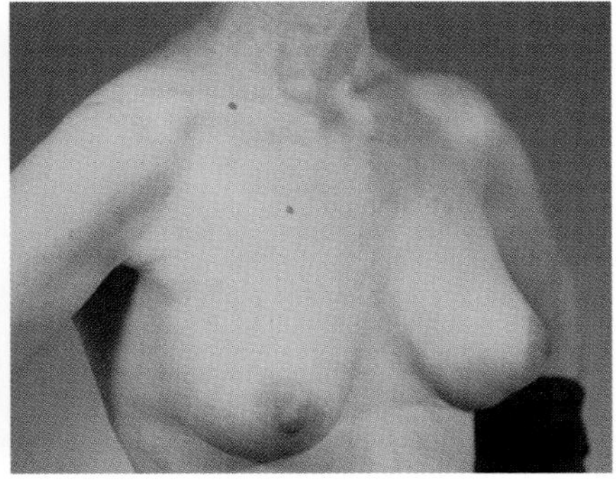

**F.**

## Figure 16-9

### *Tissues:*

Two pregnancies, but minimal stretch of the skin envelope, moderate amount of breast tissue, envelope already relatively full (note upper breast is relatively full in side view before surgery).

### *Problems:*

Patient desires more cleavage, larger, fuller breasts to improve balance with hips and torso, overall figure balance.

### *Corrections, Limitations, Tradeoffs:*

Dramatic improvement in cleavage was possible because the gap between the breasts was narrower prior to surgery, the breast tissue was wider (to cover the edges of the implant), and the patient's skin was thicker in the gap between the breasts. All of these factors reduce the risk of seeing an implant edge between the breasts and allowed use of a wider implant to maximally improve the cleavage. Overall breast fullness improved, overall balance with figure improved.

**Figure 16-9.**

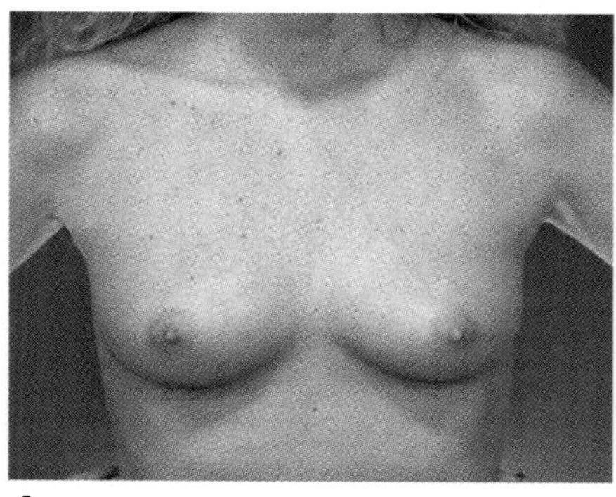

**A.**

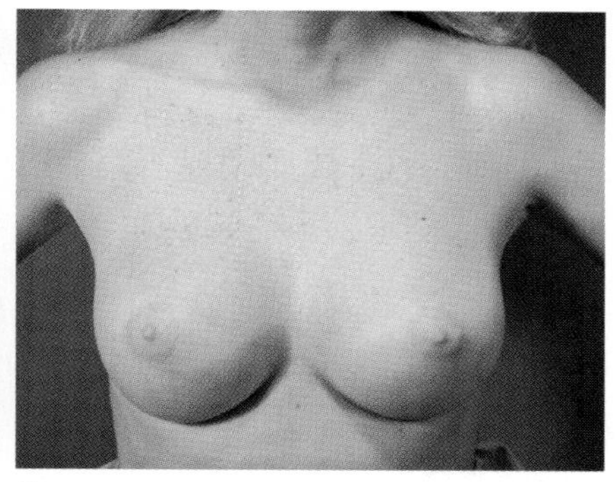

**B.**

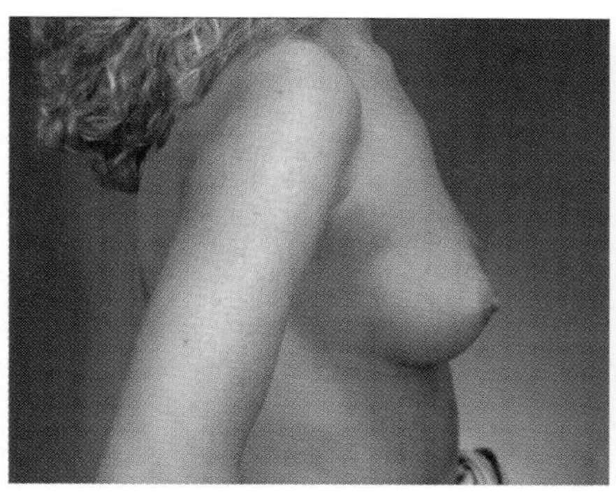

**C.**

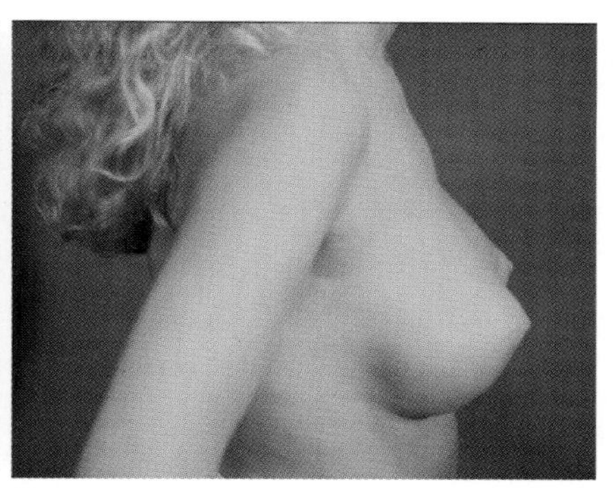

**D.**

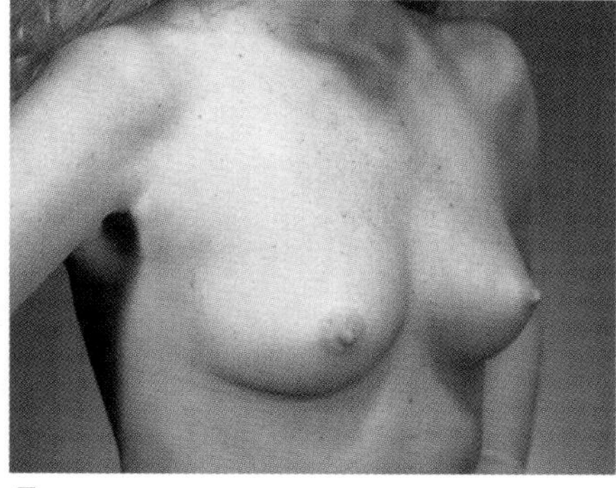

**E.**

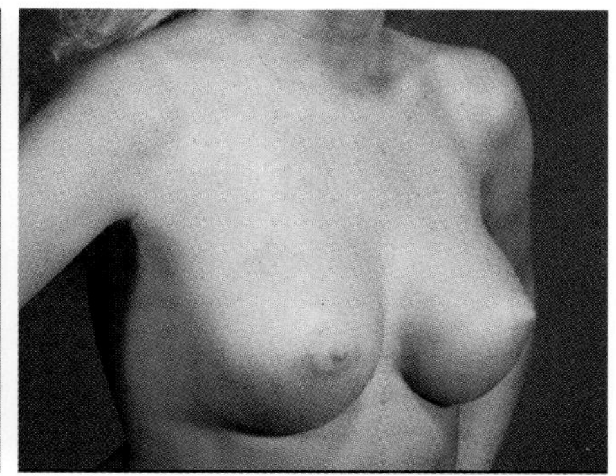

**F.**

## Figure 16-10

### *Tissues:*

No pregnancies, skin envelope not stretched by pregnancy, but stretched by gravity pulling downward on breasts over time. Moderate amount of breast tissue, located primarily in the lower portion of the skin envelope. Breast shape determined by developmental factors during puberty and by gravity over time.

### *Problems:*

Extreme down-pointing breasts, nipple-areola located low on breast mound and down-pointing, sagging appearance, inadequate fullness upper breast, inadequate cleavage or fullness in the middle area of each breast. Nipples located toward the outside of each breast mound rather than more centrally.

### *Corrections, Limitations, Tradeoffs:*

Patient declined nipple repositioning due to tradeoffs of scar around nipple-areola and possible sensory loss. Overall appearance improved but with limitations. Nipples lifted, but still somewhat down-pointing. Nipples still located toward the outside of each breast mound. Upper fullness improved, overall breast shape improved, cleavage improved. Narrowing of the gap between the breasts limited due to risk of visible implant edge under the thin skin between the breasts if a wider implant were placed.

**Figure 16-10.**

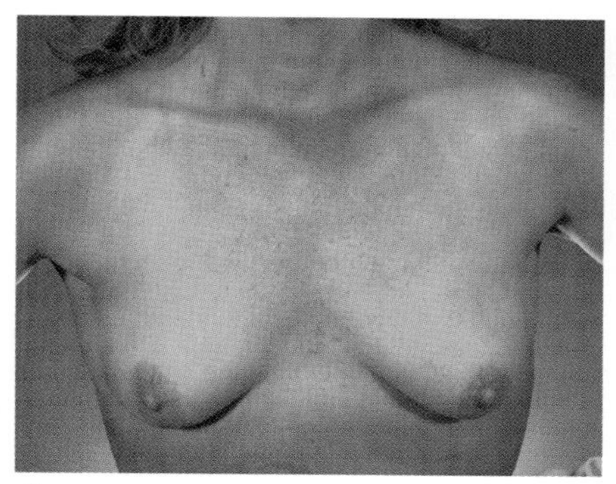

**A.**

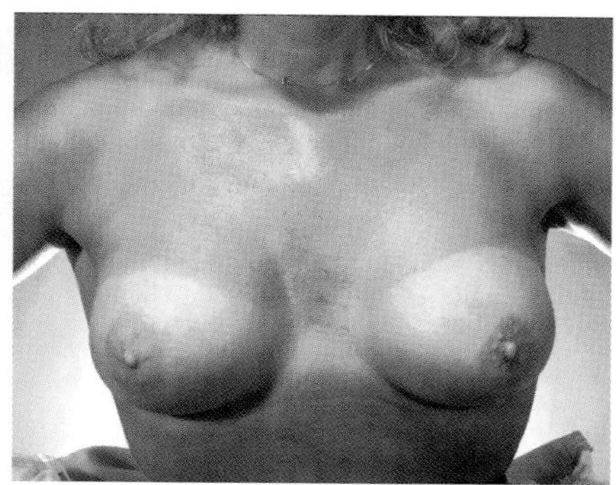

**B.**

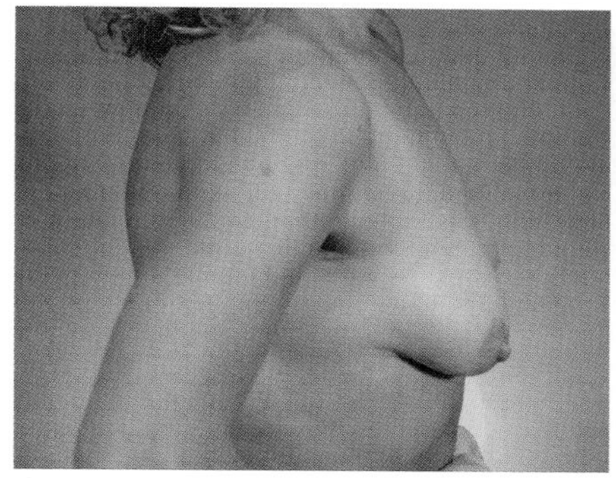

**C.**

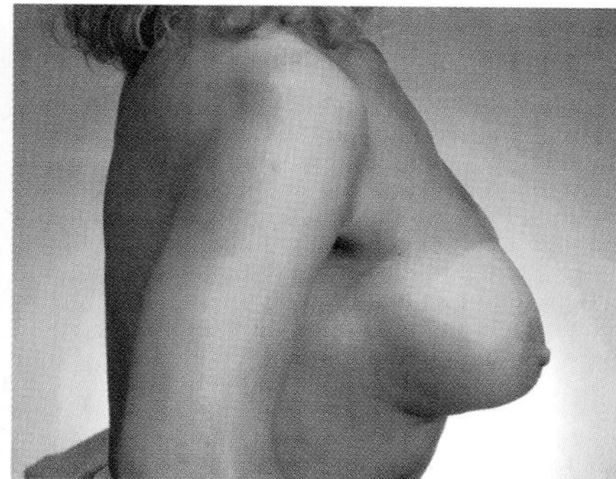

**D.**

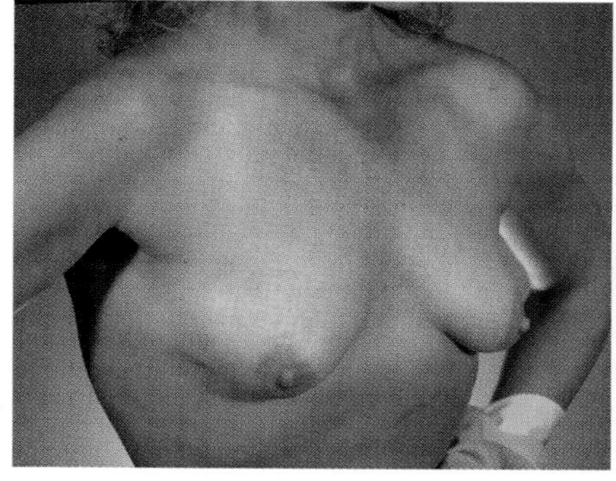

**E.**

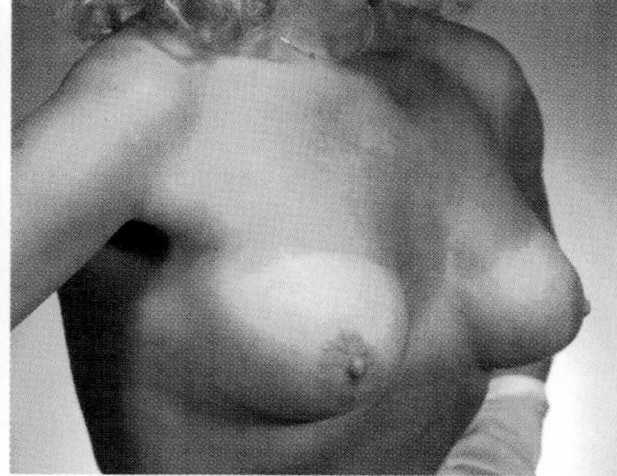

**F.**

## Figure 16-11

### *Tissues:*
Envelope thin, not stretched, virtually no breast tissue present.

### *Problems:*
Very little skin to work with, very difficult to achieve a normal appearing breast without the implant being obvious, lack of fullness in all areas of the breast, figure imbalance breasts with torso and hips, lack of cleavage with wide gap between the breasts.

### *Corrections, Limitations, Tradeoffs:*
Improved overall breast shape and fullness, natural appearing breast, implant not obvious, improved cleavage and narrowing of gap between breasts but limited due to thin skin between breasts and risk of implant edge visibility. Note the visible ribs and breast bone between the breasts. Using any larger implant would produce visible implant edges in this area.

**Figure 16-11.**

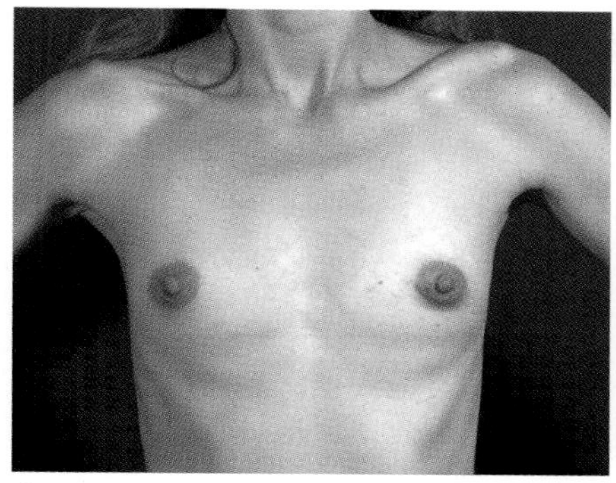

**A.**

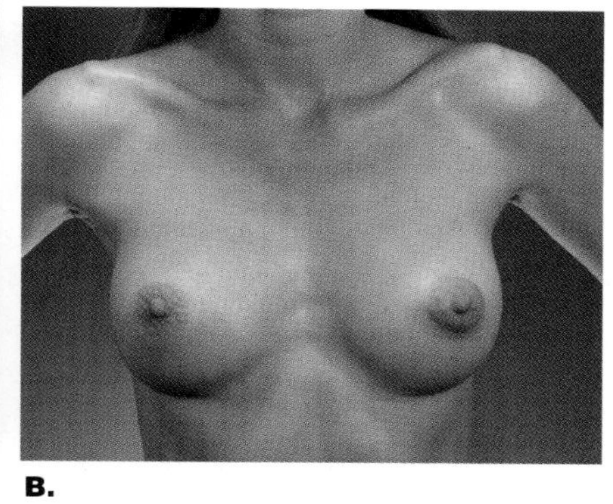

**B.**

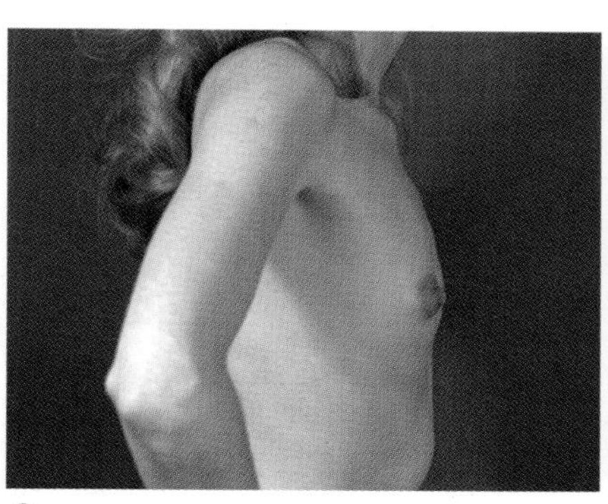

**C.**

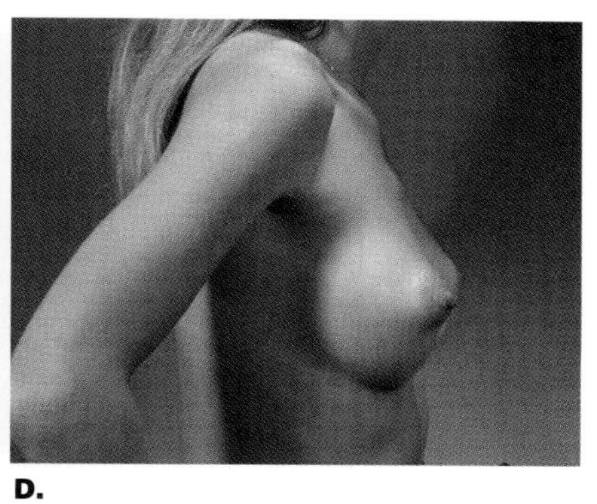

**D.**

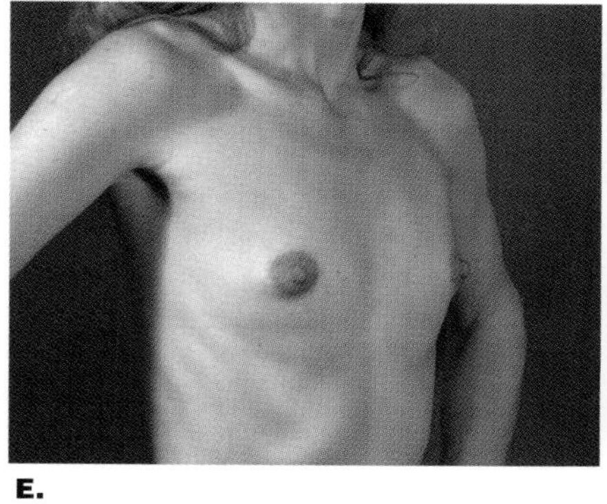

**E.**

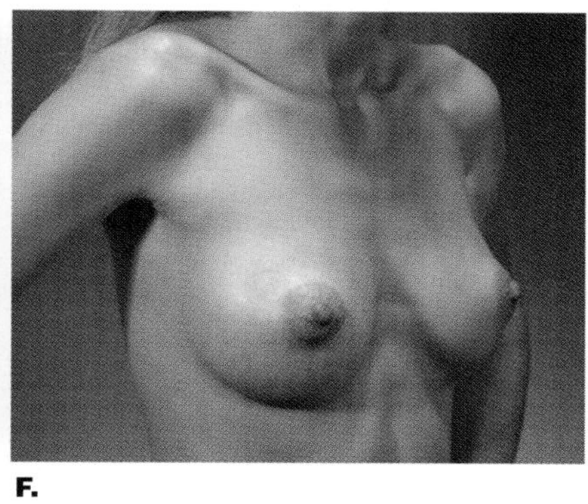

**F.**

## LESSON 3:
### What is enough, and what is too much?

The ideal size of implant is different from one woman to another, depending on the size of the woman's skin envelope before augmentation. If we could insert a funnel into the top of the breast, as we pour fluid into the funnel, the bottom of the breast would fill first, but the top would not be adequately filled (Figure 16-12, A). As we continue to add fluid, at some point, the upper breast would be full, but still have a natural appearance (Figure 16-12, B). If we continued to add fluid, the upper breast would begin to bulge outwardly, with an excessively full and somewhat unnatural appearance (Figure 16-12, C).

**Figure 16-12.**

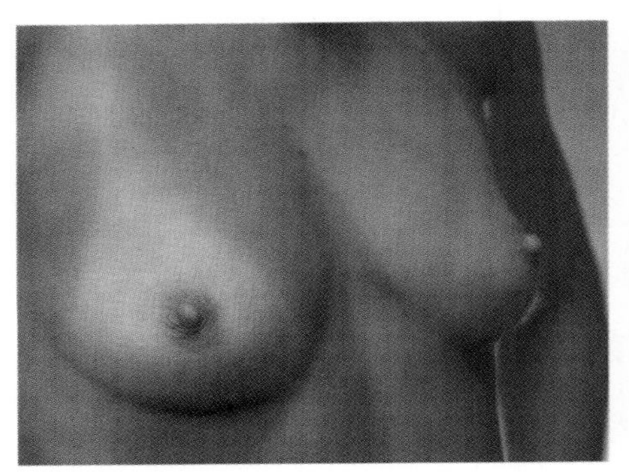

**A.**

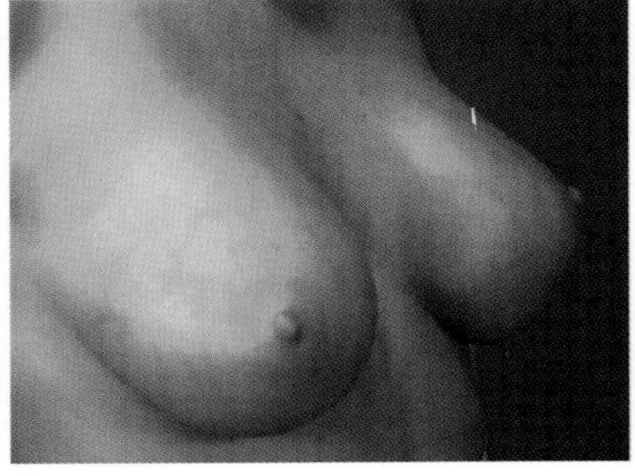

**B.**

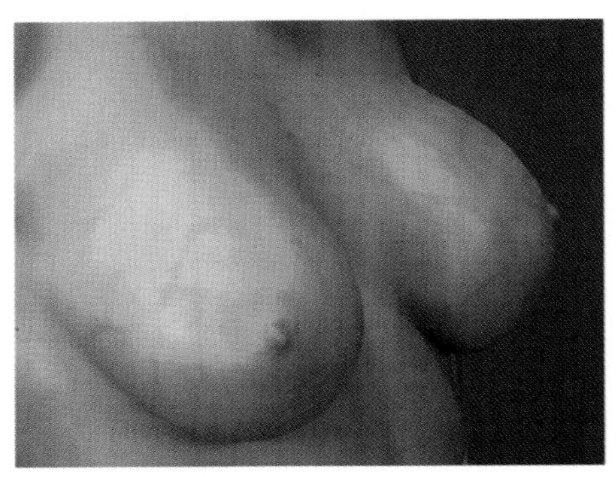

**C.**

The ideal size implant for any breast is the implant that will adequately fill the breast, but not overfill it— "just enough." A surgeon can always put a larger-than-ideal implant in a breast, and many patients request implants that are too large for their tissues. Many patients actually prefer the appearance of an excessively full upper breast with outward bulging—the "too much" look *without* a bra. When any implant that is larger than ideal for a specific patient's tissues is placed in a breast, the patient will pay a price in the future. The skin envelope will stretch and thin, the breast will sag, and all of the following risks increase: Feeling the implant, seeing an implant edge, loss of upper fullness, visible rippling at the top or sides of the breast from the large implant pulling downward on thin tissues, and necessity of additional surgery to correct problems.

## LESSON 4:
### You won't look like your friend.

Let's assume that two friends (we'll call them Sharon and Janet, but the names are fictitious) decide to have breast augmentation. Sharon (Figure 16-13, A-B) has her augmentation first (Figure 16-13, C-D).

Janet sees Sharon's result, and says, "I want my result to look just like Sharon's." When we examined Janet, we found that her breasts were very different than Sharon's (Figure 16-14, A-B). Can we produce the same breast that we produced for Sharon? Of course not, because the breasts were so different *before* augmentation. Janet's result is shown in Figure 16-14, C-D.

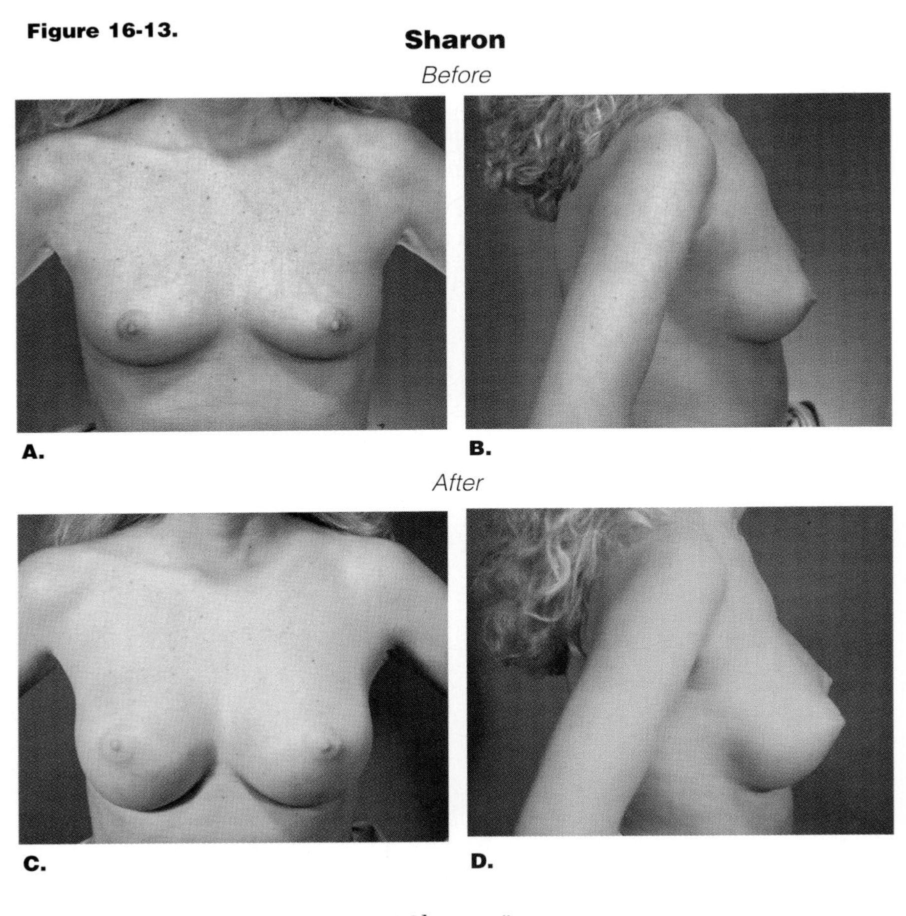


**Figure 16-13.** **Sharon**

"Sharon"
Wide breast in front view
Narrow gap between breasts
More breast tissue in skin envelope
Thicker skin envelope
Skin envelope not very stretched

Janet wants to achieve the same result that Sharon achieved. Can any surgeon match Janet's breasts to Sharon's?

**Figure 16-14.**

**Janet**

*Before*

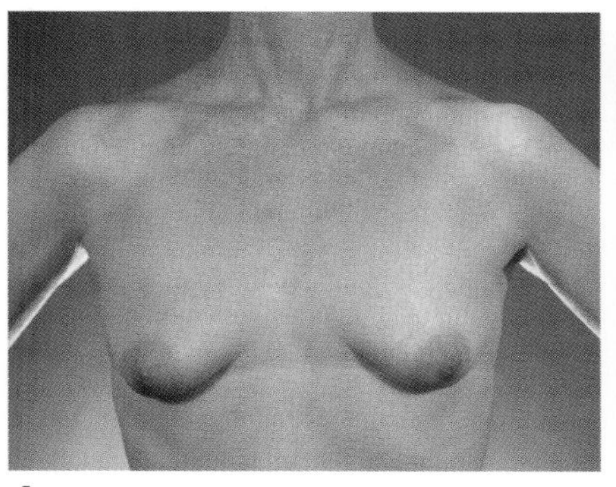

A.

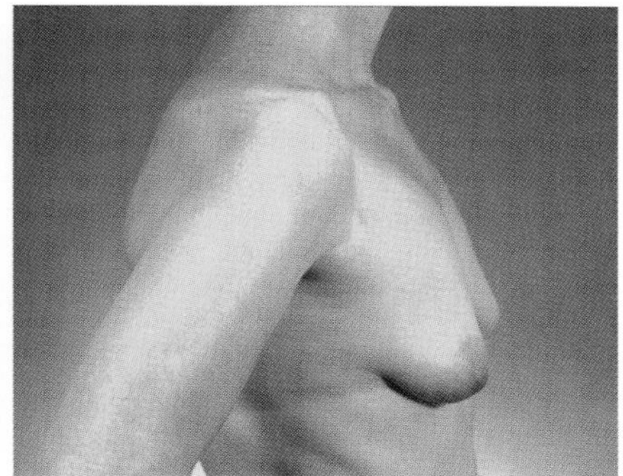

B.

*After*

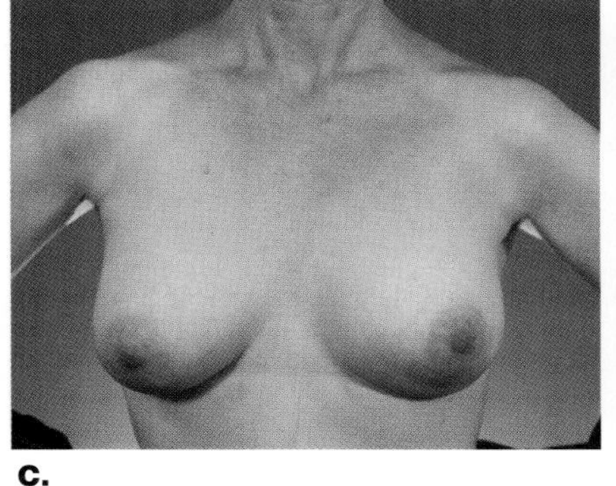

C.

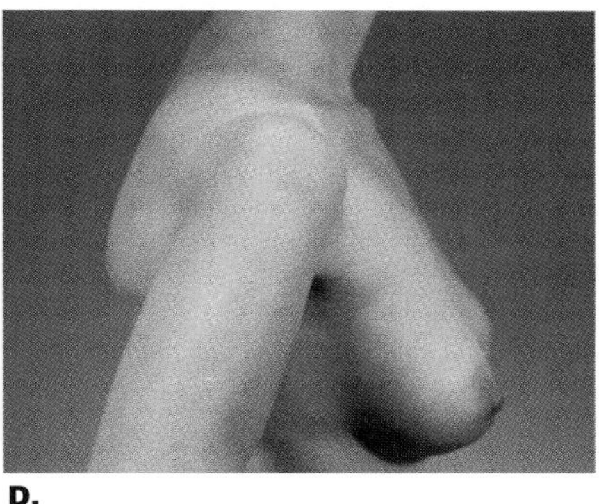

D.

"Janet"
Narrow breast in front view
Wide gap between breasts
Less breast tissue in skin envelope
Thin skin envelope
Skin envelope very stretched

Note the differences in Sharon and Janet *before* surgery:

A surgeon cannot change the *differences in these two patients' tissues before surgery*. Different tissues before surgery guarantee that their breasts will be different after surgery.

**You can't select a certain breast from a picture and realistically expect to achieve that result.**

## LESSON 5:
### A certain size implant does not produce a certain size breast.

Let's look again at our two hypothetical friends from Lesson 4 (Figures 16-15, A-D and 16-16, A-D). These friends, Sharon and Janet, requested and received exactly the same size implant. Are their breasts the same size after surgery? No. *A certain size implant does not produce a certain size breast.* Remember our formula from Chapter 4?

**Figure 16-15.**

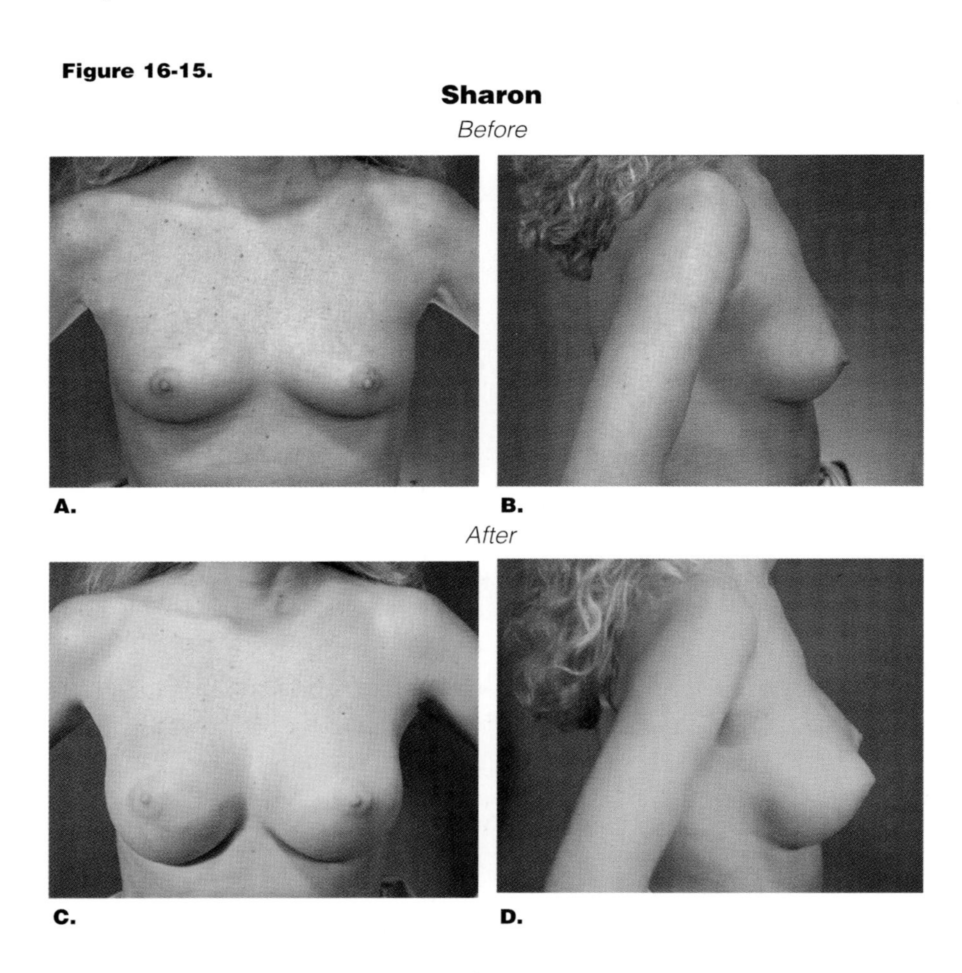


**Augmentation Result =**
**Envelope + Parenchyma (breast tissue) + Implant**

**Figure 16-16.**

**Janet**

*Before*

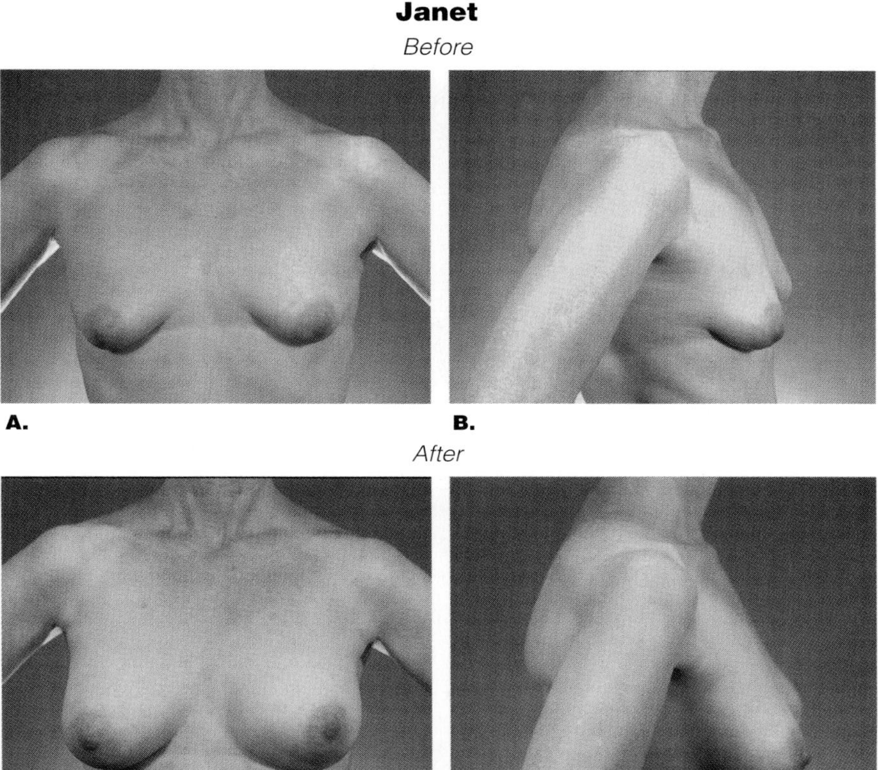

A. B.

*After*

C. D.

Sharon had more breast tissue *before* surgery than Janet, so with the *same size* implant, Sharon's breasts will be larger than Janet's breasts *after* surgery. The size of implant required to achieve the breast size you want *after* surgery depends on how much breast tissue you have *before* surgery.

We frequently see patients who have a certain size implant in mind, based on what a friend had or what they may have heard, read in magazines, or learned from a chat group on the Internet.

**Many women believe that a certain size implant (in ccs) is required to achieve a certain cup-size breast. This lesson clearly illustrates that a certain size implant does not produce a certain cup-size breast.**

You should know that when you request a certain size implant, the *easiest* thing for a surgeon to do is fulfill your request rather than try to explain to you why that size implant may not be the best for you long-term. If you want the best result and the least risk of problems and additional operations as you age, discuss your wishes with your surgeon, but ask your surgeon to help you make the best decisions about implant size. Remember that "excessively large" carries a price as you get older.

## LESSON 6:
### Cleavage-what makes it and how much can I get?

Normal breasts don't cleave. Bras make breasts cleave. As breasts develop during puberty, the breast tissue develops on a curved surface, the chest wall. Gravity pulls the breasts outward slightly, so most breasts point slightly outward. Very few women's breasts point straight ahead. The width of the gap between the breasts depends on two factors: 1) The width of the woman's breast in front view, and 2) the total width of the torso. For a specific width *torso,* the wider the breast, the narrower the gap between the breasts. Stated another way, for a specific width *breast,* the wider the torso, the wider the gap between the breasts.

When the gap between the breasts is wide (Figure 16-17, A), two factors determine how much the gap can be narrowed: 1) The width, amount, and consistency of the patient's own breast tissue, and 2) the width and size of the breast implant. The wider the implant (Figure 16-17, B), the more the gap narrows, but distinct tradeoffs and risks exist. If the implant is wider than the patient's breast tissue (Figure 16-17,C), the breast tissue no longer covers the edge of the implant, and the edge rests beneath only the thin skin in the gap between the breasts. When thin tissues cover an implant edge, the patient must accept a higher risk of the implant

**Figure 16-17.**

**A.**

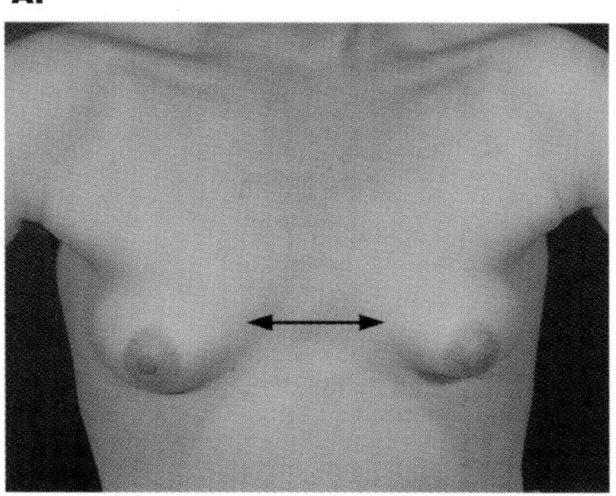

**B.**

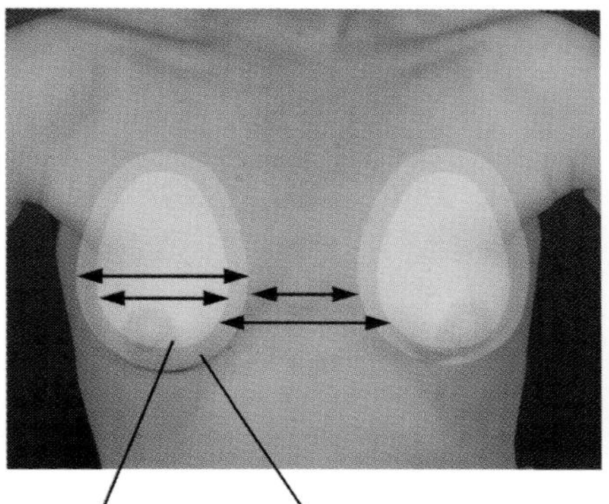


**C.**

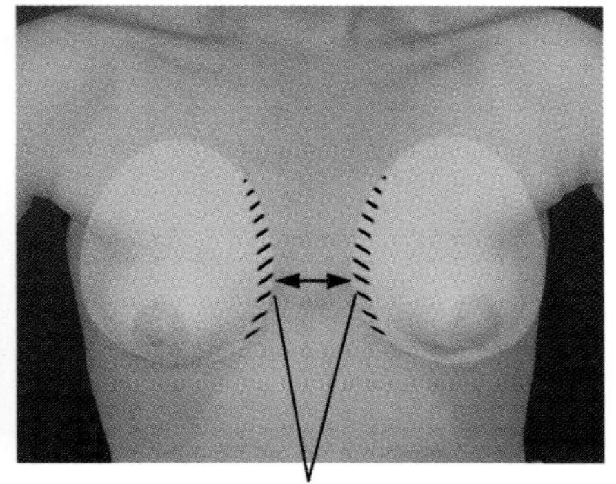


being visible in the cleavage area. What is the message to remember? If you request narrowing of the gap between your breasts, ask your surgeon to demonstrate how much the gap can be narrowed without risking edge visibility of your implant. If you want more narrowing than the surgeon demonstrates, be prepared to sign an informed consent document that confirms your acceptance of the risk of implant edge visibility.

**Figure 16-18.**

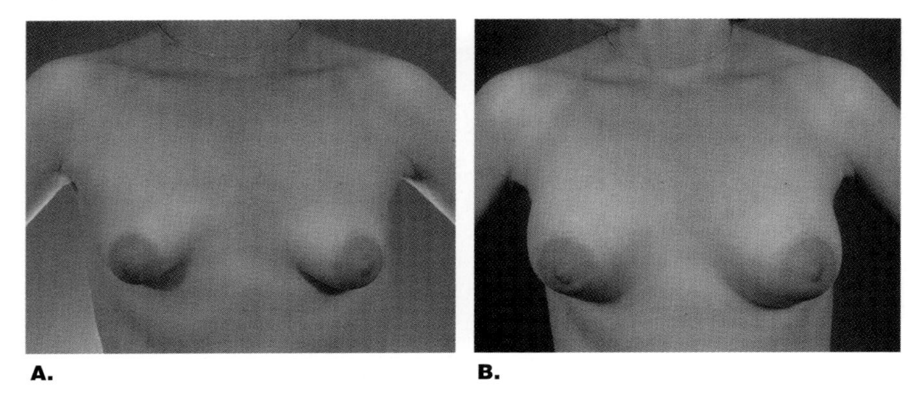

**A.** **B.**

The patient above (Figure 16-18, A) has extremely narrow breasts and a wide gap between the breasts. Following augmentation (Figure 16-18, B), the gap between the breasts is narrower, but not extremely narrow. Notice in the picture after augmentation that the sternum (the central chest bone) is visible under the thin skin between the breasts. If a wider implant had been used to narrow the gap further, the edge of the implant would be just as visible as the breastbone and ribs. More fullness in the middle would further emphasize the already outwordly pointing nipples.

## LESSON 7:

**A certain incision location or pocket location (beneath breast or beneath muscle) does not produce a specific appearance in the result.**

If you looked through our extensive before-and-after pictures in our office, you absolutely cannot tell by looking at a picture whether an implant is placed above muscle (behind breast tissue only) or beneath the pectoralis muscle. An experienced augmentation surgeon can produce almost exactly the same result above or below muscle, provided the surgeon has adequate experience with both locations.

Look at the following results following augmentation (Figure 16-19). Which are over muscle and which are under muscle?

**Figure 16-19.**

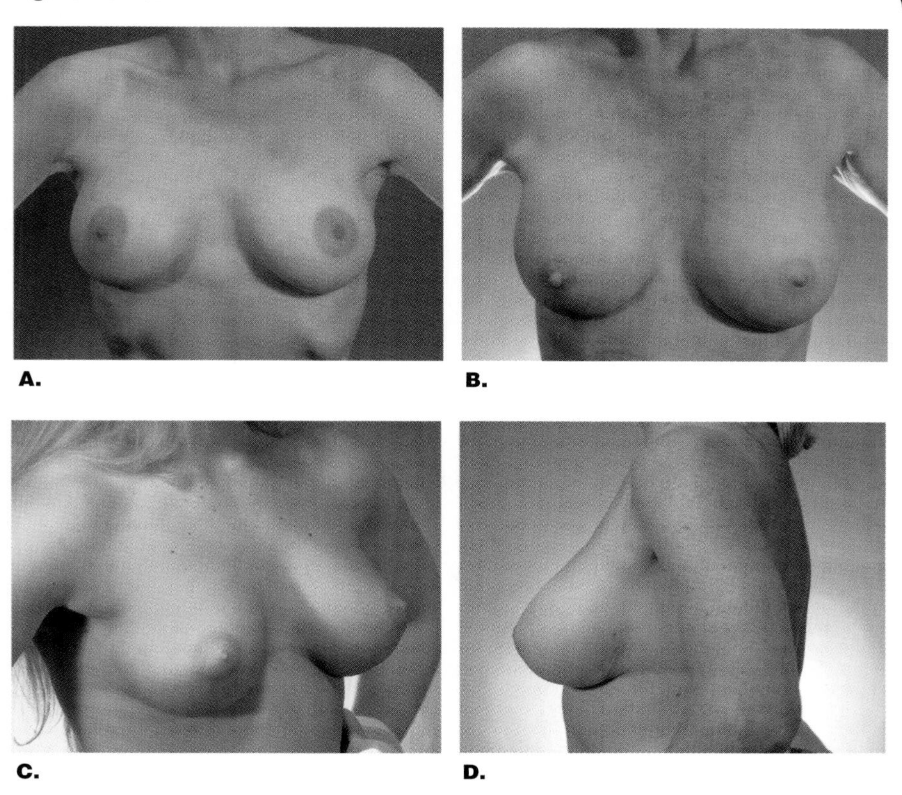

**A.** **B.** **C.** **D.**

The implants are under muscle(A), over muscle(B), over muscle(C), and under muscle(D). Incision locations are under the breast(A), in the armpit(B), in the armpit(C), under the breast and around the areola(D). Each incision location and pocket location have advantages and tradeoffs that are described in detail in Chapter 6.

## LESSON 8:

### Nipples point where they point. Surgically repositioning nipples involves substantial tradeoffs.

Ideally, the nipple, surrounded by the pigmented skin called the areola, is located in the middle of the breast mound when viewing the breast from the front. In reality, nipple-areola position is extremely variable woman to woman. In the pictures that follow

(Figure 16-20, A-D), notice the wide variation in the position of the nipples from patient to patient as well as the differences in nipple position from side-to-side in the same patient.

Following augmentation, notice that the nipples basically point in the same direction as before surgery. Although the implant can be positioned to change nipple tilt and position slightly, any major correction of nipple position requires surgical repositioning. When the nipple-areola complex is repositioned surgically, the patient must accept the following tradeoffs: Increased risk of sensory loss, possible interference with ability to nurse, and visible scar around the areola. Every woman has differences in nipple position, but surgical repositioning should be reserved for very significant differences and for patients willing to accept the tradeoffs.

**Figure 16-20.**

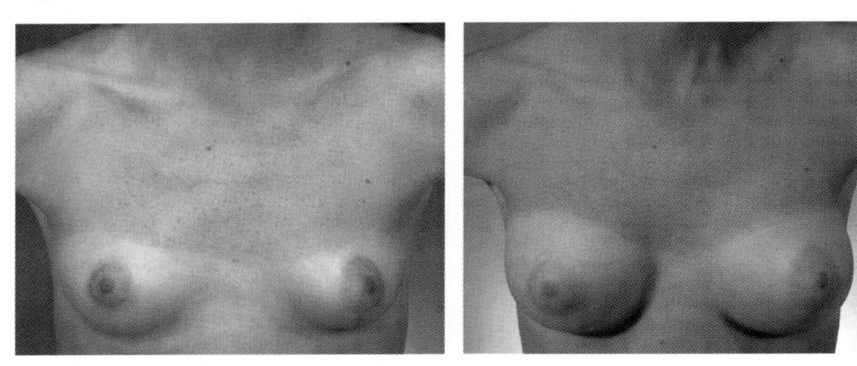

**A.** *Left nipple-areola larger and more outwardly pointing.*

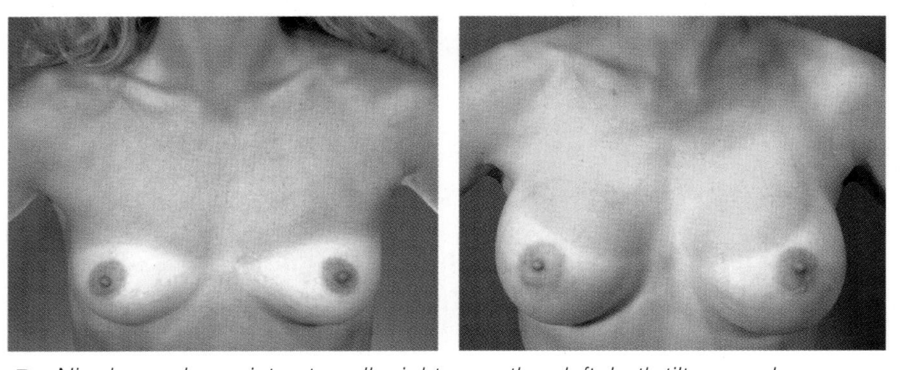

**B.** *Nipple-areolas point outwardly right more than left, both tilt upward.*

**Figure 16-20. (continued)**

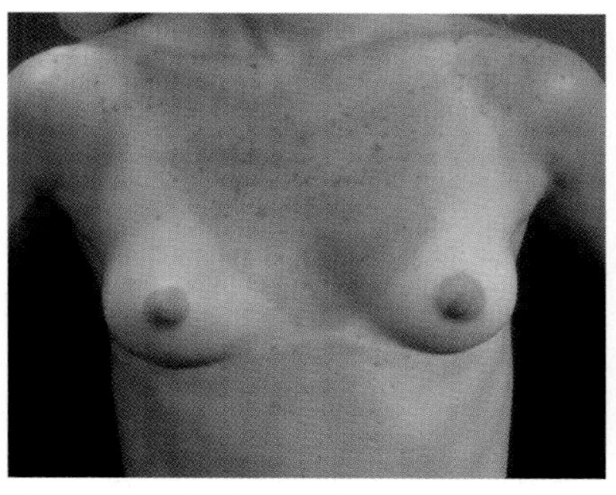
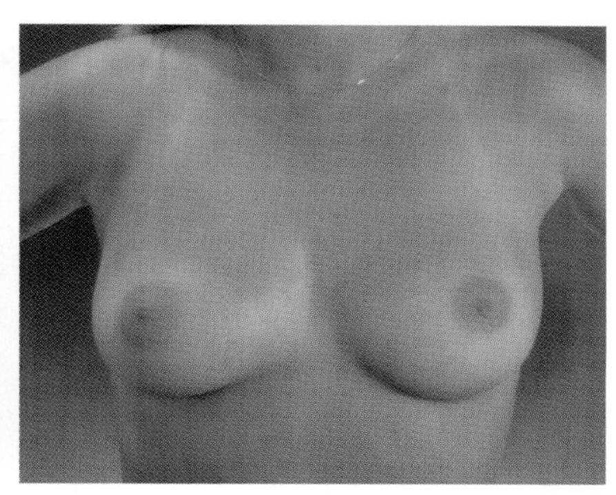

**C.** *Right nipple-areola smaller than left, left higher than right.*

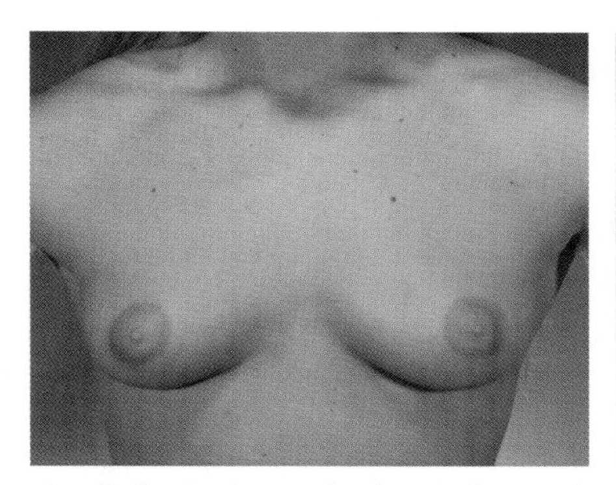
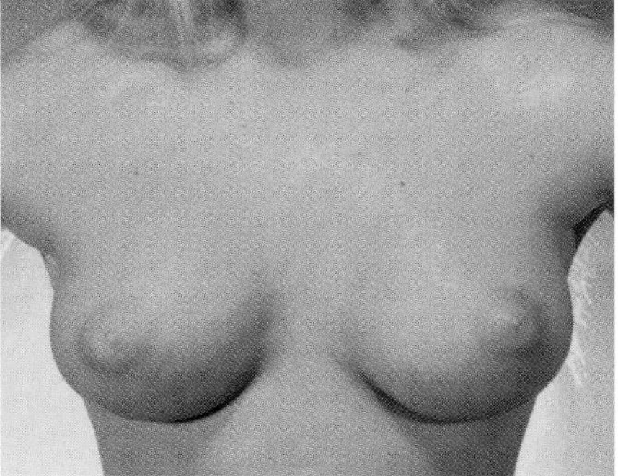

**D.** *Both nipple-areolas located toward outside of breast mound, left higher than right.*

## LESSON 9:

**A round implant can produce a breast that looks good but may have a folded implant shell that can fail earlier. An anatomic-shaped implant can be filled adequately to protect the shell and still achieve a natural appearing upper breast.**

If a breast looks natural following augmentation using a round implant (Figure 16-21, A-B), chances are that the shell of the round implant has collapsed vertically and the upper shell is folded (Figure 16-21, C). A folded shell risks early shell failure and implant rupture and requires additional surgery to replace the implant. If the round implant were filled enough to protect the shell and prevent collapse with the implant in the upright position (Figure 16-21, D) in the breast, the implant would usually cause excessive upper bulging or an excessively globular appearance (Figure 16-21, E).

**Figure 16-21.**

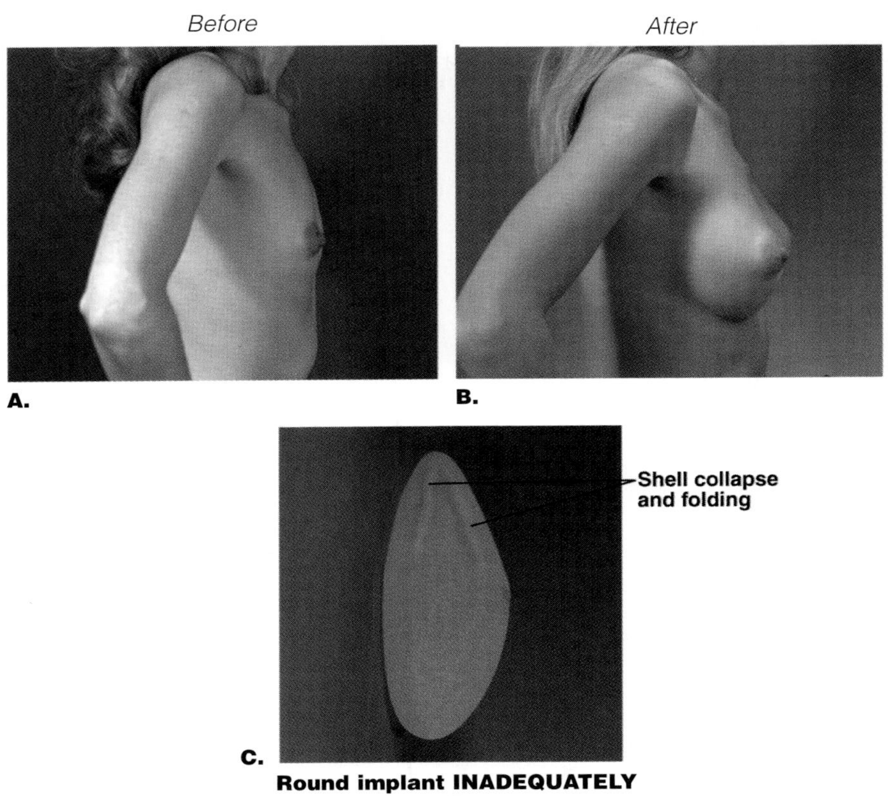


**Round implant INADEQUATELY FILLED (even filled to current manufacturer's recommendations)**

**Figure 16-21. (continued)**

**D.**

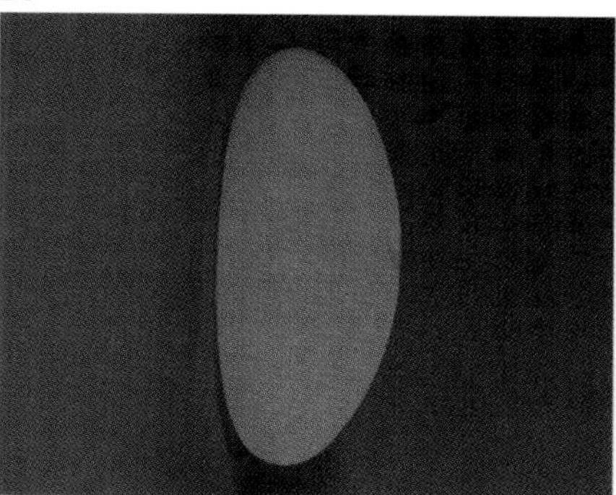

**Round implant ADEQUATELY FILLED to prevent shell collapse and folding**

**E.**

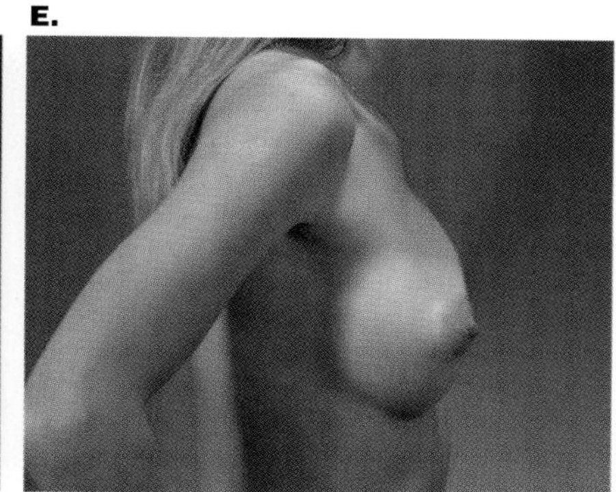

**Unnatural upper bulge that is more likely to occur with an adequately filled ROUND implant**

An anatomically-shaped implant (Figure 16-22, A) can be filled adequately to prevent upper shell folding (Figure 16-22, B) with the implant upright, protecting the shell against shell collapse, shell folding, and early shell failure. When an adequately filled anatomic implant is placed in the breast (Figure 16-23, A-D), the tapered shape of the upper portion of the anatomic implant does not cause excessive upper breast bulging. The result is a natural appearing breast and an implant without a folded shell that could fail sooner.

**Figure 16-22.**

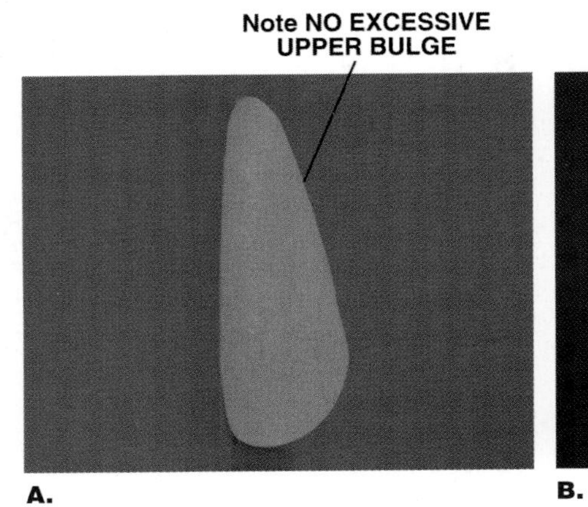


**A.**

**Anatomic implant ADEQUATELY FILLED to prevent shell collapse**

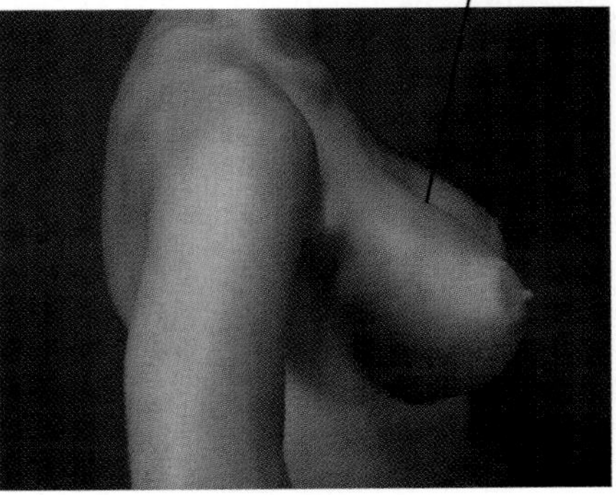


**B.**

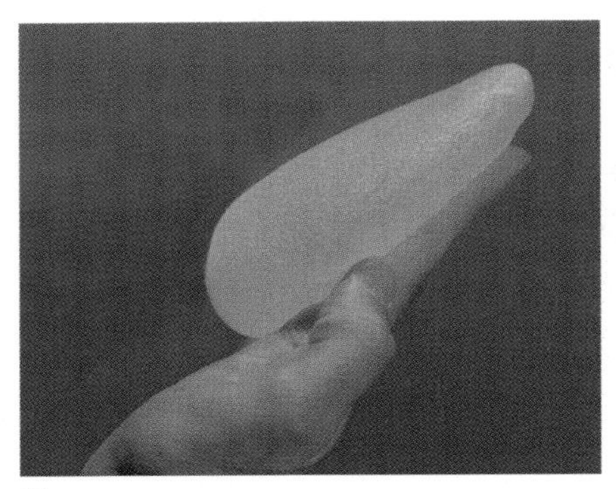

**C.**

**Figure 16-23.**

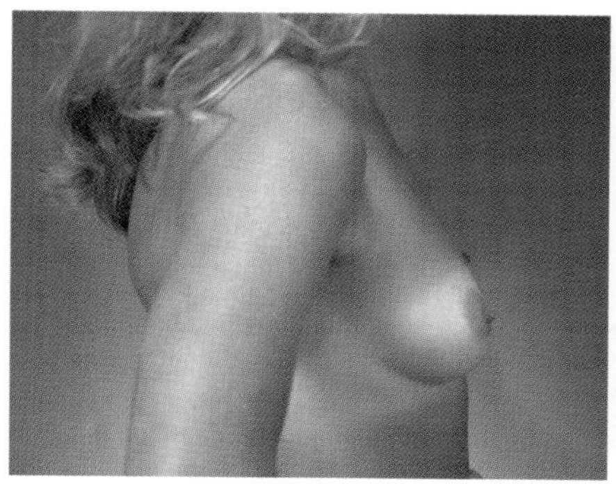

**A.**

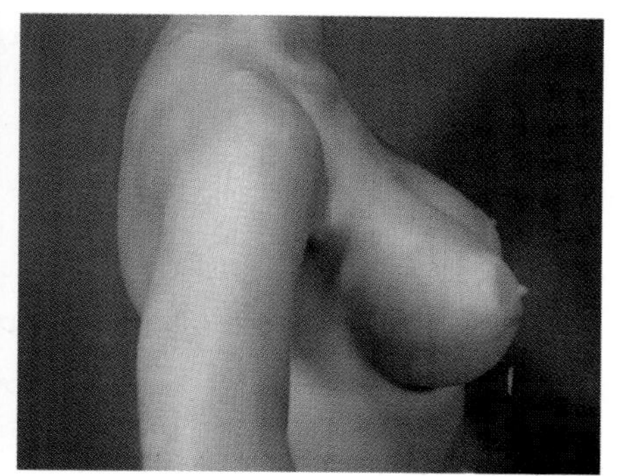

**B.**

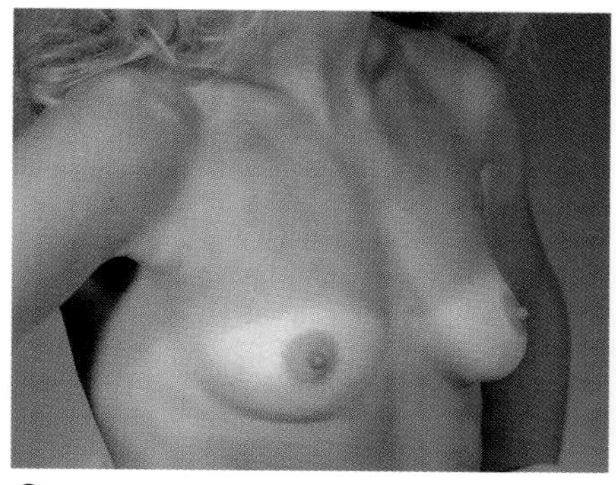

**C.**

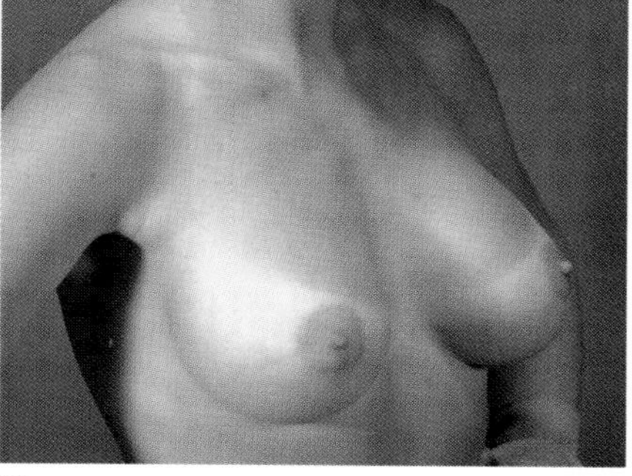

**D.**

## LESSON 10:
### The prices you can pay for selecting an excessively large implant

The skin envelope of the breast stretches to accommodate the enlargement of the breast during pregnancy and nursing, but this enlargement is a natural, physiologic process that occurs over several months and is usually limited to a moderate amount of enlargement. Breast augmentation enlarges the breast very rapidly, and the amount of enlargement depends on the patient's wishes and her tissues.

When a woman selects excessively large implants, she may enjoy the result for a while, but she is choosing long-term risks that she may not like. The skin envelope of the breast does not improve as a woman ages. Visualize your grandmother's breasts. Skin usually gets thinner and stretches as gravity pulls on the breast over time, with or without an implant. The larger the implant, the heavier the implant, the more stretch and thinning of tissues occurs, and the more rapidly it occurs. Excessively large implants can cause any or all of the following problems:

- Excessive skin stretching
- Sagging of the breast
- Loss of upper breast fullness as the lower breast stretches
- Thinning of the skin envelope
- Shrinkage of the patient's own breast tissue from pressure by the implant
- Visible implant edges
- Visible rippling caused by the heavy implant pulling downward on the skin envelope (Figure 16-24)
- Distortion of breast shape

**Figure 16-24.**

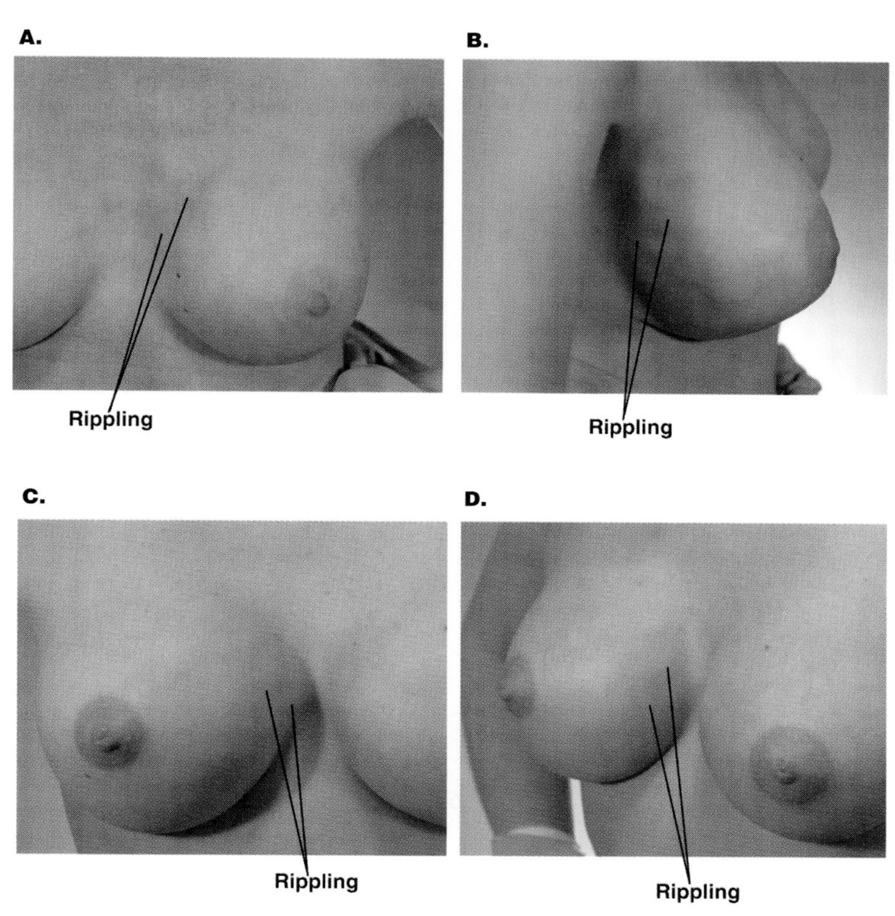


What implant size is safe and what is excessive? In part, the answer depends on a patient's tissues. *The thinner the tissues, the more a large implant can affect those tissues.* The rule of thumb that we follow is that any breast implant larger than 350cc to 400cc can produce the problems listed above. Special circumstances may require larger breast implants, but whenever a patient needs or selects an implant larger than 350cc, we advise the patient of the increased risks of the problems listed above.

The following patients (16-25, 16-26) had larger breasts that had been significantly stretched by pregnancy and nursing, requiring larger implants to adequately fill the envelope. The tradeoffs of breast lift (mastopexy) were unacceptable to both patients, and both accepted the tradeoffs of placing large implants. Both were fully aware that they might well require breast lifts in the future, with removal of the large implants, and either no implant replacement or replacement with a much smaller implant. Remember, as you age, your tissues won't support weight as well.

**Figure 16-25.**

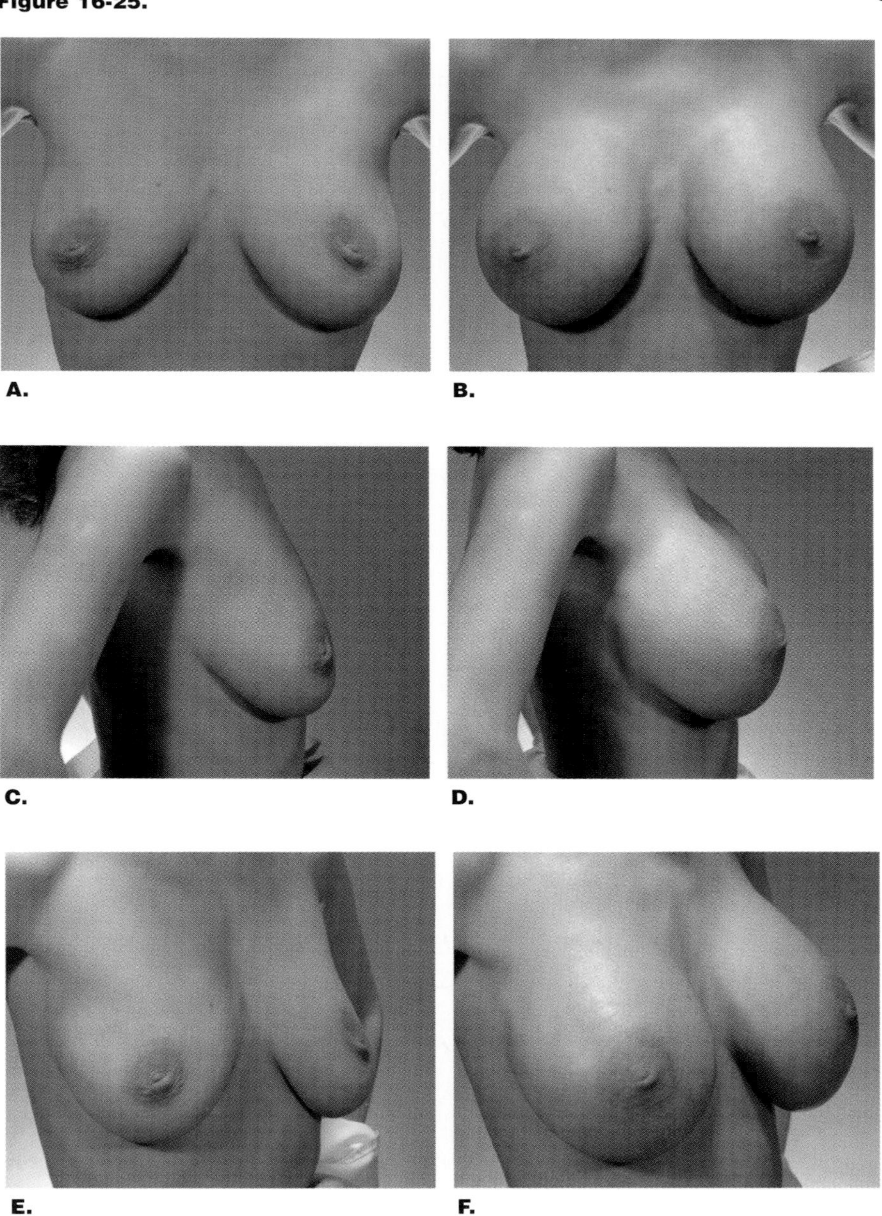

**A.** **B.**

**C.** **D.**

**E.** **F.**

**Patient with markedly stretched tissues who refused breast lift (mastopexy) and requested very large implants.**

**Figure 16-26.**

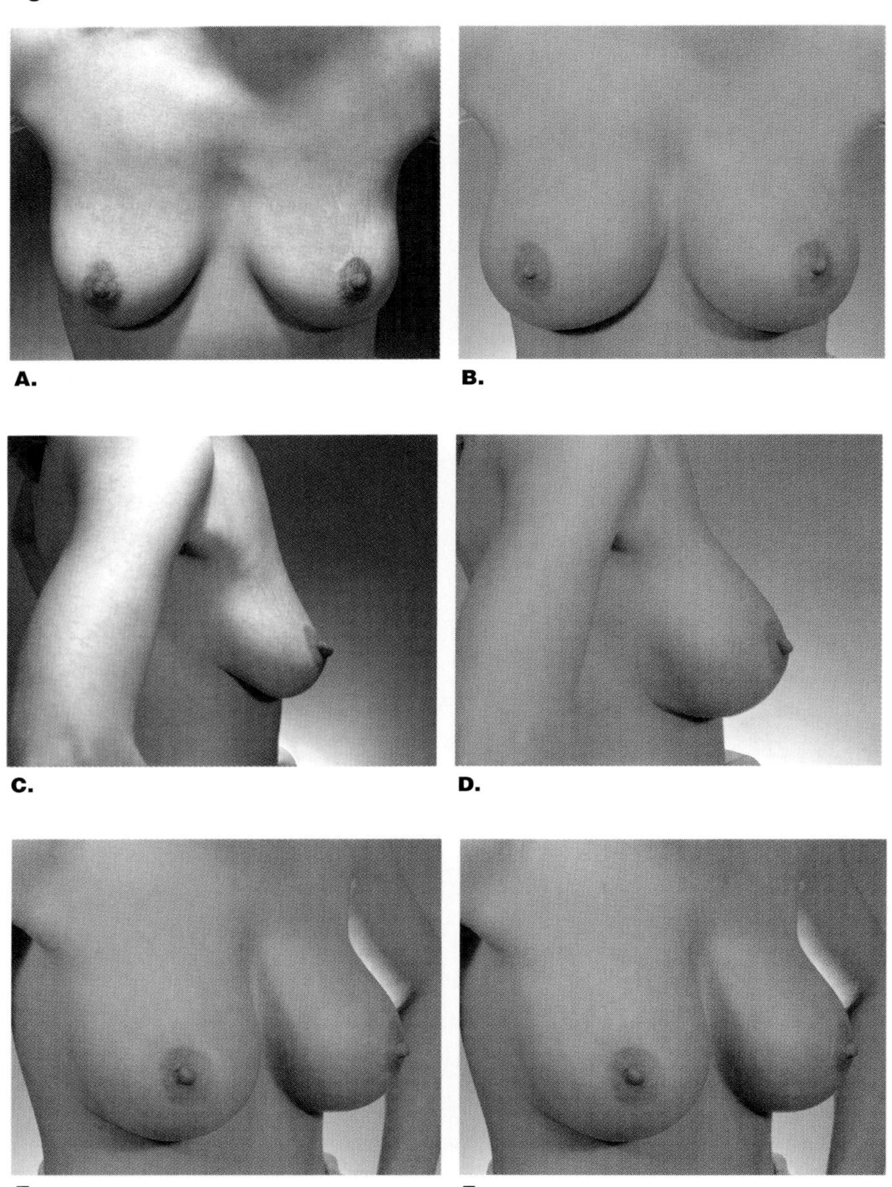


**Patient with stretched envelope and sagging following pregnancy, who required a large implant to adequately fill her envelope.**

## LESSON 11:
### What is capsular contracture?

When a medical device is placed in the body, the body forms a tissue lining around the device. This lining, called a capsule, forms around every breast implant in every patient. In most patients, the lining surrounds the implant but does not cause any problem. In a small percentage of patients, the capsule contracts or tightens excessively, squeezing on the implant, making the implant feel too hard, and often pushing the implant out of position and distorting breast shape.

The risk of capsular contracture varies with the type of implant, implant shell characteristics, and type of filler material, but the average risk is 2-5 percent for textured shell, saline-filled implants. This means that from two to five patients in 100 will develop a capsular contracture on one or both sides.

Figure 16-27, A-F illustrates a patient who developed a capsular contracture of the right breast. As the capsule tightens excessively around the implant, it often displaces the implant upward (A), making one breast appear higher than the other. In side view (B), as the implant is pushed upward by the contracting capsule, the upper breast bulges, and the breast feels very firm compared to the left breast. After correction (D, E, F), the breasts appear more symmetrical (D), the excessive upper bulging is corrected (E), and both breasts have a very natural appearance (F).

Another patient who has severe capsular contractures on both sides is illustrated in Figure 16-27, A-F. Both breasts are displaced upward (A), producing excessive upward bulging and down-pointing nipples (B,C). The middle portion of the left breast is flattened and distorted (A), and both breasts feel extremely hard. After removal of the capsules and implant replacement (D, E, F), the breasts appear much more symmetrical and natural, with normal contours, a natural slope to the upper breast, and a softer feel.

**Figure 16-27.**

**A.**

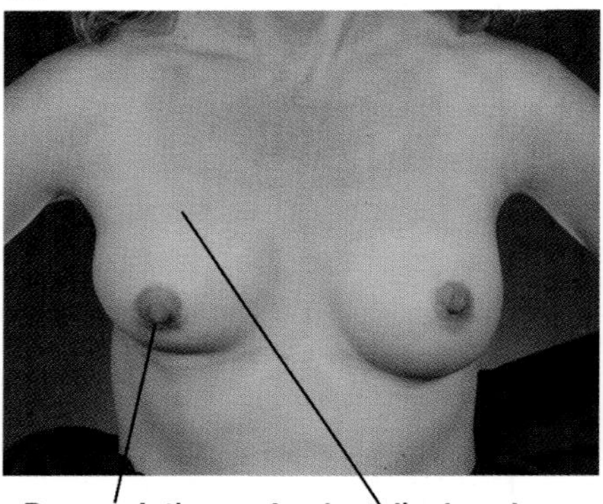


**Right breast developed capsular contracture following augmentation**

**D.**

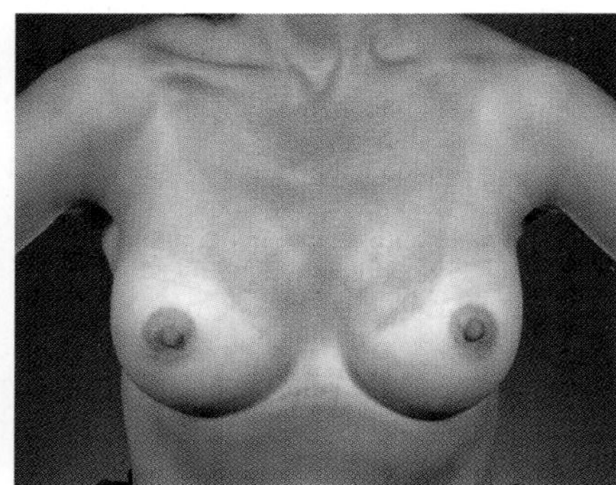

**B.**

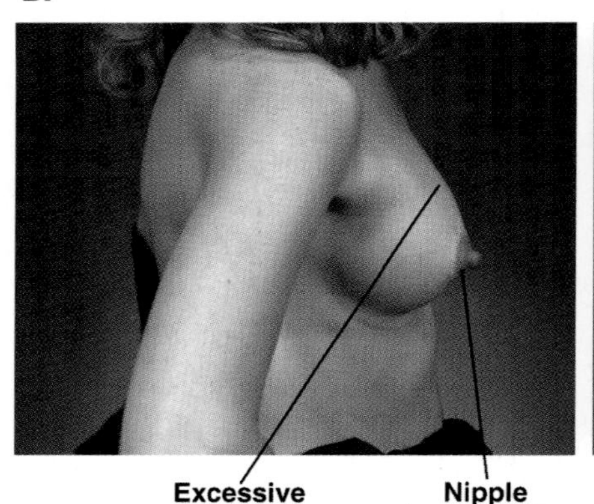


**Before correcting capsular contracture**

**E.**

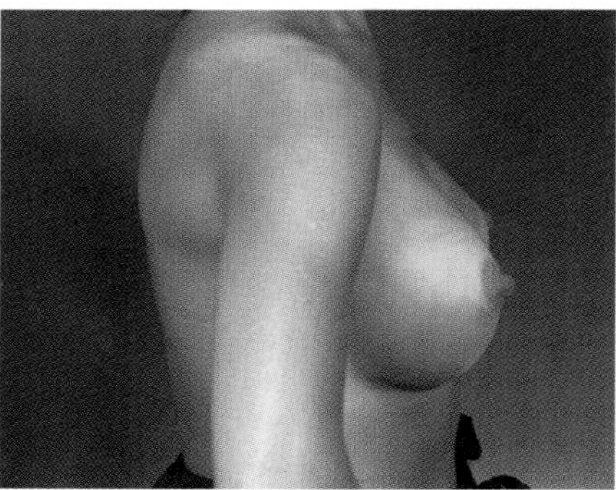

**After correcting capsular contracture**

**C.**

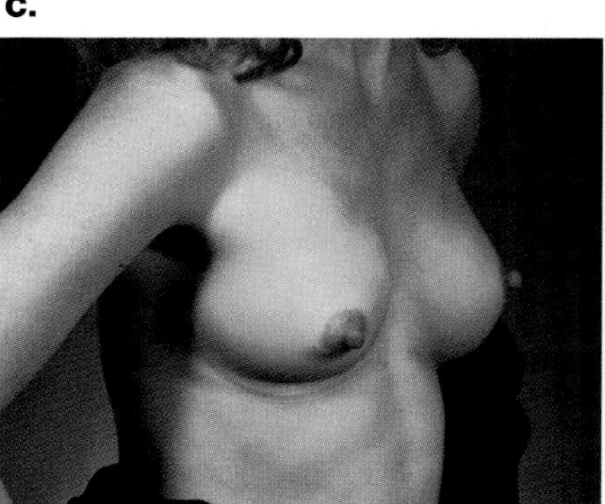

**F.**

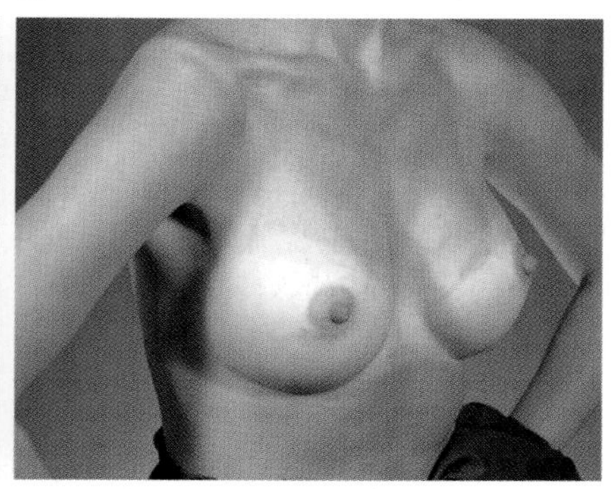

**Figure 16-28.**

**A.**

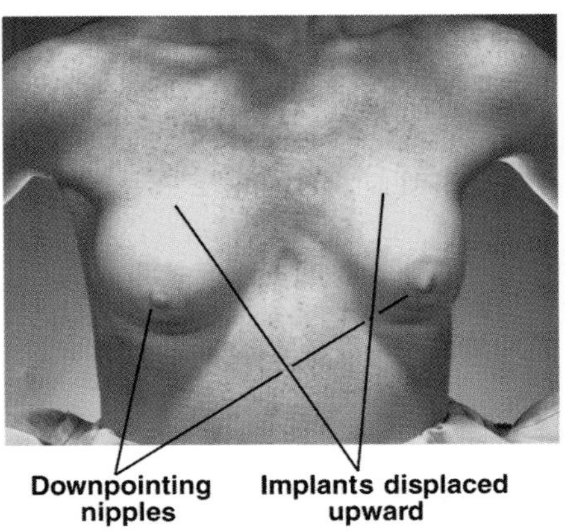


**Breasts developed capsular contracture following augmentation**

**D.**

**B.**

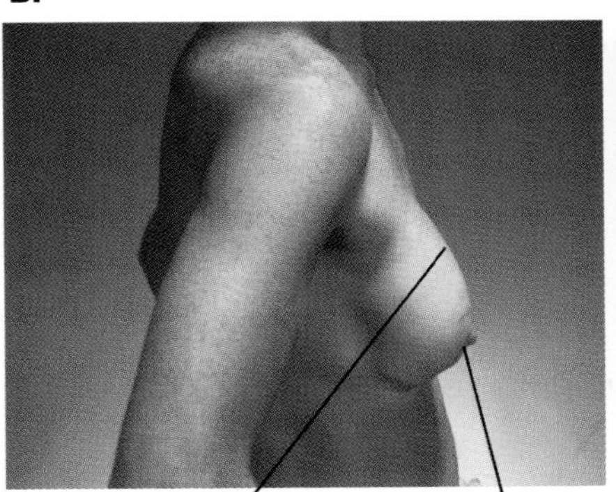


**Before correcting capsular contracture**

**E.**

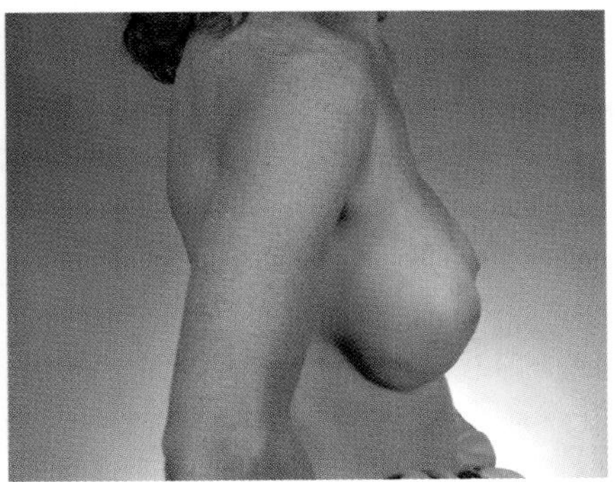

**After correcting capsular contracture**

**C.**

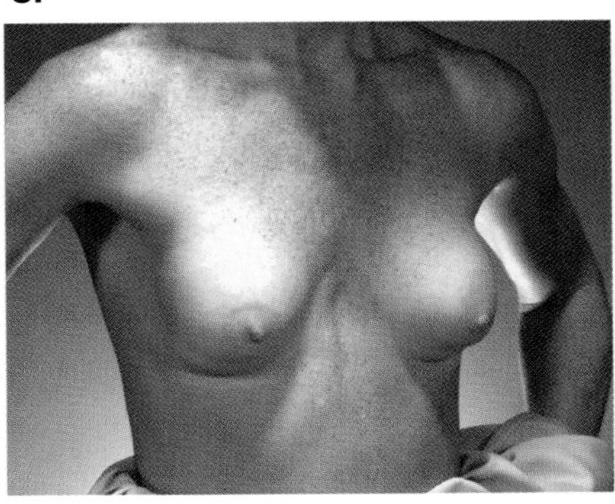

**F.**

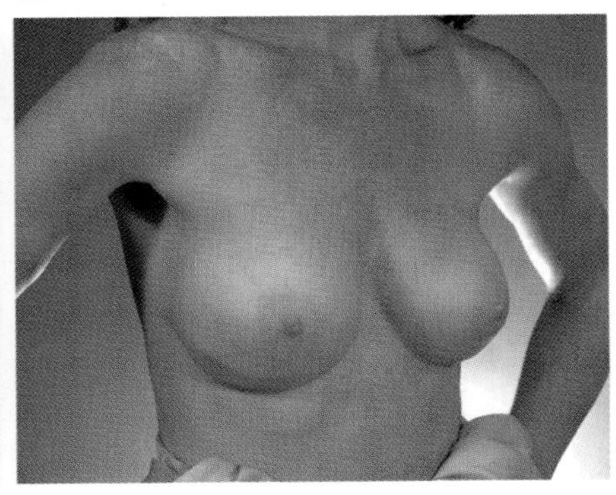

[APPENDIX 1]

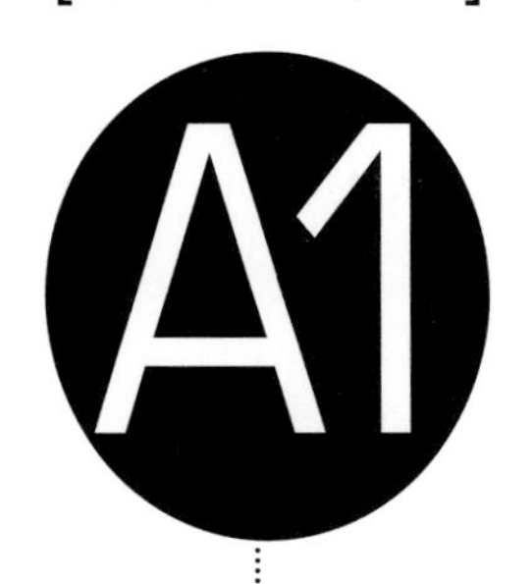


# U.S. AND INTERNATIONAL STUDIES OF BREAST IMPLANTS AND BREAST CANCER

The following is a summary of the epidemiology studies of breast implants and breast cancer conducted by prominent researchers at prestigious institutions. Unlike the reports of individual women (often called "case reports" or "case series"), these studies were designed to make comparisons between groups of women with and without breast implants. These more rigorous epidemiology studies provide the opportunity to determine whether breast cancer among women with implants is occurring more frequently than might be expected.

**International Epidemiology Institute, Karolinska Institute,** and the US National Cancer Institute, McLaughlin, PhD; Nyren, MD; Blot, PhD; et al; Rockville. MD. - 1998 Breast Implants/Breast Cancer
This nationwide Swedish study included 3,473 women who had cosmetic breast implant procedures from 1965 through 1993. Followed for an average of 10.3 years, 18 women developed breast cancer compared to 25 expected cases. The authors concluded, *"Our study showed a statistically nonsignificant reduction in the incidence of breast cancer that may be due to concomitant risk factors (e.g., lower age at first pregnancy and decreased glandular density)."*
In an earlier publication (1995), McLaughlin and colleagues reported similar findings based on 1,756 women with cosmetic breast implants in Sweden.

**University of Southern California School of Medicine,** Deapen, DrPH; Bernstein, PhD; Brody, MD; Los Angeles, CA - 1997 Breast Implants/Breast Cancer
This study reports continued follow-up of more than 3,100 women in Los Angeles County who received cosmetic breast implants between 1953 and 1980. Followed for a median of 14.4 years, 31 women with implants subsequently developed breast cancer compared to 49.2 expected cases of breast cancer. The authors concluded, *"In Los Angeles County, augmentation mammaplasty patients experience a significantly lower than expected risk of breast cancer and no delay in breast cancer detection..."*
In two earlier publications (1986, 1992), Deapen and colleagues reported similar conclusions based on following these same women for a median of 6.2 and 10.6 years, respectively.
Directly funded by Dow Corning Corporation.

**Danish Cancer Society; International Epidemiology Institute; and the US National Cancer Institute,** Friis, MD; McLaughlin, PhD; Mellemkjaer, MSc; et al; Copenhagen, Denmark - 1997 Breast Implants/ Breast Cancer
This nationwide Danish study included 1,135 women who had cosmetic breast implant procedures between 1977 and 1992. Followed for an average of 8.4 years, 8 women developed breast cancer versus 7.8 expected cases. The authors stated, "*In summary, breast implants were not related to an excess risk of breast or other cancers in our population-based cohort study.*"
In an earlier publication (1994), McLaughlin and colleagues reported similar conclusions based on 824 women with cosmetic breast implants in Denmark.

**Hartford Hospital,** Kern, MD; Flannery; Kuehn, MD; Hartford, CT - 1997 Breast Implants/Breast Cancer
These authors reported on subsequent cancers in 680 Connecticut women who had breast implant surgery compared to 1,022 women who had tubal ligation surgery and no breast implants. No woman had a prior history of cancer. Women were followed for an average of 4.6 years after implant surgery and 5.4 years after tubal ligation surgery. Women with breast implants had a nonsignificantly lower rate of breast cancer compared to women without implants. The authors stated, "*Based on these data, it was concluded that silicone breast implants are not carcinogenic, because they are not associated with increased rates of either breast or nonbreast cancers.*"

**US National Cancer Institute,** Brinton, PhD; Malone, PhD; Coates, PhD, et al; Bethesda, MD - 1996 Breast Implants/Breast Cancer
This study included 2,174 women who had breast cancer and 2,009 women without breast cancer. Breast implants were reported by 36 women with cancer versus 44 women without cancer. This study found that the risk for breast cancer was lower among women who had breast implants. Furthermore, the decreased risk for breast cancer persisted as the time since implantation increased. The authors stated, "*In this study, we found*

*that women who had received breast implants were not at an excess risk for developing breast cancer. This finding agrees with all the other analytical studies that have examined the relationship."*

**Alberta Cancer Board,** Bryant, MD; Brasher, PhD; Alberta, Canada - 1995 Breast Implants/Breast Cancer
This study was a re-analysis of data presented by Berkel, Birdsell, and Jenkins (1992) who reported a lower risk for breast cancer among women with breast implants in Alberta, Canada. Among the 10,835 women included in this re-analysis who had undergone breast augmentation surgery, 45 women subsequently developed breast cancer compared to 59 expected cases of breast cancer. Although the number of cancer cases was lower than expected and consistent with other research studies, since the results were not statistically significant, the authors concluded, *"...the apparent risk of breast cancer cannot be said to be either higher or significantly lower than that of the general population."*
Birdsell and colleagues (1993), in an earlier study of this general group of women, investigated the survival experience of women with breast cancer diagnosed after breast augmentation. Among the 11,670 women with cosmetic breast implants included in this report, 4l developed breast cancer after augmentation. The survival experience for these 41 women was compared to the survival of all women diagnosed with breast cancer during the same time period (1973-1990 inclusive). The researchers concluded, *"In summary, our study shows that women with a breast tumor diagnosed after having had an implant survive as long as women with breast cancer without implants. We did not find that the tumors in women with implants were diagnosed at a later stage and in fact, these tumors were smaller at diagnosis. This...allows in our opinion the conclusion that cosmetic breast augmentation is not a cause of concern in regard to breast cancer."*

**Institut Gustave Roussy,** Petit, MD; Le, MD; Mouriesse, MSc; et al; Villejuif, France - 1994 Breast Implants/Breast Cancer
The researchers studied 146 patients with breast cancer treated by mastectomy who received a gel-filled silicone implant between 1976 and 1984 for reconstruction compared to 146 matched controls with breast cancer who were treated in the same

center without reconstruction. The risks of distant metastasis and death due to breast cancer were significantly lower in the breast reconstruction group than in the control group. The risk for second breast cancer did not differ between the two groups of women. The researchers stated, "*In conclusion, our results do not support the hypothesis of a detrimental effect of gel-filled silicone implants either in the course of breast cancer or in the risk of death due to other diseases.*"

**Fred Hutchinson Cancer Research Center,** Malone; Stanford; Daling, PhD; et al; Seattle, WA - 1992 Breast Implants/Breast Cancer The authors compared the incidence of breast implants among women with breast cancer to the incidence of implants among women without cancer. For their two study groups of women with cancer (women aged 21-44 years and women aged 50-64 years), compared to women without breast cancer, there was no apparent risk for breast cancer due to silicone breast implants.

**Centers for Disease Control and Prevention,** Glasser, PhD; Lee; Wingo; Atlanta, GA - 1989 Breast Augmentation/ Breast Cancer Researchers compared 4,742 women with breast cancer (12 of whom had breast augmentation prior to their disease) to 4,754 women without breast cancer (8 of whom had breast augmentation). They found no association between breast augmentation and breast cancer.

# BIBLIOGRAPHY FOR U.S. AND INTERNATIONAL STUDIES OF BREAST IMPLANTS AND BREAST CANCER

Berkel H, Birdsell DC, Jenkins H. Breast Augmentation: A Risk Factor for Breast Cancer? *N Engl J Med* 1992;326:1649-1653.

Birdsell DC, Jenkins H, Berkel H. Breast Cancer Diagnosis and Survival in Women With and Without Breast Implants. *Plast Reconstr Surg* 1993;92:795-800.

Brinton LA, Malone KE, Coates RJ, Schoenberg JB, Swanson CA, Daling JR, Stanford JL. Breast Enlargement and Reduction: Results From a Breast Cancer Case-Control Study. *Plast Reconstr Surg* 1996;97:269-275.

Bryant H, Brasher P. Breast Implants and Breast Cancer-Reanalysis of a Linkage Study. *N Engl J Med* 1995;332:1535-1539.

Deapen DM, Bernstein L, Brody GS. Are Breast Implants Anticarcinogenic? A 14-Year Follow-Up of the Los Angeles Study. *Plast Reconstr Surg* 1997;99:1346-1353.

Deapen DM, Brody GS. Augmentation Mammaplasty and Breast Cancer: A 5-Year Update of the Los Angeles Study. *Plast Reconstr Surg* 1992;89:660-665.

Deapen DM, Pike MC, Casagrande JT, Brody GS. The Relationship Between Breast Cancer and Augmentation Mammaplasty: An Epidemiologic Study. *Plast Reconstr Surg* 1986;77:361-367.

Friis S, McLaughlin JK, Mellemkjaer L, Kjoller KH, Blot WJ, Boice JD, Fraumeni JF, Olsen JH. Breast Implants and Cancer Risk in Denmark. *Int J Cancer* 1997;71:956-958.

Glasser JW, Lee NC, Wingo PA. Does Breast Augmentation Increase the Risk of Breast Cancer? The Epidemic Intelligence Service Conference, April, 1989.

Kern KA, Flannery JT, Kuehn PG. Carcinogenic Potential of Silicone Breast Implants: A Connecticut Statewide Study. *Plast Reconstr Surg* 1997;100:737-749.

Malone KE, Stanford JL, Daling JR, Voigt LF. Implants and Breast Cancer. *The Lancet* 1992;339:1365.

McLaughlin JK, Nyren O, Blot WJ, Yin L, Josefsson S, Fraumeni JF, Adami HO. Cancer Risk Among Women with Cosmetic Breast Implants: A Population-Based Cohort Study in Sweden. *J Natl Cancer Inst* 1998;90:156-158.

McLaughlin JK, Fraumeni JF, Nyren O, Adami HO. Silicone Breast Implants and Risk of Cancer? *JAMA* 1995;273:116.

McLaughlin JK, Fraumeni JF, Olsen J, Mellemkjaer L. Re: Breast Implants, Cancer, and Systemic Sclerosis. *J Natl Cancer Inst* 1994;86:1424.

Petit JY, Le MG, Mouriesse H, Rietjens M, Gill P, Contesso G, Lehmann A. Can Breast Reconstruction With Gel-Filled Silicone Implants Increase the Risk of Death and Second Primary Cancer in Patients Treated by Mastectomy for Breast Cancer? *Plast Reconstr Surg* 1994;94:115-119.

[APPENDIX 2]

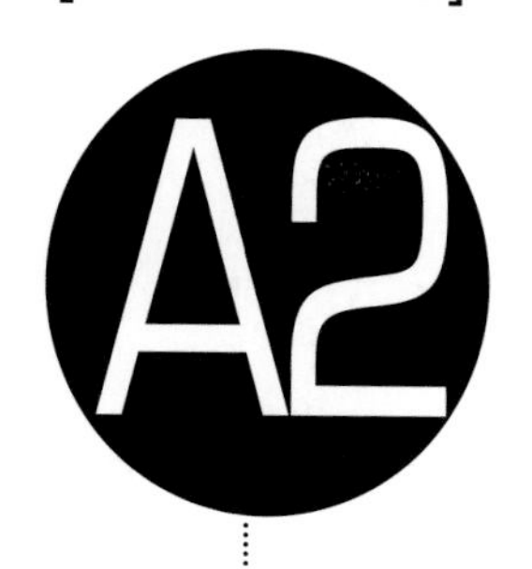


# U.S. AND INTERNATIONAL EPIDEMIOLOGY STUDIES OF BREAST IMPLANTS AND CONNECTIVE TISSUE DISEASE

The following is a summary of the epidemiology studies of connective tissue disease (CTD) and breast implants conducted by prominent researchers at prestigious institutions. Unlike the reports of individual women (often called "case reports" or "case series"), the following studies were designed to make comparisons between groups of women with and without implants. In contrast to case reports, these more rigorous epidemiology studies provide the opportunity to determine whether CTD among women with implants is occurring more frequently than might be expected.

**University of Michigan, School of Public Health,** Lacey, MPH; Laing, MD, Gillespie, PhD; et al.; Ann Arbor, MI-1997
Breast Implants, Environmental Exposures/Scleroderma
This large-scale, population-based study looked at all women in the state of Ohio diagnosed with scleroderma (SSc) between 1985 and 1992. The analyses compared the 189 women diagnosed with scleroderma to the 1,043 women in a control group who did not have scleroderma. The authors stated, "There was no association between SSc and silicone gel breast implants [adjusted odds ratio (aOR) 1.01, 95% confidence interval (CI) 0.13 to 8.15], any breast implants (aOR 1.48, 95% CI 0.34 to 6.39), or all silicone breast and facial implants (aOR 1.44, 95% CI 0.33 to 6.22)." These investigators conducted a comparable study in Michigan and found similar results (see Burns et al. 1994 in this summary). Directly funded by Dow Corning Corporation.

**University of Maryland, School of Medicine; University of Pittsburgh, School of Medicine; University of California San Diego, School of Medicine;** Hochberg, MD; Perlmutter, MSc; Medsger MD; et al.; Baltimore, MD-1996
Breast Implants/Scleroderma
This multi-center study compared the frequency of augmentation mammoplasty among 837 women with scleroderma to 2,507 women without scleroderma (SSc). The authors concluded, "These results fail to demonstrate a significant association between augmentation mammoplasty and SSc, and are consistent with those reported from other epidemiologic studies."

Funded in part by the Plastic Surgery Educational Foundation. Dow Corning has contributed money to this foundation but has no control over what research the foundation chooses to fund.

**Brigham & Women's Hospital, The Women's Health Cohort Study, Harvard Medical School,** Hennekens, MD, DrPH; Lee, MBBS, ScD; Cook, ScD; et al., Boston, MA-1996
Breast Implants/Reports of Connective Tissue Disease
This study of female health professionals assessed self-reported data on six connective tissue diseases and breast implants. It included 10,830 women with breast implants and 384,713 women without breast implants. The authors concluded that based on the self-reported data, the study's major contribution was to exclude large risks of connective tissue disease following breast implant surgery. Although the research raised the possibility of a small increased risk for women with implants, the investigators said the study could not reliably distinguish between this possibility and no risk. The study also found no difference in risk according to how long an implant was in place. According to Dr. Charles Hennekens, the lead investigator, "Considering all available evidence, women with breast implants should be reassured that there is no large risk of connective tissue disease." The authors stated that the next phase of this study will attempt to validate the self-reported diagnoses of connective tissue diseases by independent medical record review.
Funded by the National Institutes of Health and Dow Corning Corporation.

**University of Michigan, School of Public Health,** Laing, MD; Gillespie, PhD; Lacey, et al.; Ann Arbor, MI-1996
Breast Implants, Medical Devices/UCTD
This study identified 206 women in Michigan and Ohio with undifferentiated connective tissue disease (UCTD) and compared them with 2,239 women without the condition. No association was found with silicone breast implants. When considering medical devices in general, however, (both those containing silicone and not containing silicone, including breast implants), the authors found a statistically significant association with this condition. UCTD is a condition with signs and symptoms that may

evolve over time to a recognizable connective tissue disease, may never progress, or may disappear.
Directly funded by Dow Corning Corporation.

**Brigham and Women's Hospital, Nurses' Health Study, Harvard Medical School,** Sanchez-Guerrero, MD; Colditz, DrPH; Karlson, MD; et al.; Boston, MA-1995
Breast Implants/Connective Tissue Disease, Signs, Symptoms, and Laboratory Tests
This study examined the incidence of connective tissue disease and 41 signs, symptoms, or laboratory findings of connective tissue disease among registered nurses followed from 1976 to 1990. Funded by the National Institutes of Health, the study compared the findings in 1,183 women with implants to the findings in 86,318 women without implants. The authors concluded, "In a large cohort study, we did not find an association between silicone breast implants and connective-tissue diseases, defined according to a variety of standardized criteria, or signs and symptoms of these diseases."

**Emory University,** Goldman, MD; Greenblatt, MD; Joines, MD; et al.; Atlanta, GA-1995
Silicone Breast Implants/Connective Tissue Disease
A study of 4,229 women with and without breast implants from a rheumatology clinic found "no evidence that women with breast implants are at an increased risk for having rheumatoid arthritis or other diffuse connective tissue disease."
Directly funded by Dow Corning Corporation.

**University of Kansas,** Arthritis Center, Wolfe, MD; Wichita, KS-1995
Silicone Breast Implants/Rheumatoid Arthritis
This study compared 637 women with rheumatoid arthritis to 1,134 controls (479 women with osteoarthritis and 655 women selected at random from the general population). The author stated, "No associations between SBI [silicone breast implants] and RA [rheumatoid arthritis] were identified."

**Mayo Clinic,** Gabriel, MD; O'Fallon, PhD; Kurland, MD; et al.; Rochester, MN-1994
Breast Implants/Connective Tissue Diseases and Other Disorders
This study looked at medical records for all women in Olmsted County, Minnesota, who received breast implants between l964 and 1991, identified 749 women who had received breast implants and compared them with 1,498 women who had not received implants. The investigators stated, "We found no association between breast implants and the connective-tissue diseases and other disorders that were studied."
Funded in part by the Plastic Surgery Educational Foundation. Dow Corning has contributed money to this foundation but has no control over what research the foundation chooses to fund.

**Mayo Clinic,** Duffy, MD; Woods, MD; Rochester, MN-1994
Breast Implants/Connective Tissue Diseases and Other Disorders
These women may be included in the Gabriel Mayo Clinic study noted previously. This study looked at the medical records for 200 women who had 681 implants replaced or removed between 1970 and 1992. Eighty-five percent of the implants were intact. The investigators stated, "In our 30-year experience with silicone gel breast implants for augmentation mammaplasty or breast reconstruction, the data from this study suggest that no clinically evident adverse health problems were incurred by those women who subsequently experienced a silicone gel implant failure."

**University of Michigan, School of Public Health,** Burns, PhD; Schottenfeld, MD; et al.; Ann Arbor, MI-1994
Breast Implants, Environmental Exposures, and Family History/Scleroderma
This large-scale, population-based study looked at all women in the state of Michigan diagnosed with scleroderma between 1980 and 1991. Most of the analyses compared the 274 women diagnosed with scleroderma between 1985 and 1991 with the 1,184 women in a control group who did not have scleroderma. The 1994 dissertation by Burns stated, "There was no association between any contact with silicone and scleroderma." Their subsequent 1996 publication of this work concluded,

"Consistent with other studies, we found no increased risk of [scleroderma] among women with silicone breast implants." Directly funded by Dow Corning Corporation.

**University of South Florida, College of Medicine and College of Public Health,** Wells, MD; Cruse, MD; Baker, MD; et al.; Tampa, FL-1994
Breast Implants/Symptoms and Diseases
The authors examined the incidence of 23 symptoms and four connective tissue diseases among 222 women with breast implant surgery compared to 80 women with other cosmetic surgery procedures. While the symptoms of tender and swollen glands under the arms were more frequent among the women with breast implants, the symptom of change in skin color was more frequent among those with non-breast implant cosmetic surgery. The study reported, "No cases of scleroderma or lupus were found, and the incidence of arthritis was not significantly different between the implant and control groups."

**University of Pennsylvania, School of Medicine,** Strom, MD; Reidenberg, MD; Freundlich, MD; et al.; Philadelphia, PA-1994
Breast Implants/Systemic Lupus Erythematosus
The researchers interviewed 133 women with systemic lupus erythematosus (SLE) and 100 age-matched friend controls who did not have SLE. From this study, the authors concluded, "No association was seen between silicone breast implants and the subsequent development of SLE."

**University of Texas M. D. Anderson Cancer Center,** Schusterman, MD; Kroll, MD; Reece, MD; et al.; Houston, TX-1993
Breast Implants/Autoimmune Disease
Results from this study of 603 patients (250 with breast implants and 353 with reconstruction from their own tissue) showed, "The incidence of autoimmune disease in mastectomy patients receiving silicone gel implants is not different than in patients who had reconstruction with autogenous tissue."

**The Johns Hopkins Medical Institutions,** Wigley, MD; Miller; Hochberg, MD; et al.; Baltimore, MD-1992
Breast Implants/Scleroderma
This is part of the Hochberg study conducted at the University of Maryland School of Medicine noted previously. Among 210 Baltimore respondents and 531 from Pittsburgh with scleroderma (SSc), the frequency of breast implants was about the same as that estimated for the U.S. adult female population. The investigators concluded, "These data fail to support the hypothesis that augmentation mammoplasty with silicone gel-filled prostheses is a risk factor for the development of SSc."

**University of Washington, Fred Hutchinson Cancer Research Center,** Dugowson, MD; Daling, PhD; Koepsell, MD; et al.; Seattle, WA-1992 Silicone Breast Implants/Rheumatoid Arthritis.
A population-based study of 300 women with rheumatoid arthritis and 1,456 similarly aged control women showed, "These data do not support an increased risk for rheumatoid arthritis among women with silicone breast implants."

**University of California,** Weisman, MD; Vecchione, MD; Albert, MD; et al.; San Diego, CA-1988
Breast Implants/Connective Tissue Disease
The authors followed a group of 125 women from a plastic and cosmetic surgical practice in San Diego and stated, "Our survey did not reveal a single subject with an inflammatory rheumatic disease or condition following breast augmentation." They added, "It does not appear likely that augmentation mammaplasty is a significant or major inducer of inflammatory connective-tissue diseases in general."

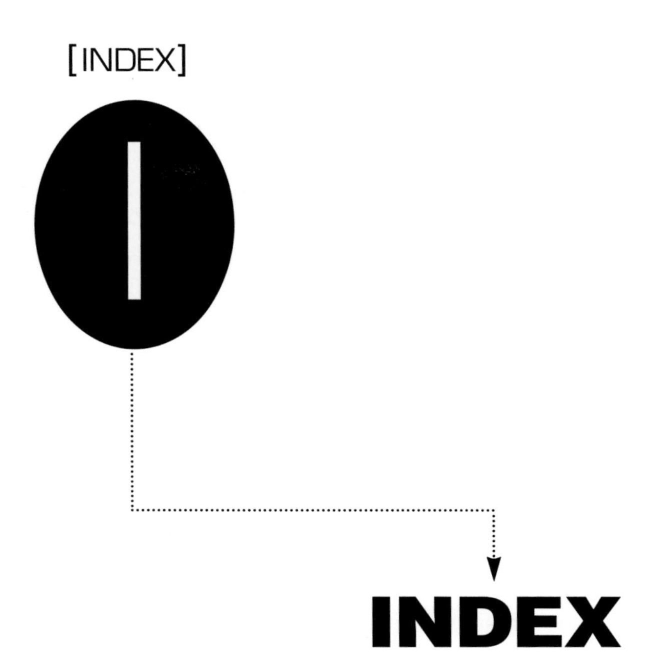


# INDEX

* indicates related illustration or photograph

## A



## B

## S

## T

[CARDS]

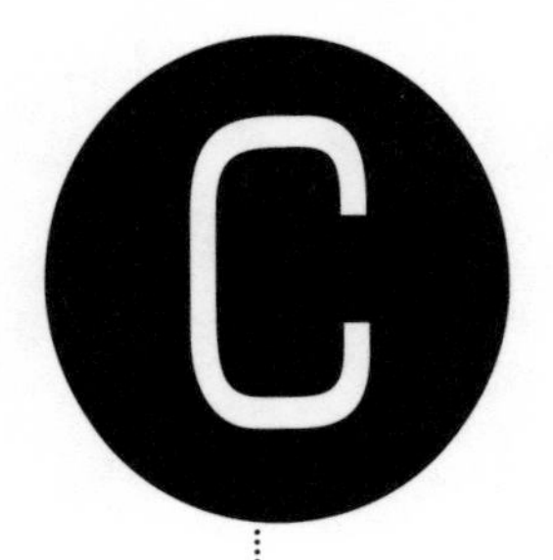


# IT'S IN THE CARDS

## ...40 cards with essential information for every woman considering breast augmentation

**...excerpted from**

***The Best Breast***

**By John B. Tebbetts, M.D. & Terrye Tebbetts**
**2801 Lemmon Avenue West**
**Suite 300**
**Dallas, Texas 75204**
**(214)220-2712 office**
**(214)969-0933 fax**

**thebestbreast.com**
**plastic-surgery.com**
**email: email@thebestbreast.com**

1

## Steps in the Quest for the Best Breast

**I- PREPARATION**

Whether to even consider augmentation

**II- KNOWLEDGE**

Arming yourself with information

**III- THE BEST DECISIONS**

Consulting surgeons and making decisions

**IV- THE BEST BREAST**

Finalizing decisions and preparing for surgery



2

## WHAT'S IN THIS FOR YOU?

***If you decide to become a breast augmentation patient, you will get what you deserve...***

*What you get depends on how much you know and how well you make decisions.*

***It's your choice...and your responsibility.***



3

## Does It Make Sense to Even Think About It?

**First, answer these questions...**

- *Is the procedure medically safe?*
- *Are there specific issues in my medical history that I should consider before proceeding?*
- *Am I just being vain?*
- *Can I achieve the changes I want any other way?*

**Then, turn this card over and answer the "Am I , Can I" questions...**



4

## CHOICES

**Every woman deserves them, choices of...**

- *Surgeon*
- *Implant type and size*
- *Implant pocket location*
- *Incision location*

**A surgeon can only offer you choices that surgeon knows how to deliver.**

## Does It Make Sense to Even Think About It?

**The "Am I , Can I" questions...**

- *Am I willing to do my homework and make my own decisions?*
- *Am I willing to realistically accept the tradeoffs and risks?*
- *Can I handle the costs or the financial burden?*
- *Am I willing to use common sense when making my decisions?*
- *Am I willing to remove my implants if necessary?*

***If you can answer "yes" to all of these questions, proceed...***



## A Logical Sequence of Steps to the Best Breast: Chapters in the Book





## ABOUT CHOICES

***No choice or combination of choices is perfect.***

**Every choice has tradeoffs — be sure you know them.**

***The choices you make now you will live with your entire life.***
**CHOOSE CAREFULLY.**



## WHAT'S IN THIS FOR YOU?

**The more you are willing to learn...**

**The more you will know...**

**And the better chance you'll make good decisions.**

5

## What You Need to Know
## *BEFORE Consulting a Surgeon*

1) What do I want, and what will my body allow me to have?
2) Implant types and options: Shape, smooth or textured shell, type of filler material
3) Possible complications, risks, tradeoffs
4) Implant pocket location: over muscle (retromammary), or partially under muscle (partial retropectoral)
5) Incision location options
6) Implant size
7) Options and tradeoffs: Sorting them out
8) Complications and tradeoffs: Things you and the surgeon can't control
9) Recovery: Ask about it up front, because what you hear can tell you a lot
10) Organizing your information to use it effectively



6

## Inescapable Truths about Breasts and Breast Size

1. Cup size is not even a consistent fashion measurement, let alone a medical term that can accurately and consistently define breast size.
2. Cup size is extremely variable and inconsistent from one brand of bra to another.
3. Women buy a bra that they can fill, not necessarily a bra that fits.
4. Women buy bras to push breast tissue where they want it to go to create a specific appearance.
5. Women don't necessarily buy bras that fit their breasts!
6. A certain number of cc's in an implant does not make a certain cup size breast. The final size of the breast depends on the amount of breast tissue the woman had prior to surgery plus the size of the implant that was placed.
7. A surgeon can only work with the tissues that you bring the surgeon.

***Turn the card over for more...***



7

## Defining what you don't like and what you want— a list

1) List the things you dislike about your breasts.
2) List how those dislikes affect your feeling of being normal, or how those dislikes affect your lifestyle.
3) List the basics of what you would like to have, based on what you know now.
4) Learn about what your body will allow you to have from Chapter 4, reconcile desires with reality, then refine you "want" list.
5) Look at your list carefully, and ask yourself if you're willing to live with your choices long term.
6) Finalize your list of "wants" that you'll discuss with surgeons you'll visit.
7) Don't let your window shopping (looking at pictures in magazines and surgeon's "brag books") fool you about reality and the future. Think about your own tissues.



8

## Golden Rules for Good Results— Short and Long Term

- For optimal results, the surgeon must adequately fill the existing breast envelope.
- Any more fill than the least amount of fill required for an optimal aesthetic result will detract from the long-term result.
- The size of implant that will be required to fill a larger, stretched envelope will be larger than the size required to fill a smaller, less stretched envelope.
- The smaller and tighter (unstretched by pregnancies) the envelope, the less implant the envelope can accept and give an aesthetically optimal result.
- No implant will produce the same result in two different patients.
- Regardless of your personal choices and choices dictated by your tissue characteristics, you should be informed and aware of the potential long-term implications of those choices before surgery.
- Perfection is not an option. Human surgeons can only produce improvement.

## How NOT to define your expectations or what you want

- ***Cup size alone***
(using cup size as the only description of what you want)

  Try explaining to yourself what a cup size really is…

  If you can't explain it to yourself, how do you expect a surgeon to produce it?

- ***Implant size in cc's*** (cubic centimeters)

  Do you really know what a certain number of cc's produces?

  Will your tissues accommodate that? How will it look?

  How will that many cc's affect your tissues as you age?



## How to Go About Getting The Best Breast

**1)** List what you need to know (the topics).
**2)** Review each topic and learn more details.
**3)** Armed with knowledge, prepare for surgeon consultations
**4)** Consult surgeons and evaluate what they tell you (using what you have learned).
**5)** Choose your surgeon.
**6)** Select from your options and discuss the tradeoffs with your surgeon (TEAM DECISIONS).
**7)** Think about the choices you've made and the tradeoffs you've accepted. Be sure you're comfortable.
**8)** If you have any questions, talk with your surgeon again. The time to clarify every detail is before, not after, your surgery.
**9)** Have your surgery, and follow your surgeon's instructions for recovery.



## What You Can Get Depends on What You've Got

- A surgeon can only work with the tissues you bring.
- A breast implant enhances what you have by giving you a better version of your current breast. It doesn't give you a totally different, new breast.
- Because a surgeon works with the tissues you bring, you can't pick a breast out of a book or magazine and expect that result unless the woman in the picture looked exactly like you look before surgery.



## Inescapable Truths about Breasts and Breast Size

8. No woman has two breasts that are the same, and no surgeon can create two breasts that are exactly the same.
9. The bigger the breast, the worse it will look over time (augmented or not)! Think about the woman you knew at a younger age with large breasts. How do they look now? Your tissues won't get better as you age, they will get worse! Think about your grandmother's breasts, or any woman's breasts after age 60.
10. Don't let cup size or implant size in cc's be the ONLY way you define what you want—use measurements and descriptions of appearance!
11. The bigger the breast YOU REQUEST, the worse it will look over time.
12. For the best long term result, you might want to balance what you want with what you tissues will allow you to have and what your tissues can support over time.

*Your surgeon should help you understand the characteristics of your individual tissues and which options are realistic for you.*

9

## Window Shopping 1- Pictures in Magazines

- The only picture that represents true breast characteristics is a picture totally without clothing, standing or lying down.
- If a surgeon looks at a picture and says, "Sure, we can make that breast! No problem!" RUN THE OTHER WAY!
- On the other hand, if the surgeon replies, "Let's look at your tissues and compare you as best we can to the person in the picture," BETTER!
- If the surgeon replies, "I'll use the pictures to help me understand what you'd like, and then I'll try to help you understand our best options and tradeoffs, given your tissues, GREAT!



10

## Things You Might NOT Want to Hear About Breast Implants — BUT REMEMBER WE TOLD YOU!

- **Breast implants are not perfect**
- **Breast implants don't last forever**
- **Breast implants may require some maintenance**
- **If you can't accept the imperfections of implants or if you're unwilling to have maintenance, don't have a breast augmentation.**



11

## Window Shopping 3- Computer Imaging

- Any trained technician can produce changes on a computer that no surgeon can produce with living tissue. Beware of marketing versus substance.
- If the surgeon uses the imager to help you understand some points, fine. If a technician or the surgeon uses the imager to try to sell you something that doesn't make sense or sell you other non-breast operations, BEWARE.
- If the surgeon morphs (changes the appearance of) your breasts on the computer and prints you a simulated before and after picture, don't look at it too much, and try not to fix the image in your mind. Your result definitely won't match the image exactly.



12

## Surgeons' Opinions about Implants

1. **The best opinion about implants is an opinion based on experience.**
   *If a surgeon has minimal or no experience with a certain type of implant, the surgeon should preface any opinion with, "I've never used that implant, but here's what I think of it."*
2. **If your only tool is a hammer, the whole world looks like a nail.**
3. **If a surgeon has experience with only one type of implant, that's likely the implant the surgeon will recommend.**
   *Hopefully. It's scary to think about the alternative.*
4. **The more experience a surgeon has with a variety of implant types, the more options the surgeon can offer you, and the better the surgeon can put those options into a realistic perspective for you.**

## Window Shopping 4 — The Internet

- Read the cards for Window Shopping 1, 2, and 3. Apply all the same principles to images on the Internet.
- Almost all images on the Internet are low-resolution images, and cannot compare to images you should see in a surgeon's office.
- All images on the Internet could have easily been modified — you have no way of knowing.
- Never select a surgeon based on images you see on the Internet. You MUST do ALL YOUR HOMEWORK described in **The Best Breast** if you expect to get the best result.

***Calling a surgeon's office using the checklist we give you, and examining the surgeon's written information will always tell youmore than a visit to a surgeon's website.***



## Window Shopping 2- Before and After Books

- If you can find a patient in the book that looks very much like you BEFORE her augmentation, it's possible that you MIGHT be able to look SOMEWHAT like her result AFTER your operation.
- If the surgeon doesn't have pictures to show you, consult other surgeons.
- If every result looks good, consult other surgeons.
- If the book does not contain a wide variety of breasts with some results better than others, consult other surgeons.
- A surgeon's habits are reflected in the quality of the pictures as well as the quality of the results. Are the pictures consistent and well-lighted, or taken with a Polaroid?



## Previous Patients' Opinions about Implants

1. **Most patients who have had an augmentation will tell you that the type of implant they have is best — otherwise, why would they have it?**

   *When a patient tells you her type of implant is best, ask why.*

2. **The more a previous patient knows, the more in-depth information you'll get. But don't be disappointed if you don't get much.**

   *Many patients are never offered options. Many patients don't learn about options on their own.*



## What You Can't Change About Implants and Your Tissues

1. **If you are thin and you can feel your ribs beneath your breast with your fingertip, you will probably be able to feel the edges or shell of any state-of-the-art implant in the world today, regardless of its shell thickness.**
2. **If you have thin tissues, you have thin tissues. You can't change that. Your surgeon can't change that.**
3. **The thinner you are, the more likely you'll feel some portion of your implants after your augmentation.**
4. **Since you can't change your thin tissues (gaining weight won't change them enough), if feeling your implant is unacceptable to you, don't have an augmentation.**

13

## Implant "Naturalness" versus Durability

**1. The longer an implant lasts, the fewer reoperations you will need during your lifetime. Reoperations increase risks and costs.**

**2. There are definite tradeoffs between naturalness and durability when it comes to breast implants given today's biomaterials and technology.**

**3 If you want your implant to last longer, you'll need to accept some tradeoffs in naturalness.**

**4. The only natural breast is a natural breast. Natural breasts don't contain a breast implant. If you want a TOTALLY natural breast, don't have an augmentation.**

**5. Naturalness is relative. Naturalness depends on what a woman HAS, what a woman WANTS, and what a woman is WILLING TO ACCEPT in tradeoffs.**



14

## Important Facts About Implant Shape and Fill Volume

### *ROUND Implants*

- **All of today's ROUND implants are UNDERFILLED if filled to manufacturer's recommendations.**

  *With virtually all of today's ROUND implants, regardless of the filler material or the size of the implant, shell collapse and folding occurs if the implant is filled to the manufacturer's recommendations! Watch for new designs with the SafeFill™ designation that we are currently designing to address this problem.*

- **Manufacturers believe that surgeons won't use (and therefore won't buy) ROUND implants with more fill because the surgeon feels that the implant is too firm.**

  *Manufacturers historically respond to the pressures of their market, like most successful companies.*



15

## What You Can't Change About Implants and Your Tissues

**1. If you are thin and you can feel your ribs beneath your breast with your fingertip, you will probably be able to feel the edges or shell of any state-of-the-art implant in the world today, regardless of its shell thickness.**

**2. If you have thin tissues, you have thin tissues. You can't change that. Your surgeon can't change that.**

**3. The thinner you are, the more likely you'll feel some portion of your implants after your augmentation.**

**4. Since you can't change your thin tissues (gaining weight won't change them enough), if feeling your implant is unacceptable to you, don't have an augmentation.**



16

## Important Facts About Implant Shape and Fill Volume

### *ANATOMIC Implants 1*

- ANATOMIC shaped implants are shaped more like a breast, fuller at the bottom, tapering at the top.
- Because of the tapering upper pole, an ANATOMIC implant can be FILLED ADEQUATELY TO PREVENT THE SHELL FOLDING—without producing an unnatural appearing upper breast.
- McGhan Medical has defined the fill volumes of their ANATOMIC implants higher at the outset—so there is no need for the surgeon to overfill the implant to protect the shell!

**Continued on back of this card...**

## Why is the Amount of Filler in Your Implant Important?

1. **The more filler you place in the implant, the less risk of shell folding and premature shell failure.**
2. **Any folding or collapse of an implant shell should worry you if you want the shell to last as long as possible.**
3. **The more filler you place in the implant, the firmer the implant- slightly firmer is a tradeoff for durability.**
4. **Exceeding the capacity of an implant shell by a larger amount can cause distortions of the shell.**



## What Affects How Natural An Implant Feels?

### 1. The thickness of the implant shell

The thicker the shell, the more durable, but the easier to feel.

### 2. The thickness of your tissues that cover the implant

The thinner your tissues, the more you will feel any implant.

### 3. The amount of filler material in the implant

The less filler in the implant, the softer it will feel, but the greater the risk the shell will fold or ripple, causing premature shell failure.



## Important Facts About Implant Shape and Fill Volume

### *ANATOMIC Implants 2*

1) **With an anatomically shaped implant, it is possible to adequately fill the implant to prevent shell collapse and folding, and still produce an optimal aesthetic result.**
2) **For most first time augmentation patients, anatomics seem SAFER (less risk of shell folding and early rupture) and MORE EFFECTVE (a more natural result with a full but not excessively bulging upper breast).**
3) **With McGhan Style 468 (saline filled) AND 410 (silicone cohesive gel filled) ANATOMIC implants, you get shell protection without filling past manufacturer's recommendations, AND you keep your warranty—no choosing between the two! No Catch 22!**

*With ROUND saline implants, you must overfill to prevent shell folding, and overfilling voids the warranty.*

**Continued on next card...**



## Important Facts About Implant Shape and Fill Volume

### *ROUND Implants*

- **Surgeons feel that firmer implants (even a tiny bit firmer), are unacceptable to patients...**

  *... Often without ever having used a significant number of the firmer implants or asking patients which they would prefer, slightly more firmness, or a reoperation sooner?*
- **When ROUND implants are filled adequately to prevent shell folding, they look very ROUND, and the upper breast can look excessively bulging, even having a sharp and bulging stepoff.**

  *Although some patients request an unnatural, excessively bulging upper breast, most don't.*
- **These principles apply to all ROUND implants, regardless of the filler material in the implant.**

17

## Important Facts About Implant Shape And Fill Volume

### *ANATOMIC Implants 3*

**4) A major anatomic implant advance is a filler material (cohesive gel) that does not migrate following disruption of the implant shell.**

**5) The McGhan Style 410 cohesive gel anatomic makes three significant advances:**
**1) adequate fill to maximally protect the shell,**
**2) a filler that doesn't migrate, and**
**3) optimal aesthetic results.**

**6) An ANATOMIC IMPLANT can maintain fill in the upper breast BETTER THAN A ROUND IMPLANT because:**

***The upper pole of the anatomic implant doesn't collapse — it maintains its vertical height.***



18

## About NEW implant designs...

- When betting on implant materials and fillers, don't place your bets on a horse until the horse has a track record.

***If you do, you likely won't be collecting money at the winners' window.***

- Don't discard SILICONE and SALINE filled implants (in that order) until there is an alternative that has at least 5 years of followup in a LARGE number of patients.
- Just because a breast implant design or filler is NEW, it's NOT NECESSARILY BETTER—no matter how promising it may seem.

***If it's really good, it will stand the test of time.***



19

## Facts About Smooth and Textured Shell Implants

- Textured silicone shell implants were developed as an alternative to smooth shell implants to reduce the risk of capsular contracture.
- Textured surface implants have a lower risk of capsular contracture than smooth shell implants.
- The difference between smooth and textured implant capsular contracture rates is more pronounced with silicone gel filled implants than with saline filled implants.

**For criteria to choose smooth or textured, see back of this card**



20

## Facts to Remember about All Surgical Options

- **No single set of surgical options is best for every patient. *If you are offered only one set of options, consult other surgeons.***
- **Every patient tends to think that the options they chose are also the best options for someone else.** *That isn't true, because no two women are alike in body or soul. Your tissues are definitely different.*
- **No surgical option is perfect. No surgical option is without tradeoffs.** *The question is whether you know the relative benefits and tradeoffs, and pick the options that best maximize the benefits and minimize the tradeoffs.*
- **If you choose surgical options without thinking about your tissues, you'll need to blame something or someone for the consequences.** *You'll probably blame the implant or the surgeon, when it's really you who are largely responsible.*

## Choosing A Textured or Smooth Implant

1) **If you choose an ANATOMIC implant, it should be TEXTURED.**
2) **If you choose a ROUND implant, and you want the least risk of capsular contracture, choose a TEXTURED surface.**
3) **Three good reasons to choose a ROUND, SMOOTH IMPLANT:**
   You are having a reoperation- not a first time augmentation.
   Your surgeon has little or no experience with anatomic implants.
   You are not concerned about the risk of capsular contracture.
4) **Two MYTHS that are NOT BASED ON FACTS:**

   Textured surface implants have thicker shells and are more easily felt in the breast. *Not true! The thickness of your tissues over the implant is much more important than the minimal differences in shell thickness.*

   Smooth shell implants have less rippling than textured surface implant *Not true! Rippling is the result of underfilling or traction, not the shell surface.*



## Important Facts About Implant Shape And Fill Volume
### *ANATOMIC Implants 4*

7) **Some surgeons find the additional demands of anatomic implants too technically challenging or time consuming, and hence don't offer their patients anatomic implants.**
8) **Anatomic implants may NOT be the best option for REOPERATION cases until a surgeon has gained considerable experience.**
9) **Anatomic implants may NOT be the best option for THIN patients who request EXCESSIVELY LARGE IMPLANTS larger than 350cc.**
10) **Anatomic implants are ideal for the majority of first time augmentation patients.**



## In Front of, or Behind Muscle — the Facts

- **Partial retropectoral placement means that the upper portion of the implant is partially covered by the pectoralis major muscle. *Total muscle cover, although possible, is rarely the best option for a first time augmentation. The closer the implant is to the tissues it is trying to shape, the more accurate and predictable the result.***
- **An implant placed IN FRONT OF THE MUSCLE (behind breast tissue, retromammary) will always more predictably control breast shape. If a surgeon tells you otherwise, I would respectfully disagree and ask how much experience the surgeon has with both types of placement.**
- **A more perfect aesthetic result is usually possible when an implant is placed in front of the muscle. *But in thin women, behind muscle is preferable because adequate tissue cover age is most important.***



## About the Manufacturer of Your Implants...

- **The company that manufactures your breast implants doesn't matter until you need to replace their implants. Will they be there?**
- **It's easier to assure that you'll have a company's guarantee and support when you need it BEFORE you put their product in your body.**
- **Look into the company that manufactures your implants BEFORE you have an augmentation, or don't complain later.**

21

## In Front of Muscle (Retromammary) — The Advantages

1) More precise control of cleavage — the distance between your breasts.
2) More precise control of upper breast fill — especially upper fill toward the middle of your chest.
3) Less chance of muscle pressure pushing your implants to the side over time, widening the distance between your breast.
4) Less chance of distorting your breast shape when you tighten (contract) your pectoralis muscle.

***See the back of this card for the tradeoffs...***



22

## In front of...or behind muscle — How do you choose?

- **If you are extremely THIN (less than 2 cm. pinch thickness above your breast), you should put the implant BEHIND muscle to assure adequate tissue cover over the implant. *If you don't, you run more risks of seeing the edges of your implant, and risk other long-term problems.***
- **If you have adequate thickness of tissues (more than 2 cm. pinch thickness above your breast tissue), weigh the advantages and tradeoffs listed on other cards and choose above or below based on your preferences and your surgeon's recommendations.**



23

## Behind Muscle (Retropectoral) — The Advantages

1) The major advantage of placing an implant behind muscle is to prevent implant edge visibility. *This does not mean that you may not feel portions of the implant, especially in the fold under the breast and the outside portion of the breast.*
2) A second stated advantage of subpectoral placement is better reduction of risks of capsular contracture compared to retromammary placement. *This difference is more marked with silicone gel implants than with saline implants. With saline implants, risks are about the same.*
3) Better mammograms. *Many radiologists feel that mammograms are more accurate with the implant behind muscle.*

**See the back of this card for the tradeoffs...**



24

## The Inframammary (under the breast) Incision

- **The greatest advantage of an incision beneath the breast is the degree of control it allows the surgeon in a wide range of breast types.**
- ***More augmentation patients have had this incision location than all other incision locations combined!***
- **The greatest tradeoff of an inframammary incision is the presence of a scar in the fold beneath the breast.**

## Behind Muscle (Retropectoral) — The Tradeoffs

- **Distortion of breast shape when you tighten (contract) your pectoralis muscle.**
- **Shifting of the implants to the side over time, widening the distance between the breasts.**
- **Less control of upper breast fill, especially upper and toward the middle.**
- **More stretch of the lower breast tissues over time. Usually not a big issue, but the muscle puts pressure on the upper implant, transmitting more pressure to the lower envelope.**
- **Increased risk of upward displacement of the implant if muscle origins are not adjusted along the fold.**

***See the front of this card for the benefits...***



## In Front of Muscle (Retromammary) — The Tradeoffs

**1) If you are extremely thin, this location may not provide adequate soft tissue cover to prevent your seeing the edges of your implant**

**2) This location may make your mammograms more difficult.**

***See the front of this card for the benefits...***



## The Periareolar (around the nipple -areola) Incision

- **The greatest advantage of an incision around the areola is that it's located in thinner skin that usually heals well, provided the areola is large enough for access.**
- **The greatest tradeoffs of a periareolar incisions are increased exposure of the implant to bacteria normally found in the breast, and (if you develop a bad scar) a scar located on the most visible location on the breast.**



## Incision Location — Important Facts

1) Most patients worry far more about incision location before the surgery than they care after the surgery (provided they have a good result).
2) If you have a beautiful breast and normal healing, neither you nor anyone else will care where the incision is located.
3) Every patient thinks that the incision location that she has is best.
4) Incision location is a common way that surgeons use to market their augmentation practice. *They may only know how to use one incision.*
5) If a surgeon is experienced with all incision locations, the surgeon will offer you all options.
6) No incision location is always best — each location has advantages and tradeoffs.

***See additional cards for advantages and tradeoffs of each incision location...***

25

## The Axillary (in the Armpit) Incision

- **The greatest advantage of an incision in the armpit is that it's location makes it the least visible of all scars for augmentation.**
- **The greatest tradeoff of axillary incisions is that a surgeon must be experienced, and the operation time is usually slightly longer(if the surgeon uses state-of-the-art techniques).**
- **The armpit incision is best for first time augmentation — if a procedure is necessary later, another approach is better.**



26

## Basic Facts about Risks

- **The more you know about what to expect and what is normal, the less confused or frightened you will be when it occurs.**
- **It's a TEAM JOB to assure that you know what to expect after surgery.**
- **It's your surgeon's and your surgeon's staff's responsibility to provide information for you. It's your responsibility to use it!**
- **Every breast augmentation operation carries inherent risks. Medical complications are not totally preventable by you or your surgeon.**
- **Do not have an augmentation mammaplasty unless you thoroughly understand and accept the potential risks and tradeoffs of the procedure.**



27

## Surgical Techniques for Creating the Pocket

**BLUNT DISSECTION** techniques for creating the implant pocket create *more tissue trauma, tear tissues, create more bleeding, and result in a longer recovery time.* State-of-the-art **ELECTROCAUTERY DISSECTION** techniques are less traumatic and have a shorter recovery time.

Dissection technique is a major factor that affects your recovery. ***The more trauma (blunt dissection), the longer and more difficult the recovery.***



28

## Questions to Ask About Recovery — Before You Choose a Surgeon!

- **What will my recovery be like?**
- **Will I have bruising?**
- **Will I have drain tubes coming out of my body?**
- **When can I return to normal activities? Drive my car, lift normal objects, arms above my head?**
- **When can I bathe?**
- **Do I need special bandages, bras, or binders?**
- **When can I return to athletic activities?**
- **The better the answers to these questions, the better you'll like your recovery...and likely your result!**

## If Problems Occur: Deal with Them

- **The best way to deal with a problem is to deal with it — now!**
- **There isn't a surgeon alive who wants an unhappy patient. Keep your lines of communication open!**
- **No surgeon can solve a problem unless the surgeon is aware that a problem exists!**
- **Most of the best surgeons will encourage you to seek another opinion — don't hesitate to ask!**



## The Umbilical (in the belly button) Incision

***The main advantage*** of an incision in and around the belly button is that the incision is located off the breast.

***The main disadvantages*** of the umbilical incision compared to other incisions are: *It offers the surgeon the LEAST CONTROL of all incisional locations, the LEAST PREDICTABLE RESULTS, and causes the MOST TISSUE TRAUMA* because more normal tissues are disturbed to get to the breast.

Access to the breast is created by bluntly pushing a one-inch diameter tube from the umbilicus to each breast, through the tissues of the upper abdomen.

***The pocket for the implant is developed BLINDLY, inserting an expander and tearing tissue to create a pocket***. Most surgeons who use the umbilical approach do not offer implant placement behind muscle. If you are thin, behind muscle is better long term.



## RECOVERY: WHAT IS POSSIBLE?

- **No bruising, no bandages, no special bras, no drain tubes coming out of your body, no limitation of normal activity from day 1.**
- **Resume full normal activity the first day after surgery — arms above your head, lift normal weight objects, drive your car.**
- **Shower and wash your hair immediately.**
- **All of the above true in over 90 percent of our patients, even if the implant is behind muscle.**



## Tradeoffs and Surprises

**TRADEOFFS** always depend on the details of each specific case. The characteristics of your tissues can significantly affect the tradeoffs.

The experience of your surgeon with different options can significantly affect the tradeoffs.

After a surgeon examines you, be sure to ask about specific tradeoffs and how they relate to your specific tissues and the surgeon's experience with different options.

**SURPRISES:** If it's a surprise, it's a problem.

A surprise can be something you don't know about that confuses or frightens you, OR ...

A surprise can be a medical complication that causes untoward medical events.

29

## CHOOSING YOUR SURGEON IS YOUR RESPONSIBILITY!

- **Many patients spend more time shopping for a car than they spend selecting a plastic surgeon!**
- **It's your body...you'll be looking at it for the rest of your life.**
- **It's your job to select your surgeon. Don't complain later if you neglect your responsibilities.**
- **Selecting your surgeon is the single most important thing you can do to assure an optimal result!**



30

## THREE THINGS TO LISTEN FOR WHEN YOU CALL A SURGEON'S OFFICE

***Listen for three things in your first call to the office:***

***COURTESY, KNOWLEDGE, SERVICE***

***"I want to make this easy for you. Let's get started!"***



31

## A Checklist for Surgeon Credentials

**Essentials:**

_ Board certified by the American Board of Plastic Surgery
_ Completed an approved residency training program in plastic surgery
_ Member of ASPRS and ASAPS (see professional societies above)
_ Has hospital privileges to do breast augmentation at an accredited hospital
_ Curriculum vitae documents scientific presentations and publications

**Cream on top of the essentials:**

_ Subspecializes in cosmetic surgery
_ Subspecializes in breast augmentation
_ Listed in Who's Who
_ Listed in Best Doctors in America
_ Recommended by a knowledgeable friend or physician

**Not as reliable:**

_ Advertisements
_ Media coverage
_ General physician referral services (most are paid by the surgeon to refer you)
_ Recommendations from anyone without in-depth knowledge about augmentation

**Red flags:**

_ Completed residency training in a specialty other than plastic surgery
_ Certified in an unrelated specialty
_ Not board certified by ABPS
_ No hospital privileges
_ If you obtain any false or misleading information — claims that aren't true
_ Unwilling to answer questions about credentials
_ Unwilling to provide access to curriculum vitae

## When You Call a Surgeon — A List of Basic Questions

*When you ask the following questions, stop talking and listen carefully to the answers! Take notes, and keep the answers organized by surgeon. The answers are key to your making good decisions when selecting a surgeon:*

1) I'm interested in getting some information about breast augmentation. Does Dr. X do breast augmentation?
2) How does Dr. X do breast augmentation?
3) Could you send me some information about breast augmentation and about Dr. X and your practice?
4) What are the risks involved in having breast augmentation?
5) Do you offer free consultations?
6) Do you have before and after photographs that I could see?
7) Would it be possible to speak with other patients of Dr. X who have had augmentations?
8) How long has Dr. X been in practice?
9) How many augmentations does Dr. X do every year?
10) Does Dr. X limit his practice to cosmetic surgery?
11) Where does Dr. X have hospital privileges?
12) Is Dr. X board certified? By which board?
13) How much will my augmentation cost?



## How to Locate Surgeons Certified by the American Board of Plastic Surgery

- The *American Society of Plastic and Reconstructive Surgeons* at:

  **www.plasticsurgery.org/findsurg/finding.htm**,
  or call at **1-800-635-0635**.

- The *American Society of Aesthetic Plastic Surgery* at:

  **www.surgery.org/enhanced**
  or call **1-888-272-7711**.

©1999 All rights reserved - CosmetXpertise May not be reproduced without permission. (214)220-2712 www.thebestbreast.com

## RED FLAGS WHEN YOU CALL A SURGEON'S OFFICE

- ***Not courteous***
- ***No knowledgeable***
- ***Not willing to spend time with you***
- ***Not telling you what you need to know***
- ***Telling you all fluff, no substance***
- ***No offer to send information***
- ***No offer for consultation with patient educator for no charge***

©1999 All rights reserved - CosmetXpertise May not be reproduced without permission. (214)220-2712 www.thebestbreast.com

32

## How to Evaluate Written Information You Receive

**A surgeon's habits are reflected in everything a surgeon does—all you need to do is notice!**
*Informational materials reflect a surgeon's habits and commitment to educating patients.*

**Is the information generic, or did the surgeon write the information personally?**
*If it's generic, you can tell...you'll probably see the same thing from other surgeons.*

**Does it appear and sound distinctively different compared to other surgeon's information?**
*If it doesn't sound different, it probably isn't much different! What might that say about your result?*

**What do the informational materials tell you about the surgeon's habits?**
*Is the surgeon compulsive enough to be different? Better? What might that say about your surgery?*

**Does the information contain substance, or just fluff?**
*If you took away the fancy look, what does it SAY? Fluff with little substance? What might that say about the surgeon?*

**Does the information address most or all of your questions and concerns? How well?**
*If only 50% of the answers are there, what might that say about the percent of knowledge?*

**Is the information written in language that is easy to understand? At the same time, is it informative?**
*If not, why not?*



33

## Are You Ready for a Consultation?

*If you can check all of the items on the following checklist, you're ready to consult with a plastic surgeon!*

- ❒ **I've read Chapters 1 through 10.**
- ❒ **I made a list of surgeons and verified credentials.**
- ❒ **I called surgeons' offices and requested informational materials.**
- ❒ **I evaluated surgeons' staffs on the phone.**
- ❒ **I've gathered information from at least 3 surgeons with solid credentials, good informational materials, and knowledgeable staffs.**
- ❒ **I took advantage of visits with patient educators.**
- ❒ **I've made a specific list of questions I want to ask the surgeon.**



34

## Pricing and Costs: Key Tips

- **If a surgeon offers a "package price", always insist that the price be broken down into the categories listed on the back of this card**
- ***If you don't, you won't be able to analyze what you're paying for and compare to other surgeons! See Chapter 13.***
- **Always ask for a written quote for costs, signed by the surgeon or a staff member.**
- ***And ask how long the prices on the quote apply!***

## Preparing to Consult a Surgeon

**If you have an opportunity to consult a patient educator before consulting the surgeon—DO IT! *The best surgeons will almost always offer this service — they want you to know as much as possible.***

**The more PREPARED you are BEFORE meeting with a surgeon, the better you'll understand the surgeon, and the better you can evaluate the surgeon.**



## Costs: A Checklist of Questions to Ask

_ Surgeon fees
_ Laboratory fees (for lab work prior to surgery)
_ Electrocardiogram fees (if needed)
_ Mammogram fees (if surgeon requires mammogram)
_ Surgery facility fees
_ Costs of implants
_ Anesthesia fees
_ Medications fees or costs (for before and after surgery)
_ Any other fees



## Seeing What They Don't Tell You — Things to Notice

**You're not going to a museum or estate — you're going to see a surgeon.** *Statues, art, and expensive furniture don't tell you a thing about the quality of surgery you'll get—but guess who gets to pay for the décor —you!*

**A quiet, comfortable atmosphere that reflects good taste is all that's required—anything more, and you're paying extra for the décor.** *You want to spend your money on the surgeon, not the decorator.*

**If the office looks like it may not belong to a plastic surgeon—there's a message.** *An overly "medical" appearing office is not typical of cosmetic surgery office s —do you want someone operating on you that doesn't do those procedures very often?*

**The organization, function and flow of every surgeon's office is a reflection of the surgeon's habits.** *Ask yourself if you want someone with these habits operating on you!*

***Are they trying to inform me, or trying to sell me?***

## Evaluating Surgeons You Consult— Key Questions

**You'll recognize a great surgeon without the surgeon having to tell you!** *How much substance is behind what you see and hear!*

**Caring, thoroughness, and substance definitely contribute to what you'll get in the operating room.** *How much of each did the surgeon have?*

**Remind yourself: This person will be changing my body forever, and I'll look at it every day!** *Are you comfortable?*

**Were you offered options? A surgeon can't offer what the surgeon doesn't know how to do!** *There is definitely NOT one best way to do an augmentation if you know all the different ways!*

**Were you told there was only one best way?** *Ask yourself why!*

**Did you honestly and frankly discuss complications and what would be done?** *If the worst occurred, would you want this person to take care of you?*

35

# QUESTIONS TO ASK EVERY SURGEON DURING A CONSULTATION

- ❒ In what specialty was your residency training? How many years? Are you board certified? By whom?
- ❒ How long have you been in practice?
- ❒ Do you have hospital privileges? Where?
- ❒ How many breast augmentations have you done, and how many do you perform each year?
- ❒ What are the three most important things you'd advise me to think about with regard to breast augmentation?
- ❒ What is your preferred incision location? Why? How many of each location have you done? Can you show me pictures?
- ❒ Which do you prefer, over or under muscle? Why? Do you do both? How many of each have you done?
- ❒ What is your preferred implant? Why? Do you offer all different types of implants?
- ❒ Do you prefer round or anatomic implants? Why? Do you offer both? How many of each have you done?
- ❒ If you prefer round implants, how do you deal with the fill issue?
- ❒ Are round implants adequately filled (saline or silicone) to prevent shell folding?
- ❒ Do you think shell folding can affect the life of the shell?
- ❒ If we overfill a round implant, are you willing to guarantee the implant if the manufacturer does not?



36

## QUESTIONS TO ASK EVERY SURGEON DURING A CONSULTATION (continued)

- ❒ What are the three worst things that can happen following my augmentation? What are the chances they will happen? Exactly what do we do in each case if they happen? What are the costs involved? Time off work, worst possible scenario?
- ❒ Would you ever recommend implant removal without replacement? If so, why? What affects how my breast will look if we had to remove implants?
- ❒ Does the size of the implant we choose affect my tissues as I get older? How?
- ❒ Do you charge me to replace my implant if it ruptures? Is there anything that can occur that you would charge me for in the future, including followup visits or surgery?
- ❒ Will anyone else be performing any part of my surgery? Are they more qualified than you?
- ❒ When can I lift my arms above my head, drive my car, and lift my children or other objects?
- ❒ Will I have drains?
- ❒ Will I have bruising?
- ❒ Will I wear special bandages, bras, or binders? For how long?
- ❒ Why should I choose you to do my surgery?

# Putting It All Together: Finalizing Your Choices

## The decisions and the sequence

***Who is my surgeon?***

- ❐ Dr. X
- ❐ Dr. Y
- ❐ Dr. Z

***What type and size implant?***

- ❐ Smooth
- ❐ Textured
- ❐ Round
- ❐ Anatomic
- ❐ Size

***Which pocket location?***

- ❐ Retromammary (behind breast tissue only)
- ❐ Partial retropectoral (behind the pectoralis muscle)
- ❐ Total muscle coverage (behind pectoralis and serratus muscles)

***Which incision location?***

- ❐ Inframammary
- ❐ Periareolar
- ❐ Axillary
- ❐ Umbilical



# Surgical Arrangements Checklist

- ❏ Select a date for surgery.
- ❏ Review surgeon's financial policies and policies for refunds.
- ❏ Pay scheduling deposit if surgeon requires.
- ❏ Sign informed consent documents and operative consent forms.
- ❏ Review and sign implant manufacturer's documents.
  - ❏ Implant package insert
  - ❏ Terms of implant guarantee
  - ❏ Verify that surgeon will register your implants with the national implant registry.
- ❏ Schedule lab tests and mammography.
- ❏ Review medications to avoid and medications to take before surgery.
- ❏ Review instructions for the night before surgery.
- ❏ Review instructions for the day of surgery.

# Before Surgery Checklist

- ❏ Read all informed consent documents and operative permits carefully—well in advance of your surgery.
- ❏ Be sure that your surgeon is aware of all medications that you are taking!
- ❏ Avoid all medications that contain aspirin for at least two weeks prior to surgery.
  *Read the labels carefully for all over-the-counter medications—many contain aspirin.*
- ❏ Be very careful about herbs and herbal medicines.
  *If you are using any herbal preparations, discuss them with your surgeon!*
- ❏ Never eat or drink ANYTHING after midnight the night before surgery.
  *If you do, material in your stomach can cause you to regurgitate, aspirate, and possibly die during surgery!*

37

## The day of surgery...a checklist

- ❑ Wear very comfortable clothing (like a jogging suit) that buttons or zips up the front.
  *You won't enjoy tugging something on over your head!*
- ❑ Make arrangements for someone to drive you home from the surgery facility and be with you overnight.
  *You'll receive medications that make driving yourself unsafe!*
- ❑ Leave off your eye makeup—otherwise you'll wake up with it in your eyes!
  *Protective eye lubricants during surgery make a total mess of makeup!*
- ❑ Leave your jewelry and valuables at home!



38

## Recovery: The Most Important DO'S

- ❑ Follow your surgeon's instructions—to the letter! Don't try to outthink your surgeon!
- ❑ Stay hydrated! Drink plenty of fluids for the first few days after surgery.
- ❑ Eat! And eat well! You need nutrition to heal!
- ❑ Never take any pain medication on an empty stomach—it'll get even emptier!
- ❑ Resume normal activity as soon as possible, following your surgeon's instructions.

***Continued on the back of this card...***



39

## The Essentials of Recovery

- **Your individual pain tolerance, motivation, and ability to follow instructions will affect your recovery.**
- ***Adopt a positive attitude, follow instructions, and get well sooner!***
- **The easier your surgeon expects your recovery to be, the shorter the list of postoperative instructions!**
- ***The more the surgeon can do in the operating room, the less you'll be burdened with after surgery!***
- **Don't try to outthink your surgeon! Follow your surgeon's instructions!**
- ***Don't follow your friend's postoperative instructions if she had a different surgeon.***



40

## What's not Normal—CONTACT YOUR SURGEON

***If you develop any of the following, you should contact your surgeon:***

- ❑ **Fever higher than 102 degrees, or fever with chills**
- ❑ **One breast that is much, much larger than the other**
- ❑ **One breast that appears much more bruised than the other**
- ❑ **Noticeable redness and tenderness in any area of the breast**
- ❑ **Any drainage from your incision area after three days**
- ❑ **Any unusual discomfort**
- ❑ **Any other symptoms that your surgeon advises you to call about**

## Recovery: The Most Important DONT'S

*Your surgeon may give you a longer list of things to avoid, but the following is a basic checklist of don'ts that we use following augmentation:*

- ❑ **Avoid any type of aerobic activities (anything that creates a significant increase in your pulse) for two weeks—walking is o.k., fast walking is not; sex is o.k.; olympic sex is not!**
- ❑ **Don't lift heavy objects (over 30-40 lbs.) or strain hard for two weeks (and watch those pain pills, they can constipate you!)**
- ❑ **Avoid whatever else your surgeon tells you to avoid.**



## Durability and Implant Rupture...

- **You don't need to "baby" your implants — they should withstand any type of normal, vigorous activity!**
- ***However, your implants were not designed to withstand closed capsulotomy — the practice of forcefully squeezing your breast to correct capsular contracture!***
- **If you ever have any type of problem with implant deflation or rupture, insist on a qualified surgeon.**
- ***Implant deflation or rupture is no big deal if your surgeon knows how to deal with it!***



## What to Expect That's Normal

*If you know what to expect that's normal, you'll be less frightened or concerned!*

- ❑ They don't match! My breasts are different size and shape! And they're different every day!
- ❑ They're too high! ❑ They're too big! ❑ They're too tight!
- ❑ They're too swollen! ❑ They're too firm!
- ❑ I hear sloshing inside my breasts!
- ❑ They don't move!
- ❑ They're numb or they're too sensitive or I have weird sensations!
- ❑ I can't lay on them—they feel like basketballs!
- ❑ My waist has disappeared!
- ❑ The magic time when they'll feel like they belong to me is 3 months!



## Recovery: The Most Important DO'S (cont'd)

- ❑ Read your postoperative instruction sheets. They'll help you expect what's normal!
- ❑ Expect to be frustrated that your tissues don't change according to your schedule.
- ❑ Expect to be too big, too high, and too tight for a few weeks.
- ❑ Expect differences and constant changes in size and shape of your breasts for 3-6 weeks.
- ❑ Get out of the house and do something — staring does not reduce swelling and tightness.
- ❑ If anything seems wrong, check your written instructions and information, then call your surgeon!